Perinatal Psychiatry

Edited by
JOHN COX
JENI HOLDEN

Perinatal Psychiatry
Use and Misuse of the
Edinburgh Postnatal Depression Scale

GASKELL

Gaskell is an imprint of the Royal College of Psychiatrists,
17 Belgrave Square, London SW1

British Library Cataloguing-in-Publication Data

A catalogue record for this book is available from the
British Library

ISBN 0-902241-68-0

Distributed in North America
by American Psychiatric Press, Inc.
ISBN 0-88048-631-7

Publication of this book was supported by an educational grant from
Dista Psychiatric Education Services – a subsidiary of Lilly Industries.

Phototypeset by Dobbie Typesetting Limited, Tavistock, Devon
Printed by Bell & Bain Ltd, Glasgow

Contents

Part III. Workshop reports

Contributors

Philip Boyce, Associate Professor of Psychiatry, University of Sydney, Nepean Hospital, Penrith, NSW, Australia

John Cox, Professor, Department of Psychiatry, School of Postgraduate Medicine, Keele University, Staffordshire

Sandra A. Elliott, Clinical Psychologist, Clinical Psychology Service, Maidstone Priority Care Trust, Maidstone, Kent

David Foreman, Senior Research Fellow, Department of Psychiatry, School of Postgraduate Medicine, Keele University, Staffordshire

Josephine M. Green, Senior Research Associate, Centre for Family Research, University of Cambridge, Free School Lane, Cambridge

Brian Harris, Senior Lecturer in Psychological Medicine, University of Wales College of Medicine, Department of Psychological Medicine, Sully Hospital, Cardiff, Wales

Alison E. Hipwell, Research Associate, Winnicott Research Unit, Department of Psychiatry, University of Cambridge

Jeni Holden, Lecturer in Psychology, Department of Management and Social Science, Queen Margaret College, Edinburgh

Nahla Jamil, Consultant Psychiatrist, East Glamorgan Hospital, Pontypridd, Mid Glamorgan, Wales

R. Channi Kumar, Professor of Perinatal Psychiatry, Institute of Psychiatry, London

Chris Lawson, Senior Registrar, Maudsley Hospital, London

Declan Murray, Consultant Psychiatrist, St Ita's Hospital, Portrane, County Dublin, Republic of Ireland

Margaret Oates, Senior Lecturer in Psychiatry/Honorary Consultant Psychiatrist, Queen's Medical Centre, Nottingham

Shaughn O'Brien, Professor and Head of Department, Obstetrics and Gynaecology, School of Postgraduate Medicine, Keele University, Staffordshire

Michael W. O'Hara, Professor, Department of Psychology, University of Iowa, USA

Brice Pitt, Professor of Psychiatry, University of London

Mike Watson, Psychodrama Psychotherapist, Department of Psychotherapy, Richmond Complex, Shelton, Stoke-on-Trent

Preface

This book is about improving the quality of the lives of childbearing women and their families. It is also about the use, and misuse, of the Edinburgh Postnatal Depression Scale (EPDS), a 10-item self-report screening questionnaire introduced in 1987 (see Chapter 8) in clinical practice and research. The recent Government White Paper *The Health of the Nation* has set targets for mental health services which include improving the quality of life for people suffering from mental illness and reducing the suicide rate by the year 2000. The consequences of perinatal mental disorders are costly, not only in terms of personal suffering, but in their potential for increasing long-term demands on health care services. Depression is not only an extremely unpleasant personal experience but can jeopardise the survival of the family; an infant's emotional and cognitive development may be affected and a 'rejected' and dejected partner may leave home. A desperate mother may decide to end her own life and/or that of her children.

Women's contact with health care services is greater around the time of childbirth than at any other time and they are a readily identified at-risk group. One of our aims in compiling this book therefore was to provide information about the growing body of research which suggests that carefully planned changes in the delivery of health care services, including informed use of the EPDS, may lead to greater ability to meet the emotional needs of families with infants and other young children, and to prevent the onset of mental disorder.

At a conference held at Keele in October 1991, sponsored by the Marcé Society and the Centre for Reproductive Psychological Medicine, our main agenda was to discuss the increasing use of the EPDS in the United Kingdom and overseas within the context of strategies for prevention. This conference generated considerable enthusiasm and ideas about how to meet the emotional needs of childbearing women and in particular focused on practical aspects of the use and misuse of the EPDS.

We decided that it was important to share the resulting information with all those whose work or concern brings them into contact with women at this time. Health professionals in primary care settings or in hospital, including general practitioners, midwives, health visitors, obstetricians, psychiatrists, clinical psychologists, psychiatric nurses, social workers, researchers, as well as voluntary bodies such as the National Childbirth Trust, Newpin, Homestart, Meet-a-Mum Association and the Association for Postnatal Illness, should all find this book relevant to their work.

A common strand running through most of the work in this book is that it has been guided by personal enthusiasm and by the wish not only to extend knowledge, but to find practical ways of helping women. Our contributors are mostly clinicians whose research has been initiated and informed by their direct experience in working with women perinatally. It is encouraging to realise that both research and practice in this field are now extending beyond traditional boundaries, to become increasingly multi-disciplinary. Psychiatrists, psychologists, obstetricians and nurses are not only working together but researching and writing together.

The book falls into three parts. The first section deals with research findings of factors associated with mental disorders and emotional distress around the time of childbirth (perinatal psychiatry), and interventions and/or possible reallocation of resources which may be effective in preventing such distress or ameliorating its effects. The second part is about uses and misuses of the EPDS in clinical practice and in research. There is, however, considerable overlap between these sections: some EPDS chapters contain ideas or recommendations for preventive interventions, and some of the studies reported in the first part of the book have also used the EPDS.

The third section arose directly from workshops at the conference. In Chapter 14, Elliott challenges an uninformed approach to using the EPDS. Foreman & Watson describe an unusual approach to counselling and psychodrama in Chapter 15. These chapters provide the reader with a glimpse of the creative spark which characterised the Keele meeting.

The book contains examples of innovative services which, although they may need commitment, specialist knowledge and funding to set up, can be both efficient and cost-effective. For example, Oates (Chapters 2 and 3) lucidly and convincingly argues the case for a specialist psychiatric service to deal specifically with the needs of women with postnatal mental illness. She not only provides evidence for the effectiveness of such a service, based on her pioneering work in Nottingham, but includes guidelines for how the service should be staffed and how it should operate. She goes on to provide a breakdown of monitoring, evaluation and auditing procedures.

Holden's chapter (Chapter 5) contains suggestions on how existing health services can be adapted to improve the care provided to antenatal and postnatal women, and their families. Health professionals cannot, however, meet the needs of all such women when they need help, and the work of volunteer agencies, which may be essential in the initiation and maintenance of primary and tertiary preventive services, are also described. For example, the Meet-a-Mum Association (MAMA) puts women in touch with others who may be socially isolated, and the Association for Postnatal Illness provides a telephone 'hotline' to depressed women staffed by recovered mothers. Cry-sis helps parents with crying infants, the National Childbirth Trust supports and informs pregnant and postnatal women, and Newpin and Homestart are schemes where the principle is to empower women to take control of their lives.

In the increasingly cross-cultural context of postnatal depression research, Boyce's Australian study (Chapter 6) throws new light on the complexity of interactions between women's perceived experience of being parented themselves, their relationship with their partner, and their emotional adjustment to motherhood. O'Hara (Chapter 10) describes cross-cultural aspects of postnatal depression and its measurement, including the use of the EPDS in other cultures and languages.

Screening for antenatal depression using the EPDS is described by Green and Murray (Chapter 12), who point out possible effects of depression on the developing foetus. These may include not attending for antenatal care, smoking, drinking and not eating well due to appetite loss. Their description of the relationship between antenatal and postnatal depression and associated factors provides many ideas which could be used as a basis for preventive interventions. Kumar and his colleagues (Chapter 4) have also drawn attention to the impact of perinatal mental disorder on the family and in particular the need to provide assessment for partners who may be experiencing a mental disorder.

O'Brien and Pitt (Chapter 7) examine the role of hormones and anti-depressants in the prevention and treatment of perinatal mental illness, while Cox outlines problems of classification in ICD–10 (Chapter 1) and reviews the early development of the EPDS, which was closely linked to his previous work in Edinburgh and Uganda (Chapter 8).

In Chapter 9 Holden includes a detailed account of the use of the EPDS in primary care with recommendations about frequency of administration, cut-off scores, and advice about how to cope with difficult clinical situations. The scale, together with scoring instructions, is included at the end of this chapter. Harris and Jamil (Chapter 11) report that the EPDS compares favourably with other self-report measures of psychiatric disorder, and Elliot (Chapter 14) usefully reminds the reader that the EPDS is not a 'magic wand' and recommends caution when it is used by health professionals not trained to understand the nature of mental disorder.

Foreman (Chapter 13) describes the range of other measures, including semi-structured interviews and observational methods, that are of use in assessing disturbed parents and their children. This chapter reminds the reader that underpinning the use of these interviews as well as self-report scales is a psychometric 'technology' which needs to be recognised.

We hope that readers of this book will be challenged by some of the suggestions for changes in practice and also become more confident about the use of the EPDS in primary care.

Jeni Holden
John Cox

Part I. Aspects of
perinatal psychiatry

1 Introduction and classification dilemmas

JOHN COX

This book was conceived at the Marcé Society Conference at Keele in October 1991, which brought together clinicians and researchers from different professional backgrounds to discuss the use, and misuse, of the Edinburgh Postnatal Depression Scale (EPDS) and to share their experience about the prevention of postnatal mental disorders.

The book is not intended as a manual of 'do's and 'don't's for users of the EPDS, although it does provide additional information to that contained in our initial publication (Cox *et al*, 1987). It *is* intended to describe the origin and subsequent usage of this self-report questionnaire and to provide practical assistance for primary care workers who use the scale and are uncertain either about what to say to a mother with a high score, or about whether the EPDS can be satisfactorily used in a multicultural community. The widespread use of the EPDS in other parts of the world was not fully anticipated; nor was it entirely foreseen that a scale validated in Scotland would be of use not only elsewhere in the United Kingdom but also in research and clinical settings overseas.

The reasons for the present interest in the detection of postnatal mental disorders are uncertain and to an extent are 'user driven'. There *is* a greater awareness that childbirth can indeed be followed by severe emotional disorder as well as by personal fulfilment. Changes in the structure of family life with an increased divorce rate and less evident support systems may also need to be considered when explaining the reasons for such persistent concern about postnatal depression.

It remains a paradox however that despite this greater 'user' awareness of the family impact of depression after childbirth, and increased knowledge about its causes and optimum management (Brockington & Kumar, 1982; Kumar & Brockington, 1988; Oates, 1989), the contribution of such knowledge to an understanding of the epidemiology of depression in women (whether or not childbearing) has only recently been more fully acknowledged. The raised incidence of postnatal mood disorders, for example, could partially explain the higher rates of depression in married

women with children than in married women without children reported by
Bebbington *et al* (1991).

ICD-10

Until recently, puerperal mental disorders have not been accorded the status
of separate categorisation by the World Health Organization. The new version
of their *International Classification of Diseases* (ICD-10; WHO, 1992) does,
however, go some way towards addressing this issue. Mental disorders
occurring at this time may now be categorised as puerperal, but only if they
cannot otherwise be classified (F53). It is curious that the psychiatrists who
argued for including a category of 'puerperal psychoses' within ICD-10 were
those from the developing countries. It was nevertheless suggested that
these psychiatrists, because of "very real practical problems", may have
been unable to gather sufficient details about puerperal illness for these
disorders to be classified elsewhere; the assumption is that if such information
had been available they *could* have been classified elsewhere, and the specific
category (F53) 'Mental and behavioural disorders associated with the
puerperium' (Table 1.1) would not then be required at all. Evidence
that the clinical presentation of puerperal psychoses when compared with
non-puerperal psychoses is more florid (Dean & Kendell, 1981) with greater
likelihood of perplexity (Brockington *et al*, 1982) is overlooked; childbirth

TABLE 1.1
ICD-10 classifications of puerperal disorders

F53   **Mental and behavioural disorders associated with the puerperium, not elsewhere classified**
This classification should be used only for mental disorders associated with the
puerperium (commencing within 6 weeks of delivery) that do not meet the criteria for
disorders classified elsewhere in this book, either *because insufficient information is available*,
or because it is considered that *special additional clinical features are present which make
classification elsewhere inappropriate*. It will usually be possible to classify mental disorders
associated with the puerperium by using two other codes: the first is from elsewhere
in chapter V (F) and indicates the specific type of mental disorder (usually affective
(F30–F39)), and the second is 099.3 (mental diseases and diseases of the nervous system
complicating the puerperium) of ICD-10.

F53.0 *Mild* **mental and behavioural disorders associated with the puerperium, not
elsewhere classified**
Includes: postnatal depression NOS
                postpartum depression NOS

F53.1 *Severe* **mental and behavioural disorders associated with the puerperium, not
elsewhere classified**
Includes: puerperal psychosis NOS

F53.8 **Other mental and behavioural disorders associated with the puerperium, not
elsewhere classified**

F53.9 **Puerperal mental disorder, unspecified**

From World Health Organization (1992).

is also known to increase the risk of a psychosis by at least 16-fold (Kendell *et al*, 1987) and threefold for non-psychotic postnatal depression (Cox *et al*, 1993). In addition, the findings of Wieck *et al* (1991) that a specific neuroendocrine mechanism – increased sensitivity of the hypothalamic dopaminergic system due to reduction in circulating oestrogens – may predict relapse of a puerperal psychosis is of the utmost importance. If replicated this finding would support further the separate classification of the postnatal mental disorders.

An additional reason for including postnatal mental disorder within an international classification of mental illness is to prevent the 'category fallacy' (Kleinman, 1987) of a common local 'folk' disorder being overlooked. Postnatal depression is indeed a diagnostic term regarded by most women as useful, and for this reason alone in a 'user-orientated' service it could be included in a classification, which would then reflect actual usage; most women regard postnatal depression as 'different' from depression at other times. The F53 category is useful both in estimating workload and "when decisions are made about the provision of services", but this is only so if the category is routinely used in this way. The present WHO recommendations, alas, are unlikely to encourage such use.

Training issues

The unresolved nosological debate outlined above does not give support for these proponents of a 'normalisation' approach to postnatal mental disorder. As Holden (1991) has cogently pointed out, these disorders *are* experienced by most women themselves as distressing and unexpected – and not as a time of personal growth, or purposive suffering. Experience reported from the Stoke-on-Trent Parent and Baby Day Unit suggests that a diagnostic approach is useful for the full assessment of a new referral, and that this approach is not restricted to assessment by a doctor only. All health professionals who undertake assessments of women with perinatal mental disorder need therefore to be familiar with the purpose of this approach and so to consider the possibility of an organic cause for depression such as thyroid dysfunction or even a cerebral tumour. It is to be hoped that a trend towards denigrating the diagnostic approach will be reversed and that mental health professionals may again share a common core language. Most attenders at a postnatal mental illness clinic are not only 'clients' or 'customers' but also patients – they suffer, and most seek informed medical help.

Health Service managers are more aware than formerly of the specific needs of a postnatal mental illness service. Thus three-quarters of health authorities regard a specialised mother and baby facility as a resource priority (Prettyman & Friedman, 1991) and in the Department of Health's

(1993) guidance to purchasers, the need of women with puerperal psychosis to be treated in a 'designated facility' was likewise recognised. Margaret Oates (Chapters 2 and 3) has emphatically underlined how the user-orientated NHS reforms can be an advantage to women with postnatal mental disorders. The known user demand, acknowledged need for specialist facilities and the sound research base is advantageous when negotiating service contracts between the purchaser and provider. At the present time therefore there is a need to disseminate information about postnatal mental disorder as widely as possible. The Marcé Society should not become an inward-looking organisation but an international society which can influence other professions as well as governments.

The Keele meeting was enhanced by a local link between the Departments of Obstetrics and Psychiatry and there is a need for more such 'healthy alliances'. Collaboration between mental health specialists and social service departments as well as with community units, general practitioner fund-holders and voluntary groups will similarly advance service developments and research.

The Royal College of Psychiatrists (1992) published recommendations about manpower requirements for a postnatal mental illness service from a working party invigorated by the contribution of Margaret Oates, Channi Kumar, David Foreman and Helen Anderson (see also Chapters 2–4). Another College report, "Prevention of mental illness" (1993), included a section on prevention of postnatal mental illness.

Thus the clinical and research base of this subject is now more widely recognised, and is included in more general publications. It is to be hoped therefore that these College reports will be read by managers and clinicians and not only by a research readership; it is within this broader professional setting that the prevention strategies for perinatal mental disorder described in this book, including antenatal and postnatal screening, should be undertaken.

References

BEBBINGTON, P. E., DEAN, C., DER, G., *et al* (1991) Gender, parity and the prevalence of minor affective disorder. *British Journal of Psychiatry*, **158**, 40–45.
BROCKINGTON, I. F. & KUMAR, R. (1982) *Motherhood and Mental Illness*. London: Academic Press.
——, WINOKUR, G. & DEAN, C. (1982) Puerperal psychosis. In *Motherhood and Mental Illness* (eds I. F. Brockington & R. Kumar), pp. 37–69. London: Academic Press.
COX, J. L., HOLDEN, J. & SAGOVSKY, R. (1987) Detection of postnatal depression: development of the 10-item Edinburgh Postnatal Depression Scale (EPDS). *British Journal of Psychiatry*, **150**, 782–786.
——, MURRAY, D. M. & CHAPMAN, G. (1993) A controlled study of the onset, prevalence and duration of postnatal depression. *British Journal of Psychiatry*, **163**, 27–31.

DEAN, C. & KENDELL, R. E. (1981) The symptomatology of puerperal illnesses. *British Journal of Psychiatry*, **139**, 128.

DEPARTMENT OF HEALTH (1993) *The Health of the Nation: Mental Illness Key Area Handbook.* London: HMSO.

HOLDEN, J. M. (1991) Postnatal depression: its nature, effects, and identification using the Edinburgh Postnatal Depression Scale. *Birth*, **18**, December 1991.

KENDELL, R. E., CHALMERS, L. & PLATZ, C. (1987) The epidemiology of puerperal psychoses. *British Journal of Psychiatry*, **150**, 662–673.

KLEINMAN, A. (1987) Anthropology and psychiatry. The role of culture in cross-cultural research on illness. *British Journal of Psychiatry*, **151**, 447–454.

KUMAR, R. & BROCKINGTON, I. F. (1988) *Motherhood and Mental Illness 2: Causes and Consequences.* London: John Wright.

OATES, M. (1989) *Psychological Aspects of Obstetrics & Gynaecology.* Clinical Obstetrics & Gynaecology, vol. 3, no. 4. London: Baillière Tindall.

PRETTYMAN, R. J. & FRIEDMAN, R. (1991) Care of women with puerperal psychiatric disorders in England and Wales. *British Medical Journal*, **302**, 1345–1346.

ROYAL COLLEGE OF PSYCHIATRISTS (1992) Report of the General Psychiatry Section Working Party on Postnatal Mental Illness. *Psychiatric Bulletin*, **16**, 519–522.

—— (1993) Prevention of mental disorder. *Psychiatric Bulletin*, **17**, 633.

WIECK, A., KUMAR, R., HIRST, A. D., *et al* (1991) Increased sensitivity of dopamine receptors and recurrences of affective psychoses after childbirth. *British Medical Journal*, **303**, 613–616.

WORLD HEALTH ORGANIZATION (1992) *The ICD-10 Classification of Mental and Behavioural Disorders.* Geneva: WHO.

2 Postnatal mental illness: organisation and function of services

MARGARET OATES

"The incidence of psychiatric illness following childbirth was much greater than the statistics from psychiatric hospitals would indicate, and large numbers of cases were cared for at home and never recorded." (Esquirol, 1839)

It is now well established that two out of every thousand women delivered are admitted to a psychiatric hospital suffering from puerperal psychosis. It is remarkable that the incidence has remained broadly constant for over a century and in different countries (Kendell *et al*, 1987; Paffenbarger, 1964; Brockington *et al*, 1982). It is likely therefore that this incidence will be the same in the future. This figure represents a dramatic increase in risk compared to non-childbearing women (Kendell *et al*, 1987), but nonetheless admission for puerperal psychosis remains relatively rare.

The incidence of puerperal psychosis, defined by admission alone, would seem insufficient grounds for the development of a special service. However, those women admitted with puerperal psychosis represent only the tip of the iceberg. As Esquirol noted as early as 1839, many women with severe mental illness following childbirth are not admitted, and presumably some do not even receive psychiatric care. Some studies reveal that a further two per thousand women delivered are admitted to hospital suffering from non-psychotic conditions (Kendell *et al*, 1987; Meltzer & Kumar, 1985). Not only is the rate of admission to psychiatric hospital following childbirth increased but also the rate of referral to psychiatric services (Kendell *et al*, 1987; Oates, 1988). According to the latter study, almost 2% of all women delivered are referred to a psychiatric service within a year of childbirth, the majority with serious or major psychiatric disorder. Numerous prospective antenatal and community studies reveal an incidence of postnatal depressive illness in the community, in the year following childbirth, of between 10% and 15% (Kumar & Robson, 1984; Cox *et al*, 1982). These rates would indicate a substantial morbidity in any community, despite the fact that some studies (Cooper *et al*, 1988; O'Hara *et al*, 1989)

8

suggest that this incidence is no greater than in non-childbearing women. Few of these women are known to psychiatric services and few indeed even to their general practitioner (Cox *et al*, 1982). Despite this, Cox's more recent work would suggest that a significant proportion of these women are seriously depressed and would benefit from psychiatric care.

This chapter outlines the evidence for a substantial psychiatric morbidity, part of that population already presenting to, the rest in need of, psychiatric services. These patients are sufficiently numerous, and sufficiently distinctive in terms of their clinical characteristics and health care needs, to justify the setting up of a special service. The existence of mental illness, at a time when most people would expect to be happy, and its potential impact on the relationship with the child and on marital and family relationships, further underlines the importance of this area of mental health care.

The way in which such a service will function will need to be clearly defined. Its resources, criteria for referral and the types of care that it will provide will need to be described. A system of monitoring and evaluating the service will have to be developed to ensure that not only are the needs of these patients met but also the requirements of the purchasers and referrers are satisfied. The design of the service will need to take into account the principles of health care delivery, determined both nationally (the *Health of the Nation* targets and the Patients' Charter) and locally.

Health needs assessment exercise

The purpose of this exercise is to demonstrate to colleagues, planners and potential purchasers that there is a substantial group of patients who need (i.e. will experience significant benefit from) a postnatal mental illness service. Knowledge, derived from research and best clinical practice, is combined with local statistics and socio-demographic factors to present the case of need, the case for specialisation and an estimation of the likely local morbidity and service usage.

The case of need

This can be summarised under the following seven headings: (a) substantial morbidity; (b) serious nature; (c) the fact that the need is unmet; (d) effective treatment; (e) grave consequences; (f) information available; and (g) prevention.

(a) Psychiatric morbidity associated with childbirth

This is substantial: two per thousand women delivered will require admission to a psychiatric hospital, two per thousand suffering from psychotic conditions. On an annual basis, 17 per thousand women delivered will already be referred to the general psychiatric services, and a further proportion of those women delivered, currently not referred, are likely to require psychiatric treatment. In most of the recent studies confirming a prevalence of postnatal depressive illness in the community of at least 10% (Cooper *et al*, 1988; O'Hara *et al*, 1989), their cases have been found to satisfy Research Diagnostic Criteria (RDC) for major depressive illness. It is difficult to be certain what proportion of these patients would benefit from psychiatric treatment. However, it is likely that between 3% and 5% of all women delivered will suffer from a depressive illness of such severity that they would normally be referred to a psychiatrist (Pitt, 1968; Cox *et al*, 1982). In Great Britian as a whole, an average health district, with a population of 350 000 and a standard birth-rate of approximately 5000 births a year (12.5/1000), will have, annually: 500 women suffering from major depressive illness; between 85 and 150 referrals; and a minimum rate of 20 admissions a year, of whom half will be suffering from puerperal psychosis. These figures apply if the strictest criteria of postnatal mental illness are used, that is, a new episode of illness occurring within a defined time period of childbirth. If, in addition to this, those patients suffering from pre-existing illness and those who are pregnant are included, then the numbers will be even higher. In terms of episodes, a general adult population, aged 16–60, will generate 200 to 300 new referrals a year per 50 000 of the population (Oates, 1988). It can be seen, therefore, that the numbers of new referrals generated by a delivered population of 5000 is equivalent to at least half that generated by a general adult population of 50 000, and is the same if wider criteria are used. According to Royal College of Psychiatrists' norms, in a non-teaching hospital, there should be one general adult psychiatrist per 50 000 of the population (1 to 25 000 in a teaching hospital).

(b) The morbidity is serious

Compared with age-matched controls, patients with puerperal psychosis are more seriously disturbed (Dean & Kendell, 1981; Katona, 1982). Using proxy measurements of severity in referred postnatal patients and a comparison group of new episodes of psychiatric care in other women and men, one study found that the postnatal patients were more seriously ill in that they were more likely to receive a diagnosis of major mental illness, to be seen as an emergency, and to be admitted or in receipt of intensive out-patient care (Oates, 1988).

(c) The need is largely unmet

A recent study (Prettyman & Friedman, 1991) found that under half of all health districts in the United Kingdom had facilities for admitting mothers with their babies, and even fewer could guarantee such facilities would be available when required. Of those health authorities that could accommodate mentally ill mothers and their babies, the majority did so by the occasional admission to a general psychiatric ward; few had designated facilities with specialist staff; even fewer health districts had a designated consultant with special interest, and it was rare for them to have specialised out-patient clinics or community psychiatric nurse specialists. The majority of women who become mentally ill following childbirth will, therefore, not receive specialist attention from psychiatric services, nor will they, in the event of needing admission, be admitted with their babies.

(d) Treatment is effective

As is usual for acute-onset major affective illness, treatment is effective. Indeed, it may be that puerperal affective disorders, in particular, are more responsive to treatment and are of briefer duration than non-puerperal illnesses (Dean *et al*, 1989; Oates, 1989*a*).

(e) The consequences of untreated postnatal illness may be grave

Pitt found that, without treatment, 30% of patients suffering from severe postnatal depressive illness were still ill at one year postpartum (Pitt, 1968). Recent studies (Stein *et al*, 1991; Murray & Stein, 1989) of the effects of a community-based sample of postnatal depression on infants have supported this finding. From these studies there is evidence that prolonged postnatal depression, particularly when associated with social adversity and marital conflict, exerts an adverse effect on the social attachments and cognitive development of a child. This effect may be detectable long after the resolution of the maternal illness. Postnatal mental illness, particularly if prolonged, may deter a woman from having further children or lead to marital breakdown.

(f) Information available

Information is available that will enable the prediction of *groups of patients at risk* and in particular circumstances of *individuals at risk*. The findings of epidemiological research, together with knowledge of the local annual birth-rate, enables a precise estimation of the size of local morbidity and the likely number of referrals. Studies of the psychosocial and obstetric correlates of postnatal mental illness (Kendell *et al*, 1981; Kumar & Robson, 1984; Elliott, 1989) have led to an understanding of some of the risk factors for this illness. This allows the identification of groups of women in the antenatal clinic who are at greater than average risk of developing postnatal depression. Women with a history of bipolar affective disorder, or

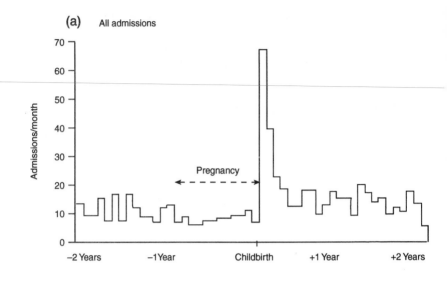

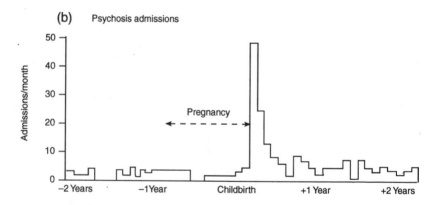

Fig. 2.1. Temporal relationship between psychiatric admission and childbirth: (a) all admissions; (b) psychosis admissions (Kendell et al, *1987)*

puerperal psychosis, are now known to be at very high risk, thought initially to be 1 : 5 (Protheroe, 1969) then 1 : 3 (Kendell *et al*, 1987) and, more recently, as high as 1 : 2 (Wieck *et al*, 1991). Unusually for mental health issues, not only are the number of likely patients known, as well as those groups most vulnerable to developing the illness, but also some of the individuals who are at high risk.

There is also much information available on the timing of the presentation of postnatal patients in relation to delivery. Numerous studies (e.g. Kendell *et al*, 1987) have shown that the majority of puerperal psychoses presented to psychiatric services within 14 days postpartum, and the majority of severe mental illnesses requiring admission presented by 90 days postpartum. Data collected by Kendell in Edinburgh are shown in Fig. 2.1.

In Nottingham, over a one-year period all psychiatric referrals from a defined catchment area, within a year of childbirth, were recorded (Fig. 2.2).

As will be seen from the figures, the histograms are remarkably similar. Despite the fact that the Nottingham data include all patients referred

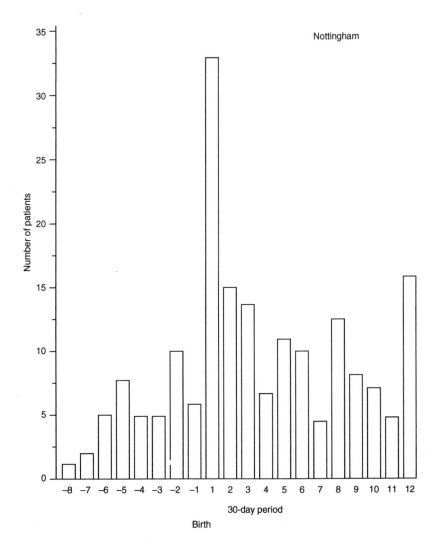

Fig. 2.2. Number of referrals in 30-day periods during pregnancy and within a year of childbirth

while the Edinburgh data include only those admitted, both show a clear peaking of admissions and referrals during the first three months following delivery. The Nottingham group was broken down into diagnostic categories, using Research Diagnostic Criteria on the case notes and clinical ICD–9 case register diagnoses. This revealed that the majority of the schizophreniform illnesses, bipolar disorders and one-third of major depressive illness had presented early in the puerperium, by 30 days postpartum, confirming the findings of Kendell and others. The minor mental illnesses did not show this peaking and presented steadily throughout the first postpartum year. It is clear that early presentation is strongly associated with a diagnosis of a serious condition. Information on the timing of the presentation of various conditions, and their likely severity following childbirth, is very useful when planning service and management strategies for individual patients.

(g) Detection and prevention

Women come under high levels of health care scrutiny during pregnancy and the puerperium. They are seen at regular intervals throughout pregnancy by both doctors and midwives, twice daily by a midwife for the first five days postpartum, and then daily until the tenth postpartum day. In many areas they are seen regularly by a midwife until 28 days postpartum, when all women are seen by health visitors. All women are examined by a doctor at six weeks postpartum for their postnatal check. This structure, which is unique in the human lifetime, provides at the very least an exciting opportunity for the identification for those at high risk, the early detection and speedy treatment of postpartum illness, and the screening at postnatal examination for postpartum depression. This can be accomplished by routinely enquiring about well-being and mental health or by using a screening questionnaire, such as the Edinburgh Postnatal Depression Scale (see Chapters 8 and 9, and Cox *et al*, 1987).

There is evidence that continuing the medication of chronic schizophrenic women during pregnancy avoids a relapse of their condition postpartum (Kendell *et al*, 1987). A non-randomised study of high-risk women receiving lithium following delivery (Stewart *et al*, 1991) has suggested that this strategy may significantly reduce the risk of a postpartum episode, although this remains to be confirmed by a randomised controlled trial. Wieck *et al* (1991) have suggested that those women identified as being at high risk of relapse, by virtue of a history of bipolar disorder or puerperal psychosis, have a D2 receptor hypersensitivity to the rapid fall of oestrogen levels postpartum. A trial on the efficacy of transdermal oestrogen in preventing subsequent postpartum episodes is currently under way. The service for postnatal mental illness could, in the not too distant future, offer a unique opportunity in mental health to prevent serious mental illness.

The case for specialisation

The case of need outlined above could be seen as merely an argument for the importance of recognising and treating postnatal mental illness. A further argument is needed to convince both psychiatric colleagues and potential purchasers that the needs of this group of patients are best served by a specialist service. The arguments which can be put forward for the development of a specialist service for postnatal mental illness are, to some extent, the same arguments that have in the past 40 years led to the development of most major specialities in medicine and subspecialities within psychiatry. In the 1960s it was commonplace for children to be treated in hospital on adult wards. It is now thought desirable that children should always be treated by specialists in child care and should always be nursed on paediatric wards, a standard which is now achieved by most health districts. Similarly, few health districts lack specialist services for care of the elderly, alcoholism, rehabilitation, forensic psychiatry or psychotherapy, all of whose patients in the recent past were treated by general adult psychiatrists. The development of these specialities has been paralleled by a recognition in education and training by the appropriate colleges. The specialised health service for a defined group of the population is justified when the following criteria are met:

(a) large group/shared characteristics
(b) distinctive needs
(c) different organisation of service
(d) general service not meeting needs
(e) sufficient workload

(a) Large group/shared characteristics

The target group is a large number of patients suffering from either a *specific condition* (e.g. diabetes, alcoholism, breast cancer) or one which is clearly defined by *age* (geriatric medicine, paediatrics), by a common *disability* (rehabilitative medicine, psychiatric rehabilitation, mental handicap) or by *gender-specific* disorders (gynaecology).

(b) Distinctive needs

The group has shared and *distinctive characteristics* which clearly distinguish them from the majority of patients dealt with by that branch of medicine. The distinctiveness may be in terms of their clinical characteristics, their special needs (medical, nursing and social), the special skills and training from health care professionals and the requirement to liaise with different agencies and other branches of medicine.

(c)   Different organisation of service

All of these distinctive characteristics will require that the service to meet their needs be *organised in a different way* to that of the general service.

(d)   General service not meeting needs

It will be necessary to show not only that the existing psychiatric services are not meeting the need adequately, but also that there is likely to be a significant health benefit to this group of patients by organising specialisation in their care. It is now widely accepted in areas such as diabetology, clinical haematology, oncology and infertility that the outcome for patients, in terms of consumer satisfaction, treatment response and survival, is better if the patient is treated in a specialist setting than if treated by a generalist – even if the same treatment protocols are used. Most health districts in Great Britain would now accept the provision of such services for their population as an efficient, valid way of meeting a health care need.

(e)   Sufficient workload

There should be a *sufficient workload* generated by a specific group of patients to justify the sessional commitment of a consultant, with supporting resources. Development of a special service should not only meet the needs of the target group but should also lead (if only by reducing the workload of other services) to an improvement in the care of people not suffering from the condition.

Postnatal mental illness satisfies all of the above criteria for a specialist health service. It represents a large group of women, united by a condition of mental illness – predominantly severe affective disorder – and the presence of a baby. The most severely ill will have a very young baby in the first few weeks of its life. The needs of these women compared with other psychiatric patients are *distinctive*. If admitted they need to have facilities for their baby to be admitted with them. They will require a different organisation of in-patient care and daily routine. They have physical needs not shared by other patients. They require skills and understanding on the part of their doctors and nurses that are not normally found in psychiatry. The professionals involved in their care will have to give a high degree of priority to the needs of the child and possess the requisite skills for their patient's care. The team involved in their care will regularly work with midwives, health visitors, obstetricians and child care social workers, and will need to have an understanding of these professional disciplines and languages, again something not generally required in general adult psychiatry. In addition, postnatal patients would appear to be distinctive clinically when compared with other psychiatric patients.

In two one-year periods in Nottingham, all patients who presented with a new episode requiring psychiatric care during the postpartum year were compared with all other new episodes of psychiatric care, in both men and women, from the ages of 16 to 50, using case register ICD–9 diagnoses (the comparison group). They were also compared with a randomly selected tightly controlled group of first onset illnesses in the same time period, in both men and women, using both ICD–9 diagnoses and RDC diagnoses (the control group). A report of the 1983/84 study is given by Oates (1988).

Using both ICD–9 and RDC diagnoses it can be seen that postpartum women are significantly more likely to be diagnosed as suffering from major depressive illness, and more likely to be suffering from depressive illness

TABLE 2.1
ICD–9 diagnosis of study group and comparison group 1985–86

| | Study group | | Women | | Men | |
	n	%	n	%	n	%
Schizophrenia	17	(12)	154	(8)	229	(14)
Mania/mixed affective state	2	(1)	29	(2)	35	(2)
Manic depression/depressed	48	(35)	104	(6)	41	(3)
Neurotic depression	16	(12)	186	(10)	87	(5)
Non-depressive neurotic	12	(9)	212	(11)	126	(8)
All others and NPD	43	(31)	1151	(63)	1086	(68)
Total	138		1836		1604	

TABLE 2.2
RDC diagnoses (postnatal referrals compared with other first onset referrals 1985/86)

| | Women with child under 1 | | Women without child under 1 | | Men | |
	n	%	n	%	n	%
Schizophrenia	5	(3.7)	6	(7.8)	7	(10.9)
Bipolar disorders	6	(4.4)	1	(1.3)	4	(6.3)
Major depression	51	(37.5)	8	(10.4)	3	(4.7)
Minor depression	22	(16.2)	21	(27.3)	5	(7.8)
Anxiety disorders	8	(5.9)	8	(10.4)	6	(9.4)
Personality disorders	5	(3.7)	7	(9.1)	14	(21.9)
Other psychiatric disorders	11	(8.1)	6	(7.8)	7	(10.9)
No psychiatric disorder	28	(20.6)	20	(26)	18	(28.1)
Total	138		77		64	

Column 1 v. (Columns 2 + 3): $\chi^2 = 42$, d.f. = 7, $P = 0.0000$.
Column 2 v. 3: $\chi^2 = 15.7$, d.f. = 7, $P = 0.0277$.

TABLE 2.3
Type of first contact of study and comparison groups 1985–86

	Women with child under 1		Women without child under 1		Men	
	n	%	n	%	n	%
Admission/day care	8	(6)	61	(3)	74	(5)
Emergency domiciliary visit	24	(17)	147	(8)	118	(7)
Ward referral	25	(18)	97	(5)	81	(5)
Attempted suicide	11	(8)	208	(11)	142	(9)
Out-patient contact	70	(51)	1323	(72)	1189	(74)
Total	138		1836		1604	

of all types, but significantly less likely to be suffering from anxiety disorders and personality disorders (Tables 2.1 and 2.2).

The same study compared the pattern of service usage between postnatal women and other men and women presenting with a new episode of care. It can be seen from Table 2.3 that postpartum women are much more likely to be seen as an emergency, either at home or on the postnatal ward. Table 2.4 shows that they are much more likely to be admitted or in frequent out-patient contact, and much less likely to be seen on one occasion only. It would therefore seem that postnatal women have a different pattern of service usage, with over half of them being seriously ill and requiring urgent assessment and intensive psychiatric care. Approximately the same proportion of the general adult population are seen on two or fewer occasions and the majority are seen for the first time in scheduled out-patient clinics. These findings were stable over the two time periods, 1983–84 and 1985–86.

Having established that postnatal patients have special needs, distinctive characteristics and different patterns of service usage from general psychiatric patients, it follows that the service to meet their needs should be organised differently from general psychiatric services. This can be accomplished in the following ways:

(a) The service will need to provide in-patient facilities for mothers and their babies. These, together with the out-patient facilities, will need to

TABLE 2.4
Level of care reached in the three months: study and comparison groups 1985–86

	Study group		Women		Men	
	n	%	n	%	n	%
Admission	33	(24)	148	(8)	171	(11)
Day care	—		49	(3)	35	(2)
4 + out-patient contacts	28	(20)	64	(3)	63	(4)
1–3 out-patient contacts	43	(31)	609	(33)	476	(30)
No further contact	34	(25)	966	(53)	859	(54)
Total	138		1836		1604	

be modified to meet the physical and emotional needs of mothers, their babies and families.

(b) The service will need to be staffed by a multidisciplinary team, whose members will need to possess special skills and understanding and be able to cope with severely mentally ill mothers, the majority of whom will have small babies.

(c) The service will need to respond rapidly to over a third of all patients referred, seeing them either at home or on the postnatal wards; many of these will be psychiatric emergencies. The majority of the patients will be seriously mentally ill, at least twice as many as among new referrals to general psychiatric services, and are three times more likely to be seen as an emergency.

(d) The team must include community psychiatric nurses with the ability to cope with severely ill women at home, many of whom have older children.

(e) The team will need to liaise not only with general practitioners but also midwives and health visitors, as well as with obstetricians and when necessary child psychiatrists.

There should also be sufficient workload (according to the size of the population and its delivery rate) generated by a delivered population to justify designated specialist consultant sessions.

Local morbidity

Information derived from epidemiological and health service research into the incidence and risk factors associated with postnatal mental illness should be combined with local health statistics, sociodemographic and ethnogeographic information to produce an estimate of the likely local morbidity. The basic local information required will be the population of the health district to be served and its annual birth-rate. It will also be important to note whether the population and birth-rate likely to be served by the team is greater than that of the health district. For example, is the annual delivery rate of maternity hospitals within the health district greater than that of the health district itself? Are there areas of adjacent health districts whose health needs have tended to be met by the health district in which the postnatal mental illness service is based? Are there potential purchasers in these areas? Using the incidence rates described previously – two per thousand deliveries admitted with puerperal psychosis – a minimum of 1.7% referred to psychiatric services, a reasonable target of 3% of all deliveries referred and a likely community morbidity of at least 10%, local incidence and morbidity figures can be produced, both for the health district and for the potential market. It should be borne in mind that these figures, particularly those above from the Nottingham studies, are derived from an area whose population pyramids, social class distribution, ethnic mix, annual birth-rate, indexes of socio-economic deprivation and contact rates with the psychiatric services are representative of the rest of the UK. It is therefore important to note whether the health district under examination is unusual or non-standard in any of these dimensions, or if parts of the area covered by the service have distinctive demographic or ethnogeographic features. This is particularly important for those areas where risk factors for postnatal mental illness are likely to be over-represented, for example, areas with high levels of social isolation, single parents, low birth-weight babies or the presence of maternity hospitals which specialise in high-risk obstetric problems.

The development and function of a service

It is not possible to prescribe one standard model for service provision. Health districts vary greatly in size of population from under 200 000 to almost a million. Some health districts lie totally within an urban conurbation, others are predominantly rural, and others consist of many small towns. Whatever its final design a postnatal mental illness service must ensure that all women suffering from psychiatric disorder associated with childbirth have access to a specialist service, a psychiatrist with a special interest in their condition, a specialist community nursing team and specialist mother and baby beds should women require admission. As outlined below, such a model requires attention to design, resources and function.

Designing the service

The rational planning and design of the service will be affected by the site of the hospitals and maternity units, existing patterns of referral to these units, 'natural' patterns of usage of centres by the population (including public transport networks), major and subsidiary concentrations of population, the proportion of urban and rural communities and concentrations of high-risk populations. The latter includes areas of high birth-rate, high socio-economic deprivation and infant morbidity. Such small-area statistics, obtained by combining health service statistics and census data with postcoding, is usually available from the Director of Public Health. It is important to note that areas usually associated with high rates of referral to general psychiatry may be different from those associated with high referral rates of postnatal mental illness. Such patients usually come from areas where their babies are born. These areas may change over a period of, say, five to ten years. The building of a new housing estate or the closure of a colliery can quickly change the 'map' of postnatal mental illness, an important consideration when planning community facilities.

Three models for designing the service will be described as follows:

(a) For a large health district of between 600 and 800 000, with a large urban conurbation, the rest of the health district being small villages.
(b) For a medium-sized health district of population of approximately 350 000, composed of many small towns, one larger than the rest.
(c) For a small health district population 200 000, containing one main town in a predominantly rural area.

Resources

Whatever the design of the service, the resources in terms of consultant sessions, nursing staff, bed numbers and out-patient sessions can be calculated in the following way:

(a) Consultant sessions. The Royal College of Psychiatrists recommends one general adult consultant psychiatrist to 50 000 of the population (1 to 25 000 of the population for a teaching hospital).
(b) A full-time consultant psychiatrist will see between 200 and 300 new referrals a year, with an annual total patient contact of approximately 2000.
(c) A delivered population of 10 000 (health district population 800 000) will generate 170 new referrals (1.7%) to 300 new referrals a year (3%), justifying a half-time commitment at the lower rate of referral or a full-time commitment at the higher rate.
(d) A delivered population of 5000 (health district population 400 000) will generate between 85 and 150 new referrals a year, justifying a 2–3 session a week commitment at the lower rate of referral to a half-time commitment at the higher rate.
(e) Extending the role of the postnatal service to include assessment and management of women with chronic mental health problems, antenatal patients and prenatal counselling (see section on prevention, p. 29) will increase the referral rate and justify a higher sessional commitment.

Beds

Two per thousand of the delivered population will be admitted suffering from puerperal psychosis, but women suffering from non-psychotic conditions, particularly severe postnatal depression, are also likely to be admitted. Some studies suggest that four per thousand women delivered will be admitted for all diagnoses. Experience in Nottingham over the last ten years (during which there have been three phases of increasing the delivered population served by the postnatal service) has shown that mother and baby bed numbers have more than adequately served the needs of the delivered population. All of those mothers requiring admission for a new episode of mental illness following childbirth have been admitted with their babies, and a reliable system of cross-checking has confirmed that no mother has been admitted without her baby. Mother and baby bed numbers are as follows:

(a) Three mother and baby beds were adequate for a delivered population of 5000 (health district size 390 000), with 16 patients admitted per year.
(b) Four mother and baby beds were adequate for a delivered population of almost 8000 (health district size 650 000), with 26 patients admitted per year.
(c) Six mother and baby beds were adequate for a delivered population of over 13 000 (two health districts with a combined population of 1 000 000), with 40 patients admitted per year.

As Nottingham is 'standard' for the rest of Great Britain in terms of psychiatric morbidity, indexes of socio-economic deprivation, socio-demographic and ethnic mix and birth-rate, it is likely that these bed requirements can be generalised to the rest of Great Britain. However, during this ten-year period there have always been community nurses attached to the service. It is likely that their involvement serves to shorten the stay in hospital and reduce the numbers of admissions, particularly those of non-psychotic patients. Therefore, if there is no community nurse involved, there would be a requirement for at least one more bed for the smaller delivered population and two more for the larger. Throughout this period of time the average bed occupancy has been over 60%, ranging from 25% to 100%.

Mother and baby beds versus mother and baby unit

It is reasonable to plan to provide one bed for every 2000 women delivered (1.5 beds per 2000 if there is no community nurse involved in their care). For small health districts with only four to eight admissions of mother and baby pairs a year, it would be difficult to provide special facilities or specially designated staff. The occasional admission of a mother and baby pair to a general psychiatric ward will not allow the special experience and skills required for their care to be developed. It may be better in such circumstances to arrange admission facilities in a larger unit as near as possible to the patient's home. This 'critical mass' argument would suggest that the minimum number of mother and baby beds needed to form a viable in-patient facility is four. A small mother and baby unit, between four and six beds, can take the form of an annexe to a general psychiatric ward, with which it is administratively linked. It would have its own designated nurse but be able to draw on the nurses from the main ward when necessary. Larger mother and baby units, of six to nine beds, could justify a separate unit with its own staff. A mother and baby unit will need single rooms for the mothers, of sufficient size to allow rooming in of infant, a nursery, a day area, a 'clean' kitchen (not used by other patients) and separate laundry and toilet facilities.

In-patient nurses

A mother and baby unit will require an establishment of 4.5 nurses to provide one nurse per shift on duty. This would be the minimum requirement for a four- to six-bed unit and will need to be increased proportionately for larger units. One of these nurses will need to be of a higher grade and designated 'the ward manager'. There will also need to be a nursery nurse on each day-time shift (an establishment of two would produce one nursery nurse).

Community psychiatric nurses

To allow bed numbers to be kept to the minimum, the avoidance of unnecessary admissions and a smooth transition from in-patient stay to community care, community psychiatric nurses are an essential part of the postnatal service. It may also be possible (Oates, 1988) for community nurses to be able to manage severely ill patients at home as an alternative to admission. A specialist community psychiatric nurse should carry no more than 25 cases at a time. Experience in Nottingham reveals that approximately one-third of all referrals will require community psychiatric nursing input. The minimum number of community psychiatric nurses for a delivered population of 8000 is three; for a delivered population of 13 000 it is five. For the larger teams, one of the community psychiatric nurses will need to be of a higher grade and designated 'team leader'.

Other professionals

The service will give a high degree of priority to the needs of the child. A large proportion of the patients seen by the service will be psychiatric emergencies. The psychiatric social worker will therefore be an essential member of the multidisciplinary team, and should be experienced in child protection and the Mental Health Act. Smaller health districts would justify a half-time social worker, the larger ones a full-time social worker. An occupational therapist and a psychologist are also desirable members of the multidisciplinary team. The mother and baby unit will require the services of a liaison health visitor for a minimum of one session a week and there should also be formal links with a designated paediatrician and child psychiatrist.

Day hospital

Experience of a unique Health Service day hospital for mothers and their babies (run by Professor Cox in Stoke-on-Trent) suggests that a day hospital can be a very useful part of a postnatal service. Its nursing staff can be flexibly deployed in the community, it can act as a team base and resource centre for the service and it can provide care for a wide variety of conditions ranging from serious mental illness to minor psychiatric disorder. It can also fulfil a function for assessment of mothers with ongoing mental health needs and allow for the care of whole families, including husbands, relatives and older children. A day hospital could be sited adjacent to the mother and baby unit – allowing for the sharing of some in-patient facilities and staffing – or in the community.

Out-patient clinics

A delivered population of 5000 will generate between 85 and 150 new referrals a year with up to 1500 total patient contacts. This is equivalent to approximately 3 new patients and 30 follow-up appointments a week, justifying one out-patient session to be conducted by a consultant and supporting junior staff. The numbers of out-patient sessions can be increased proportionately, according to the delivered population.

An outline of three examples of service design – for a large, standard and small health district – follow:

(a) **Large health district:** this would typically have a population of between 650 000 and 800 000 with an annual birth-rate of between approximately 8000 and 10 500. It will have one large urban conurbation, the rest of the health district being predominantly rural: small towns and villages. There will be large district general hospital containing the maternity unit and the natural routes will be to the centre. The most efficient use of resources would be a small mother and baby unit containing between four and six beds, together with special facilities, managed as an annexe to a general admission unit in the district general hospital. On the same site will be the out-patient clinics and the day hospital, which acts as the team base and resource centre. This allows for some flexible usage of staff and comprehensive integrated care. The community nurses will travel out to manage patients in the community. The size of the unit can be increased if it serves the needs of patients from outside the health district and if the role of the service is extended. This service will require a minimum of a half-time consultant with supporting junior staff, and between three and five specialist community nurses.

In Nottingham (population 650 000; births 7800) there has been a motherhood and mental health service in an extended role since 1984.

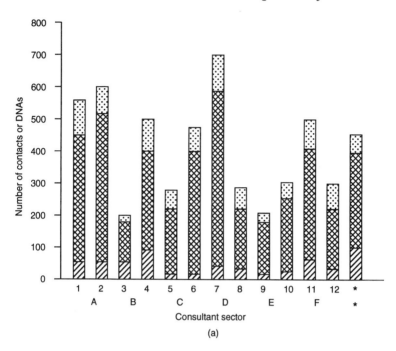

(a)

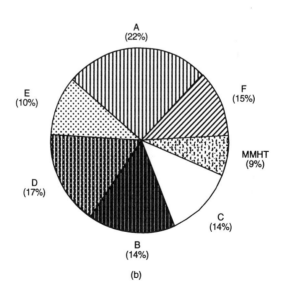

(b)

*Fig. 2.3. Acute mental health services (Out-patient contacts October–December 1992). (a) Breakdown of contacts seen (▧ new, ▨ repeat, ⬚ DNA, * Motherhood and mental health team (MMHT)). (b) Percentage of contacts by consultant sector*

It also serves an adjacent health district (population 325 000; births 3000). It has one half-time equivalent consultant (the author) with supporting junior staff, five community psychiatric nurses and a six-bed mother and baby unit. Figure 2.3a shows that the numbers of new patients and total contacts seen by the service compares favourably with those seen by other individual consultants and with those seen by the sector services – childbirth-related disorders forming 9% of total contacts with the acute mental health service (Fig. 2.3b).

(b) **Standard health district:** this will typically have a population of approximately 350 000 and an annual birth rate of under 4000 a year. It will consist of a number of small towns, the largest of which contains the district general hospital with the maternity unit. An admission rate of between 8 and 16 patients a year, and need for only two to three beds, means that there will be insufficient demand to sustain a specialist mother and baby unit for this health district alone. However, such a unit could be justified if an adjacent health district can be persuaded to use the facilities. The delivered population of this health district will generate between 68 and 120 new referrals a year, more if the role of the service is extended. This will justify designation of between three specialist sessions to a half-time consultant, and two community psychiatric nurses. A small mother and baby unit (minimum size four beds) can be sited on the main district general hospital maternity unit campus, or in-patient facilities in an adjacent health district can be used. The out-patient clinic and main team base should be sited in the district general hospital where a day hospital could also be situated. However, a day hospital and community base could also reasonably be sited in the second largest town in the health district.

(c) **Small health district:** these typically will have populations of approximately 200 000 and an annual birth rate of up to 2600 with only four to six admissions a year. The service should consider using an adjacent in-patient facility when necessary, or combine together with a number of other health districts to provide a subregional or regional service. There will be between 60 and 90 new referrals a year, justifying the designation of one or two specialist consultant sessions, one small out-patient clinic and one community psychiatric nurse.

Supra-district/regional units

It can be seen from the preceding calculations that combining health districts to provide a population of a million or more, with an annual birth rate in excess of 13 500, can justify the setting up of a specialist in-patient unit of sufficient size to be independently staffed and to provide a base for training and research. However, great care must be taken that such a centralised facility does not prejudice the essential needs of postnatal patients, which is to have comprehensive and integrated care provided as near as possible to their homes. If the health district decides to use the resources of such a unit it does not preclude provision at district level of a special interest consultant, special out-patient clinics and a community team base. In this situation a day hospital in each of the user health districts may be a very useful way of ensuring that wherever possible treatment is available locally.

Operation and function

Operational criteria for referral to the service are essential. They should be clear and unambiguous so that the referrer easily knows which patients the service will see. If the only criteria is the use of the term 'postnatal' or 'puerperal' then this will beg the issue of whether the conditions managed by the service are only those resulting from, or caused by, childbirth (aetiological criteria) or whether the service manages conditions associated with childbirth (temporal criteria). This is not only likely to lead to confusion among referrers but more importantly will lead to certain patients it is important to refer not being referred. For example, if there is an aetiological assumption of referral, women with a history of major psychiatric illness may not be referred as the referrer may assume that their condition is not caused by childbirth. Similarly, a depressed postnatal patient with marital and social problems may not be referred, because the referrer assumes that her depression is caused by her problems rather than by childbirth. The service exists to meet the needs of patients whose early motherhood is complicated by co-existing mental illness, not just those women whose illness is thought to be a consequence of childbirth.

At present the law on infanticide and DSM–III–R and ICD–9 regard the postnatal period as being one-year long. Obstetricians regard it as being six weeks long, finishing at the postnatal examination. Many studies have shown that the bulk of the excess morbidity associated by childbirth is in the first 90 days postpartum. By this time the majority of puerperal psychoses and a substantial proportion of the major depressive illnesses will have presented. However, a significant proportion of the major depressive illnesses, and the majority of the minor illnesses, will continue to present throughout the postpartum year. Whereas it is likely that postnatal mental illness has its onset within the first 90 days, there may be a delay before the non-psychotic conditions present. Having a 'cut-off period' too early in the puerperium may mean that women who would be likely to benefit from the service are excluded.

In summary, therefore, the best operational criteria for referral are administrative. This can be defined as a new episode of mental illness (having previously been well or less ill) occurring within a defined period of childbirth (between six months and a year).

The essential function of the postnatal mental illness service is therefore to oversee the following:

(a) Women suffering from puerperal psychosis and major postnatal mental illness, within a year of childbirth. It will provide mother and baby admission facilities (or obtain them) for those who require it as well as out-patient clinics and community treatment.
(b) It will accept referrals from general practitioners, psychiatrists and obstetricians.
(c) It will advise on, and manage if required, patients with continuing mental health problems who become pregnant.
(d) It will advise general practitioners and other referrers for less serious psychiatric conditions and assess or manage them when appropriate.

Extended role of the postnatal mental illness service

Once the core functions have been achieved then it is likely that the role of the service can be rationally extended.

Obstetric liaison

The service can see patients with mental health problems associated with pregnancy, miscarriage, termination of pregnancy, stillbirth and other obstetric loss, infertility and assisted reproduction.

Prenatal counselling and clinics for high risk patients

The postnatal mental illness service can see women who are at high risk by virtue of a previous major mental illness, or puerperal psychosis, on behalf of psychiatrists and obstetricians, and also see women referred by obstetricians who are concerned that they might suffer from postnatal depression.

Assessment

The service can, at the request of psychiatric colleagues and social workers (in collaboration with child psychiatrists and social services), see women with chronic major mental illness, and provide an assessment of their capacity to care for their child. Such a period of assessment can, if the patient has the potential, also serve to provide a secure and supportive environment in which the new mother can establish a relationship with her child and learn the appropriate skills.

Advice to primary health care teams

The service can provide an advice, support and supervision service to general practitioners, health visitors and midwives in their management of postnatal depressive illness and other emotional problems associated with motherhood, that would not normally require specialist psychiatric treatment.

Education

The service team can contribute to undergraduate and postgraduate medical education and to the training of midwives and health visitors.

Prevention

Puerperal psychoses

The prevailing current opinion is that biological factors (including genetic factors) are likely to be as important if not more important in the causation of puerperal psychoses than psychosocial and obstetric factors. The most plausible explanation for these conditions is that the majority of them are a variant of bipolar disorder and that the women carry this genetically determined susceptibility in childbirth, following which the illness is triggered by some factor. One recent explanation for this 'triggering' mechanism is that such patients develop a hypersensitivity of the central D2 receptors, which may be related to the effects of oestrogen withdrawal on the function of the dopamine systems. However, other steroid hormones have been implicated (Wieck, 1989). Although there has been conflicting evidence about identifiable psychosocial and obstetric risk factors for puerperal psychosis, this is in contrast to the consistent finding of major contributions to risk of having a family history of affective psychosis or a personal history of either puerperal or non-puerperal affective psychosis. The risk, for a woman, of having a family history of affective psychosis has not often been quantified but according to Reich & Winokur (1970) it may be 1 : 3. However, over the last 25 years, the risk for a woman who has a previous history of affective psychosis has frequently been estimated and is now thought to lie between 1 : 3 and 1 : 2 (Kendell *et al*, 1987; Wieck *et al*, 1991). This risk may be even higher if the patient has previously been manic.

Such a level of risk would suggest that information on family and personal psychiatric histories should be routinely gathered at the booking clinic. A woman with a personal history of affective psychosis should be referred to a specialist psychiatrist during her pregnancy. Ideally when general adult psychiatrists are managing young women with bipolar disorder, the issue of their future childbearing should be raised and the risk explained, with the advice that such a patient should get back in touch with the psychiatrist when the time arises, for further discussion and planning. It is unlikely that such a discussion will raise the patient's anxieties, as such women are highly likely to raise this issue themselves when they are pregnant and be concerned about potential risk. Preconception counselling or antenatal referral of a well woman with a history of bipolar disorder at the very least offers the psychiatrist a unique opportunity to know the patient when well and to engage in forward planning. It will enable those caring for the patient, both professionals and family, to be alert after delivery for the early signs of the illness and to ensure prompt and appropriate treatment (secondary prevention).

At best it offers the opportunity to engage in prophylactic treatment (primary prevention). There is some early and encouraging evidence that lithium carbonate, started on the first postpartum day, and aiming at a therapeutic level between day 3 and day 5, may prevent the onset of postpartum affective psychoses (Stewart *et al*, 1991). However, the usefulness of this technique remains to be confirmed by randomised controlled trials. Alternatives, particularly for breast-feeding mothers, include using small doses of neuroleptic medication such as haloperidol or chlorpromazine. This regime should also begin on the first postpartum day.

The findings of Wieck *et al* (1991) suggest a rationale of avoiding the postpartum drop in oestrogen levels. A trial of transdermal oestrogen in the prevention of recurrent postpartum psychosis is under way.

The use of progesterone, given intramuscularly before birth and rectally for a period of time afterwards, has been suggested by Dalton and has enthusiastic popular support (Dalton, 1985). However, its clinical effectiveness has not been confirmed by others.

Non-psychotic conditions

The weight of research findings and the prevailing current opinion is that psychosocial factors are at least as important, if not more important, than biological factors in the causation of most severe or major depressive illnesses and the majority of minor depressive illnesses in the puerperium. However, there may be a subgroup of very severe postnatal depressive illnesses which present early, within the first four weeks postpartum, comprising one-third of all referred severe depressive illnesses (Kendell *et al*, 1987; Oates, 1988), patients for whom biological factors are in the ascendancy. For this subgroup of early presentation of severe depressive illnesses it might appear rational to engage in primary prevention, using hormonal or psychotropic medication. However, there is little clinical or anecdotal evidence and no evidence from randomised control trials to support this strategy as yet.

In order to engage in the primary prevention of postnatal depressive illness, in which it is presumed that psychosocial factors appear to have a critical causative role, risk factors first need to be identified which prospectively distinguish those who will suffer from the condition from those who will not. Secondly, a randomised intervention study will need to be carried out in an identified high-risk group which clearly shows a reduction in the incidence of postnatal depression in the treated group compared with the non-treated group. Most major studies of the psychosocial correlates of postnatal depressive illness reveal numerous and complex risk factors, which make it unlikely that prediction in the individual case will be possible, only that groups of women at increased risk can be identified.

Leverton and Elliott (Elliott, 1989; Leverton & Elliott, 1989) devised a questionnaire for identifying risk factors for postnatal mental illness for use at the booking antenatal clinic. This questionnaire contained items on five psychological and sociable variables, including psychiatric history, previous postnatal depression, marital relationships, confiding relationships and anxiety. These items were selected because they had been frequently mentioned in previous major prospective studies of postnatal depression by other authors. They validated their questionnaire against the Present State Examination at three months postpartum. They found that the group without identified risk factors had an incidence of 16% suffering postnatal depression at three months, compared with 40% of women with identified risk factors. In the second stage of their study they designed a rational intervention programme (one that is easily replicable without major resource implications). This was based on modified antenatal and parentcraft groups with restricted membership (i.e. closed), continuity of psychologically trained staff, social support, access to individual help and anticipatory learning (focusing the group beyond childbirth and into the likely experiences of early parenthood). Throughout the programme the emphasis was on the development of social support rather than the traditional emphasis on education. Women identified at the booking clinic as being vulnerable by high scores on the questionnaire were randomly allocated to the intervention programme or standard antenatal care. They found that the vulnerable group, who had been on the intervention programme, had a reduced rate of postnatal depression at three months (19%) as compared with the vulnerable group who received standard care only (40%). These are very interesting findings and remain to be confirmed by others.

A trial is currently under way to identify those at risk of developing postnatal depression by using the Edinburgh Postnatal Depression Scale validated for use in pregnancy. Patients will receive a number of sessions of non-directive counselling by specially trained health visitors of the type that has previously been found to be effective in the treatment of postnatal depression (Holden *et al*, 1989). The results of this trial are awaited.

Secondary prevention in postnatal depression is now a practical possibility. The postnatal examination carried out on all women in the United Kingdom at six weeks postpartum should include either a brief routine clinical examination to detect depressive illness or the use of the Edinburgh Postnatal Depression Scale. Such a strategy would go a long way towards detecting the 10% of women likely to be suffering from postnatal depressive illness and would ensure early treatment of this condition, thus reducing avoidable and prolonged psychiatric morbidity and limiting the consequences for the child. Such early treatment for the more severe cases would include antidepressants and, for the less severe cases, non-directive counselling or a cognitive psychotherapeutic approach (Elliott, 1989). A better understanding of the numerous psychosocial risk factors for the development of postnatal depressive illness would enable obstetricians, midwives, health visitors and general practitioners to be more aware of the vulnerable patients that they treat and more alert to the early signs of the illness, as well as to the possibility of reducing certain risk factors, should this be possible.

Acknowledgements

The original research for this chapter was supported by a Trent Regional Health Authority grant and was carried out with the assistance of the Nottingham Psychiatric Case Register.

References

BROCKINGTON, I. F., WINOKUR, G. & DEAN, C. (1982) Puerperal psychosis. In *Motherhood & Mental Illness* (eds I. F. Brockington & R. Kumar), pp. 37–69. London: Academic Press.

COOPER, P. J., CAMPBELL, E. A., DAY, A., *et al* (1988) Non-psychotic psychiatric disorder after childbirth: a prospective study of prevalence, incidence, course and nature. *British Journal of Psychiatry*, **152**, 799–806.

COX, J. L., CONNOR, J. M. & KENDELL, R. E. (1982) Prospective study of psychiatric disorders of childbirth. *British Journal of Psychiatry*, **140**, 111–117.

——, HOLDEN, J. M. & SAGOVSKY, R. (1987) Detection of postnatal depression: development of the 10-item Edinburgh Postnatal Depression Scale (EPDS). *British Journal of Psychiatry*, **150**, 782–786.

DALTON, K. (1985) Progesterone prophylaxis used successfully in postnatal depression. *Practitioner*, **229**, 507–508.

DEAN, C. & KENDELL, R. E. (1981) The symptomatology of puerperal illnesses. *British Journal of Psychiatry*, **139**, 128–133.

——, WILLIAMS, R. J. & BROCKINGTON, I. F. (1989) Is puerperal psychosis the same as bipolar manic–depressive disorder? A family study. *Psychological Medicine*, **19**, 637–647.

ELLIOTT, S. A. (1989) Psychological strategies in the prevention and treatment of postnatal depression. In *Psychological Aspects of Obstetrics & Gynaecology*. Clinical Obstetrics & Gynaecology, vol. 3, no. 4, pp. 879–904. London: Baillière.

ESQUIROL, E. (1839) *Mental Maladies: a Treatise on Insanity* (trans. E. K. Hunt). Philadelphia: Lea & Blanchard.

HOLDEN, J. M., SAGOVSKY, R. & COX, J. L. (1989) A controlled study in the treatment of postnatal depression in primary care. *British Medical Journal*, **298**, 223–226.

KATONA, C. I. F. (1982) Puerperal mental illness: comparison with non-puerperal controls. *British Journal of Psychiatry*, **141**, 447–452.

KENDELL, R. E., RENNIE, D., CLARKE, J. A., *et al* (1981) The social and obstetric correlates of psychiatric admission in the puerperium. *Psychological Medicine*, **11**, 341–350.

——, CHALMERS, L., PLATZ, C. (1987) The epidemiology of puerperal psychoses. *British Journal of Psychiatry*, **150**, 662–673.

KUMAR, R., ISAACS, S. & MELTZER, E. (1983) Recurrent postpartum psychosis: a model for prospective clinical investigation. *British Journal of Psychiatry*, **142**, 618–620.

—— & ROBSON, K. M. (1984) A prospective study of emotional disorders in childbearing women. *British Journal of Psychiatry*, **144**, 35–47.

LEVERTON, T. J. & ELLIOTT, S. A. (1989) Transition to parenthood groups: a preventive intervention for postnatal depression? In *The Free Woman. Women's Health in the 1990s* (eds E. V. van Hall & W. Everaerd), pp. 479–486. Amsterdam: Parthenon Publishing.

MELTZER, E. S. & KUMAR, R. (1985) Puerperal mental illness, clinical features and classification: a study of 142 mother and baby admissions. *British Journal of Psychiatry*, **147**, 647–654.

MURRAY, L. & STEIN, A. (1989) The effects of postnatal depression on the infant. In *Psychological Aspects of Obstetrics & Gynaecology*, pp. 921–934. Clinical Obstetrics & Gynaecology vol. 3, no. 4. London: Baillière.

OATES, M. (1988) The development of an integrated community-orientated service for severe postnatal mental illness. In *Motherhood and Mental Illness* (eds R. Kumar & I. F. Brockington), vol. 2. London: Wright.

—— (1989a) Management of major mental illness in pregnancy and the puerperium. In *Psychological Aspects of Obstetrics & Gynaecology*, pp. 905–920. Clinical Obstetrics & Gynaecology, vol. 3, no. 4. London: Baillière.

—— (1989b) Normal emotional changes in pregnancy and the puerperium. In *Psychological Aspects of Obstetrics & Gynaecology*, pp. 791–804. Clinical Obstetrics & Gynaecology, vol. 3, no. 4. London: Baillière.

O'HARA, M. W., ZEKOSKI, E. M., PHILIPPS, L. H., *et al* (1989) A controlled study of postpartum mood disorders: comparison of childbearing and nonchildbearing women. *Journal of Abnormal Psychology*.

PAFFENBARGER, R. S., Jr (1964) Epidemiological aspects of postpartum mental illness. *British Journal of Prevention and Social Medicine*, **18**, 189–195.

PITT, B. (1968) 'Atypical' depression following childbirth. *British Journal of Psychiatry*, **114**, 1325–1335.

PRETTYMAN, R. J. & FRIEDMAN, T. (1991) Care of women with puerperal psychiatric disorders in England and Wales. *British Medical Journal*, **302**, 1345–1346.

PROTHEROE, C. (1969) Puerperal psychoses: a long term study 1927–1961. *British Journal of Psychiatry*, **115**, 9–30.

REICH, T. & WINOKUR, G. (1970) Postpartum psychosis in patients with manic depressive disease. *Journal of Nervous Diseases*, **151**, 60–68.

STEIN, A., GATH, D. H., BUCHER, J., *et al* (1991) The relationship between postnatal depression and mother–child interaction. *British Journal of Psychiatry*, **158**, 46–52.

STEWART, D. E., KLOMPENHOUWER, J. L., KENDELL, R. E., *et al* (1991) Prophylactic lithium in puerperal psychosis: The experience of three centres. *British Journal of Psychiatry*, **158**, 393–397.

WIECK, A. (1989) Endocrine aspects of postnatal depression. In *Psychological Aspects of Obstetrics & Gynaecology*, pp. 857–877. Clinical Obstetrics & Gynaecology, vol. 3, no. 4. London: Baillière.

——, KUMAR, R., HIRST, A. D., *et al* (1991) Increased sensitivity of dopamine receptors and recurrence of affective psychosis after childbirth. *British Medical Journal*, **303**, 613–616.

3 Postnatal mental illness: auditing services

MARGARET OATES

Monitoring and evaluation of a postnatal mental illness service

The function of the Postnatal Mental Illness Service is to meet the psychiatric needs of this group of patients. The monitoring and evaluation of the health care process involves the setting of standards of care and ensuring that these standards are met, an activity known as audit. Health Service audit is now a requirement laid down in the White Paper *Working for Patients* (Department of Health, 1989). Clinical and medical audit are therefore relatively recent. However, audit activities have been carried out in some areas of the Health Service for many years, although under different titles. Royal College accreditation visits to hospitals and General Medical Council (GMC) visits to medical schools are both audit activities since standards are set for training and such visits ensure that they are met. The Mental Health Act Commission visits hospitals to ensure that standards which are set for detained patients are met. The Nursing Care Plan assesses the needs of patients and the process of care ensures that these needs are met.

Health Service Audit may evaluate the performance of the whole or part of the system, the care received by a group of patients or an individual. The organisation that supports the delivery of health care can be audited (*organisational audit*). The care delivered by the multidisciplinary team can be audited (*clinical audit*) as can that part of the care which is the responsibility of individual professions (*medical audit, nursing audit*).

Setting and measuring standards

A standard is an aspect of the health care process which fulfils certain criteria. As outlined below, it should be: (a) important; (b) achievable; (c) measurable; (d) explicit; and (e) agreed.

(a) A standard should be seen as *important*. It must play a pivotal and fundamental role in the success of the whole treatment or management strategy. It should reflect the best contemporary practice (*quality*). There will be some prioritisation in an hierarchical fashion of such standards. The most important and most fundamental standards should be set first and these should be few in number. Only when these standards have been achieved should the team move on to set standards of a lower degree of importance.

(b) A standard must be *achievable* and *feasible*. It should be attainable within existing resources or those which can be reasonably expected for the team to obtain over a defined period of time (*a target*).

(c) A standard should be *measurable*. Every standard that is set should be accompanied by a *monitoring tool* which must be simple to describe, to measure and to record. A measure may be quantitative, qualitative or descriptive. The monitoring may be done on a complete sample or on a random sample. The monitoring tool should also be achievable. It should be designed so that the standard can be measured within existing or easily achievable resources.

(d) A standard should be *explicit, written* and *public*. It is insufficient for a standard to exist only in the minds of the team members. Some standards have to form the basis of contracts and only written standards can fulfil this function. Written standards are also necessary for the induction of new staff members and in providing information for potential purchasers and users.

(e) A standard must be *agreed, owned* and *shared* by all the team members. Ideally a standard should be set and monitored by those who carry the responsibility of meeting the standard.

Some standards are already set for the clinical team by the Patients' Charter, health and safety regulations, health district and mental health unit charters and policies. Other standards will be imposed upon the team by purchasers and formalised in contracts – particularly those that relate to cost and volume, response times and communication times. These standards will be audited externally by audit managers and quality assurance managers, either within the provider unit or by the purchaser (general practitioners or district health authorities).

Other standards are set internally by the clinical team and by the individual professions. These standards will reflect the best care achievable in the light of contemporary practice. They will be audited by the clinical team, who have the responsibility to act on the findings and seek remedies for those standards which are not met (*closing the audit loop*). The findings of all audit activities should be available for inspection. Most units of management and district health authorities have audit committees who are responsible for the overview of the audit activities within their remit.

Setting standards

The process of care delivered by the service can be divided into four main areas: (a) the entry to care; (b) the initial assessment; (c) the process of care; and (d) the outcome. Standards will need to be set and the monitoring tool established in each of the four categories, bearing in mind the five essential characteristics of the standard, already outlined, above.

(a) Entry to care

Standards in this part of the process of care are likely to be demanded by purchasers and by quality assurance policies of the district health authority. Particularly important aspects of this part of the care process are as follows:

(i) Information: there is no point in having a postnatal mental illness service if potential purchasers or referrers to the service do not know of its existence, the criteria for accepting patients and the mechanism of referral. In addition to publicising the service, written information should be circulated in the form of a leaflet to all potential referrers and purchasers, outlining the service and how to refer to it.

(ii) Accessibility: standards relating to this aspect of care will include signposting, ease of access by public transport and the special aspects of the organisation and facilities of the service to meet the needs of this particular group of patients, e.g. waiting areas, changing rooms, facilities for breast feeding, courtesy of reception staff, etc.

(iii) Response times: all contracts with purchasers will include standards on response times which will state that the majority of patients will be seen within a defined period of time following referral, and that letters and appointments will be sent at defined periods of time after the referral has been received.

(iv) Target or priority groups: the service will need to clearly state which group of patients it expects to assess or manage during the period of the contract, and who, by definition, should not be seen by other services (*completeness of service*). The service may decide, for example, to see all women requiring admission within a defined period of time after childbirth, and all those with serious mental illness. However, it may in addition set out to achieve a greater degree of completeness over a defined period of time (*a health target*).

(b) Assessment

(i) Communication: following the assessment in terms of response time, advice and the naming of a keyworker will usually be required by the purchaser.

(ii) Completeness of history and additional information: most teams will also regard it as very important to set an internal standard for this important aspect of work. For example, this might include past obstetric and gynaecological history, a detailed account of the childbirth, etc.

(iii) Evaluation of the mother/child relationship and a related risk assessment: also an important part of the initial assessment.

(iv) Needs assessment: a simple and agreed needs assessment of an individual patient is very important, not only for the rational planning of the treatment but also as a way of measuring outcome later in the process, in terms of the success of meeting patient needs.

(v) Treatment plan: similarly a treatment plan can be set at the time of assessment, and its outcome evaluated later.

(c) Process of care

(i) The team may wish to set standards for the preferred way of managing certain clinical conditions or situations. Such standards could involve the setting of *treatment protocols* and *management protocols*, for example, explicit directives on how to proceed in the case of non-accidental injury or permitted medication when a patient is breast feeding.

(ii) Standards for periodic review are important. These can involve defining when patients seen by individual members of the team will be reviewed by the whole team.

(iii) It is important for the team to decide what events (*occurrences*) are undesirable and should not occur. These may involve the safety of the child, accidents, infections and a variety of other occurrences which reflect adversely on the quality of care.

(d) Outcome

This will either be discharge, or, if care is continuing, outcome at a defined period of time (e.g. six months/one year, etc.).

(i) Communication: most purchasers will require standards of communication following discharge. In addition, most teams would regard it as important that such communication would contain advice regarding further pregnancies.

(ii) One standard of satisfactory outcome is that the patient has been assessed for the presence or absence of continuing mental health care needs and whether a *care programme* or a *care management approach* is necessary.

(iii) Outcome can be assessed in terms of whether the needs identified at assessment and during a process of care have been met.

(iv) Most purchasers and quality assurance managers from district health authorities will now require audit of *consumer satisfaction*. *Purchaser satisfaction* is another important standard which will need to be set.

Examples of standards

Entry to care standards

(a) **Information standard:** purchasers and referrers should know of the service, whom to refer and how to refer to it. An information leaflet containing all the relevant information should be circulated to potential referrers.

Monitoring tool: random check of GPs and obstetricians enquiring if they know of the service,

> *or* record routinely all referrers and check annually for low referrers,
>
> *or* a random check of general psychiatrists to see if they are treating any postnatal patients.

Closing the loop: discuss with the low referrers the nature of the problem, inform them of the correct procedure and re-audit.

(b) **Accessibility standard:** the service base, out-patient clinic and mother and baby unit will be clearly signposted and its facilities suitable for mothers with young children.

Monitoring tool: either a questionnaire to all patients or a visit from a quality assurance manager who would trace the path that a patient would take through the service.

(c) **Target groups standard:** the service will manage all mothers from the health district who require admission and all such mothers will be admitted with their babies. It will also see all women who are seriously mentally ill.

Monitoring tool: either a random or complete check of other psychiatric sectors to see if they have admitted any postnatal women, or a *completeness of coverage survey* to check that all women admitted within a defined period of time or suffering from a major mental illness are seen by the postnatal mental illness service. This monitoring tool will only be possible if there is a patient information system which allows for cross-reference of psychiatric referral and delivery. The resources involved mean that this type of audit can only be performed infrequently.

Closing the loop: if the standard is not met then further audit or research will be necessary to discover the reason why.

> An audit of this type was carried out in 1987 in Nottingham, using the psychiatric and obstetric case registers. During this period the Postnatal Mental Illness Service managed 78% of all women referred to psychiatric services within the postpartum year; 97% of all postnatal women with a major mental illness; 94% of all women admitted to the Psychiatric Unit (all with their babies) and 96% of all patients referred by their obstetricians.

The *loop was closed* by investigating why 22% of all postnatal referrals were not seen by the service. The reason was that they were 'out of hours' patients, seen by the emergency services. As there was no possibility of extending the cover of the service to a 7-day-a-week, 24-hour service, the loop was closed by setting a new standard that over 75% of all referrals would be seen by the team. (Oates, 1988)

(d) Response time standard: urgent telephone referrals will be seen within 24 hours, following a discussion between the referrer and the service. For non-urgent, written referrals, an appointment will be sent to the patient within a working week of receipt of the referral and the patient will be seen within four weeks.

Monitoring tool: date stamp all referrals and note the date the appointment was sent and the time of response to an urgent referral. A six-monthly complete audit of response time should be done.

Closing the loop: if the standard is not met in either group, the standard needs to be re-examined. Is it achievable within existing resources? Do all non-urgent patients need to be seen within four weeks? Should non-urgent patients be further stratified? It may be possible to meet the standard by altering working methods, or it may be that the standard is wrong and needs to be re-thought.

Assessment standards

(a) Completeness of information standard: all patients will have a complete psychiatric history taken during the assessment. This will include obstetric and gynaecological history, an assessment of mother/infant relationship, a risk assessment and a standardised diagnosis.

Monitoring tool: a criteria checklist audit six times a year by random case-note sampling by an independent clinician from outside the service.

Closing the loop: if the standard is not met, reinforce the importance to the team members and include a checklist in the case-notes. Re-audit.

(b) Needs assessment and treatment plan standard: at the end of each assessment the three most important needs of the patient will be defined according to agreed criteria and a treatment plan clearly written in the notes.

Monitoring tool: audit six times a year by random case-note sampling by an external clinician.

Process of care standards

(a) Periodic review standard: all out-patients and those managed in the community will be discussed by the multidisciplinary team at the end of the first week following referral and thereafter formally reviewed at three-monthly intervals.

Monitoring tool: the team's system for recording information from patients referred will include dates for periodic review; these will be checked every six months.
Closing the loop: those patients who have not been reviewed will be discussed immediately. Patterns of failure will be investigated.

(b) Management protocols standard: any patient who expresses a fear that she might harm her child must be discussed immediately with a senior member of the team. Any patient who discloses that they have harmed their child must be discussed immediately with the team social worker. Risk assessment and the action taken must be clearly recorded in the case-notes.
Monitoring tool: a random case-note sampling six times a year, together with case discussion, chaired by an independent clinician.
Closing the loop: occasional inappropriate action noted and corrected by including standard in the induction process of new staff.

(c) Treatment protocol standard: treatment with psychotropic medication must take account of whether the patient is breast feeding; the method of infant feeding must be clearly recorded in the notes and on in-patient prescription charts.
Monitoring tool: a periodic review of all in-patient prescription charts.
Closing the loop: it has been found that on occasions breast-feeding patients have been prescribed inappropriate medication by the duty doctor. This was remedied by attaching guidelines on prescribing in breast feeding to all in-patient prescription charts and then by re-auditing.

(d) Occurrence rating standard: set a number of important events (occurrences) which should/or should not happen during a period of in-patient care. For example, the baby *should* be admitted with the mother; babies under four weeks *should* be examined by a paediatrician within 24 hours of admission; mothers *should* receive their postnatal check at six weeks post-partum; babies *should not* be cared for primarily by the nurses once the mother's mental state has resolved, etc.
Monitoring tool: establish a list of occurrences and automatically audit all negative occurrences, or audit all in-patient cases periodically by an independent clinician.
Closing the loop: investigate individual cases or patterns of occurrences and rectify the problem.

Outcome standards

(a) Communication standard: at discharge all patients will have a discharge summary sent to their general practitioner within one

week. This will include advice on further management and future pregnancies.
Monitoring tool: random check of all discharge summaries.

(b) Needs are met standard: every three months during care and at discharge, steps will be taken to ensure that the patient's needs are being met satisfactorily and that the treatment plan is followed. This will be recorded in the case-notes.
Monitoring tool: a check by random case-note sampling that the three key problems at initial assessment are being addressed and that the treatment plan is being followed. Discuss the appropriateness of the original assessment.

(c) Consumer satisfaction standard: following discharge from the service, patients will be sent a questionnaire asking them to comment on their overall satisfaction of the service and their suggestions for improving it, and on specific issues.
Monitoring tool: annual analysis of returned questionnaires.
Closing the loop: specific problems addressed, if possible, from within existing resources by re-organisation. If it is not possible to remedy the problem, then management is informed and advised as to what resources will be necessary to correct the problem.

(d) Purchaser satisfaction standard: the referring general practitioners should be satisfied with the service in terms of the ease with which they can refer patients, the appropriateness of the response to their requests and their satisfaction with the communication received from the team.
Monitoring tool: all referrers will be circulated annually with a questionnaire on these aspects of their satisfaction.
Closing the loop: an annual analysis of the returned questionnaires. Any problems will be remedied as outlined above.

General comments on standards

The collection of standardised information and activity data is essential to inform the setting of standards and the audit process and will be necessary as a basis for research. Such information will include standardised diagnoses, socio-demographic data (see Chapter 2, Health needs assessment exercise, p. 9) as well as numbers of referrals, the referrer, the site and type of the referral (hospital, home, out-patient), the professional who assesses the patient, the type of care received (in-patient/out-patient or community care) and the method of treatment and management. The collection and recording of such information is best served by a computerised patient information system (PIS), preferably one compatible with the PIS for the health district and mental health unit. However, it is possible to set and monitor standards and collect basic patient information and activity data without information technology, using a 'ledger' system. If the monitoring tool uses 'manual methods' it will be difficult to audit 100% of cases and the monitoring of the standards will usually be done on the basis of random sampling.

The examples of standards given above is not exhaustive. Teams will wish eventually to set more sophisticated standards of outcome, particularly those relating to mother/infant relationships and standards of care. This task, like many other tasks of setting standards, may seem daunting at first but in general it is best to start with very simple standards, those that are easy to define, to describe and measure, while at the same time giving thought to developing more sensitive and complex monitoring tools for the future.

Research and audit

Research and audit are both investigative but audit, unlike research, is not experimental. Audit investigates the process of care by setting standards and checking that they have been achieved. Clinical, scientific research is experimental in design and hypothesis driven and usually employs quantitative measures. Sociological research is often comparative and descriptive and may employ qualitative as well as quantitative measures. Audit is therefore distinct from scientific research. Audit reveals problems which require further investigation and remedy. Some problems may only be clarified by research, others may require further audit. Research is essential for informing standards. It is research that provides the knowledge basis for the 'best contemporary practice' upon which standards are set. Research may also result from audit. The distinction between clinical and medical audit and health service research is important because of the resource implications. Clinical and medical audit by definition is expected to be performed from within existing resources. Clinical or health service research on the other hand cannot necessarily be conducted within existing resources and will usually require additional resources and a methodology which may be different from ordinary clinical practices.

References

DEPARTMENT OF HEALTH (1989) *Working for Patients*. London: HMSO.
OATES, M. (1988) The development of an integrated community-orientated service for severe postnatal mental illness. In *Motherhood and Mental Illness* (eds R. Kumar & I. F. Brockington), vol. 2. London: Wright.

Further reading

FIRTH-COZENS, J. (1993) *Audit in Mental Health Services*. Hove: Lawrence Erlbaum.

4 Prevention of adverse effects of perinatal maternal mental illness on the developing child

R. CHANNI KUMAR, ALISON E. HIPWELL and CHRIS LAWSON

The young infant is particularly susceptible to adverse influences arising out of the presence of mental illnesses in the mother because, during pregnancy, she *is* the environment and after delivery it is almost always the mother who nurtures the infant. One way of systematically addressing the questions of such risks to the infant is to categorise them in terms of their timing – prenatal and postnatal. In the prenatal group fall all those psychiatric disorders which predate childbirth and here the mother's psychiatric problems are in a sense complicated by pregnancy and childbirth, while at the same time posing a potential risk to the child's well-being. This group of illnesses therefore encompasses the entire range of psychiatric conditions that afflict women during their reproductive lifespan. By and large, the prevalence of a given condition in pregnancy is the same as it is in the general age-matched female population. Obvious exceptions are disorders like anorexia nervosa which, by their nature, reduce fertility. Schizophrenia is also associated with reduced fertility, an effect which is augmented by neuroleptic medication. Apart, possibly, from depression and anxiety in early pregnancy (see reviews by Kumar, 1985; Oates, 1989) there are no psychiatric illnesses which have an increased prevalence during pregnancy. Indeed, epidemiological studies (Pugh *et al*, 1963; Kendell *et al*, 1976) suggest that there may be a slight reduction in prevalence of mental illness as judged by 'contact' rates with psychiatric services during pregnancy. The second main group of maternal illnesses that may pose risks to the infant are the disorders with a postnatal onset, i.e. postpartum psychosis and postnatal depression.

Women with chronic or episodic mental illnesses who also happen to become pregnant are the poor cousins of those who develop postnatal disorders in terms of the amount of research effort and attention they receive. In this chapter, therefore, we shall emphasise measures for prevention in relation primarily to psychiatric disorders the onset of which predate

43

pregnancy. Prenatal illnesses pose a risk to the embryo and foetus in ways that are directly and indirectly linked to the maternal condition – nutrition, hygiene, infection, drugs (prescribed and non-prescribed), compliance with antenatal care, self-injury and obstetric complications are some of the main concerns, and studies of obstetric outcome as well as of infant development are needed in relation to maternal diagnosis and the penumbra of associated factors. These conditions offer a major opportunity for prevention, starting at the time the mother 'books in' for antenatal care, but ideally the process should begin with education and counselling even before conception. Anticipatory measures taken by the woman, her family and by professionals can do much to avert potential risks after the child is born. Additional resources such as family aids and day nurseries can be called upon or, at the opposite end of the spectrum of responses, counselling can begin to prepare a woman for the eventuality that an alternative carer will be needed for the baby.

The key to successful prevention of perinatal illness and its consequences is, first of all, accurate detection of the subject at risk, together with some understanding of the kinds of risks that apply in a given condition and social context. The next step is the delivery of appropriate measures at the right time and in a way that is acceptable to the mother. She may not, for example, be ill at the time or she may not perceive or accept the possibility that she is the mediator of potentially damaging influences that impinge on her child's development.

A recent report of a working party of the Royal College of Psychiatrists on postnatal mental illness (Cox *et al*, 1992) recommended that the mental health service should provide "rapid, appropriate, accessible and effective care for the mentally ill mother" and it should "place a high order of priority on the emotional and physical needs of the infants". One of the authors of this chapter and an editor of this book were, respectively, a member and chairman of the working party and must therefore bear full responsibility for appearing to ignore, even in the title of the report, the special needs of women with *prenatal* mental illness. Of course, one can argue that prenatal illness becomes postnatal sooner or later, but by then it may be too late.

There is a lack of resources that are targeted specifically to meet the needs of mentally ill, pregnant women. In comparison with resources that are generally allocated to obstetrics and midwifery services, the effort and money spent on psychiatric consultation and liaison for obstetrics is negligible. Apart from a few centres where a general psychiatrist has developed a special interest in obstetrics (e.g. Riley, 1986; Oates, 1988; Appleby *et al*, 1989) there is no evidence of a generally recognised need for a designated obstetric liaison service. Similarly, there is no provision for any special obstetric input into psychiatry. For example, it is the norm for a woman who is severely mentally ill, e.g. with a condition such as schizophrenia or manic–depressive psychosis, to remain as an in-patient in a general adult psychiatric ward until she starts labour. In a more general sense, the lack of attention paid to the needs of the pregnant, mentally ill mother is reflected by the fact that there is no requirement to record whether a female psychiatric in-patient or out-patient is currently pregnant. As a corollary, screening for psychiatric conditions in most antenatal clinics is unsystematic and is often left to junior midwives to carry out.

Scale of the problem

Prenatal illness

Community surveys (Shepherd *et al*, 1966; Bebbington *et al*, 1981; Surtees *et al*, 1983; Regier *et al*, 1988) consistently show that about 15% of women aged 18–44 are suffering from a clinically significant psychiatric disorder. About 2% are likely to have a psychotic condition (schizophrenia or affective psychosis) and the majority of the remainder will be suffering from depressive and/or anxiety states. There are, of course, differences in prevalence rates that are more precisely linked to age and to other factors such as family history, personal history and current circumstances, and what is important in the present context is to know how many of these women are detected by screening procedures in antenatal clinics.

In a study by Appleby *et al* (1989) which was carried out in a London teaching hospital, the midwife at booking in asked the expectant mother if she had at any time in the past had a course of treatment (counselling or medication) for psychological or emotional problems. If the mother responded positively, or if she said she had attended psychiatric out-patients or had been an in-patient, she was brought to the attention of the psychiatrist. One further reason for referral was the perception by the midwife of severe social difficulties, problems in important relationships or severe life stress. The decision-making about referral in relation to this domain of social risk factors was not, however, operationalised in any way. In an 18-month period, when about 3500 women passed through the obstetric service, Appleby *et al* (1989) were referred 72 pregnant women for psychiatric assessment, of whom 19 failed to keep their appointments. About half of the remaining 53 were subsequently engaged in therapeutic or preventive measures. The screening procedure was therefore able to pick out about 2% of the total obstetric clientele as being current or potential 'cases' of psychiatric disorder and about half of them either defaulted or were not offered further appointments after the initial assessment. Thus it may be concluded that despite the presence of a psychiatrist in an obstetric clinic much remains to be done to improve the sensitivity and the specificity of screening procedures for psychiatric disorder. Without such improvements, attempts at prevention will be cosmetic because they will miss the majority of subjects at risk. Closer links with the primary health care team may lead not only to better recognition of such women but also to more effective engagement with them.

Postnatal illness

There are two main kinds of postnatal disorder, postpartum psychosis, which has an incidence rate of about 0.1%, and postnatal depression, which is about 100 times more common; i.e. about one in ten mothers is likely to become depressed in the first few months after childbirth. The major 'risk' factor to look out for in relation to postpartum psychosis is a history of affective psychosis, puerperal or non-puerperal. The presence of such a history elevates the risk of becoming ill to 50% (Dean *et al*, 1989; Schopf *et al*, 1984; Marks *et al*, 1992) and the risk is greater the shorter the interval since the previous episode of illness (Marks *et al*, 1992). It should therefore be routine at booking to enquire about any history of severe mental illness and then to ensure that the mother is carefully monitored in the first few weeks postpartum, when the majority of psychoses occur; these illnesses are major psychiatric emergencies and it is essential that provisions are made in advance to admit and treat the mother should the illness recur. There are as yet no definitely proven prophylactic therapies although preliminary findings with lithium have been partially encouraging (Stewart *et al*, 1991). A study is being carried out at the Institute of Psychiatry and the Bethlem and Maudsley Hospitals to confirm an anecdotal report by Hamilton & Sichel (1992) of a study carried out many years ago suggesting that the administration of oestrogen immediately after the delivery might be effective in preventing the recurrence of psychosis.

Postnatal depression is much more common than postpartum psychosis and the main warning signs are a history of severe depression (Marks *et al*, 1992), which increases the risk about threefold, the presence of marital problems, difficulties in childhood and current relationships, social adversity and evidence of conflicts about the readiness of parenthood (see reviews by Kumar, 1982; O'Hara & Zekoski, 1988; Jermain, 1992). Studies by Cox and colleagues (Holden *et al*, 1989) have demonstrated the therapeutic efficacy of non-directive counselling delivered by health visitors *after* postnatal depression has manifested itself and Henderson *et al* (1991) have similarly shown that oestrogen treatment is superior to placebo in reducing depressive symptoms that began postnatally. There is evidence (Elliott, 1988) that counselling in pregnancy is effective in preventing postnatal depression and this work needs replication and extension. Similarly, claims of the prophylactic efficacy of progesterone (Dalton, 1989) require controlled evaluation and more research is needed (see, for example, Hannah *et al*, 1993) into biological markers which will help identify those women who may most benefit from early antidepressant therapy.

Consultation/liaison service for perinatal problems

Assuming that an effective screening procedure has been developed and that the key health professionals know of most of the pregnant women who have a history of mental illness, what kind of demands may be made of them in relation to prevention? The first prerequisite is effective communication between the relevant professionals, i.e. the GP, the health visitor, the midwife and the obstetrician, the social worker and the psychiatrist. Exactly how psychiatric liaison is established will depend upon local conditions and circumstances. One of the central recommendations of the Royal College of Psychiatrists' working party was the setting-up of district-based multidisciplinary teams led by a designated psychiatrist with a special responsibility for serving the population of women with postnatal illnesses within the district *and* for establishing links with obstetric and midwifery services and with primary health care workers and social workers to assess women in pregnancy and to advise about prevention.

Perhaps the single most important piece of information which was emphasised in the Royal College report is that it is possible to predict fairly accurately the rates and kinds of perinatal psychiatric morbidity in a given district, because reliable estimates are available of general rates of female psychiatric disorders and because the birth-rate is known. Secondly, the population at risk is expected to be in regular contact with health professionals through pregnancy and for a defined period postnatally. Very sensibly, the working party desisted from recommending a blueprint for an effective consultation/liaison service that could be universally applied. Instead it proposed that a locally appropriate service should be developed by a psychiatrist with a special interest in the subject. At a time of shrinking resources it is especially difficult to mount this kind of initiative and it will be up to individual consultants to highlight the value of prevention both for the mother and for the rest of the family, but especially for the unborn child. Research which demonstrates the value of psychiatric liaison will provide the most effective rationale for the development of such a service at the interface of obstetrics, paediatrics, primary health care and social services. Comparisons should be possible between districts which have a liaison service in place and those which do not and especially careful attention will be needed in selecting measures of outcome.

The discussion which follows assumes that such a service is in place and that it consists of three main components – a consultation clinic, a liaison service for obstetrics, and a postnatal in-patient unit with associated out-patient and community links.

Consultation clinic

Preconception counselling

The psychiatrist running a consultation clinic may be asked to advise on the risks of recurrence of mental illness after a future pregnancy and delivery, what can be done to prevent recurrence and how long a mother should wait before trying to conceive again. When is it safe to come off medication which was started after the last postnatal illness? What will be the risks to the unborn baby of remaining on the given medication? Advice may be sought about contraception and about worries over possible infertility as a consequence of current and recent psychotropic medication. Another very common worry concerns the risk that the mother's illness will be genetically transmitted to her baby.

Consultation during pregnancy

A consultation clinic for pregnant women provides a focus for discussion of particularly difficult cases that may have been 'picked up' by the liaison service or referred by the GP. Considerable forward planning may be needed to deal effectively with, for example, the problems presented by a single, unsupported, chronically ill, schizophrenic mother-to-be, who is intermittently maintained on depot neuroleptics but who has conceived despite the reported effects of these drugs on fertility.

Evaluation of current and potential risk to the infant
Some general questions about sources of risk to the child include the following:

  (a) Is there any current aspect of maternal psychopathology or behaviour that poses a threat to the pregnancy or to the foetus – e.g. suicidal ideation, self-neglect, malnutrition, ingestion of non-prescribed drugs, failure to attend for antenatal care?
  (b) Is there any hazard to the foetus from prescribed medication and, if so, what alternatives, if any, are there?
  (c) Are there significant risks of exacerbation or recurrence of illness postpartum and is there a need to plan for possible admission of the mother? If she is admitted, where will this be to and will the baby be with her? Are the family prepared?
  (d) Are there sufficient concerns about possible risks to the newborn infant, whether through impulse or neglect, to ensure that social services have engaged in anticipatory planning meetings leading on to formal conferences at which decisions may be taken under the provision of the Children Act 1989?

Liaison service

Most of the issues that have been discussed under the heading of the consultation clinic also apply to the liaison service. The method of detecting women at risk will vary from clinic to clinic but at some point it hinges on someone asking the right questions and then responding appropriately to the answers. Usually, the job of booking in is devolved to the junior or trainee midwife and perhaps this may partly explain the problem of poor sensitivity and specificity of the screening process. It is precisely here that the psychiatrist has a major role in teaching the importance of mental illness as a risk not only for the mother but also for the baby. Problems that may be seen as irritants in the otherwise smooth running of antenatal clinics can, if not adequately dealt with, subsequently present as crises on postnatal wards.

The main tasks of a liaison psychiatrist in obstetrics can be summarised as follows:

(a) He or she must set up a reliable screening procedure to detect women booking in to antenatal clinics who have histories of psychiatric illness, of severe social or interpersonal problems, or who have evidence of significant current psychopathology, drug or alcohol abuse.

(b) Good liaison with the GP, health visitor and social workers will encourage notification of 'problem' mothers as well as referral back to them as appropriate for supervision and monitoring. Midwives should also play an active part in following, monitoring and supporting individual mothers through pregnancy. The psychiatrist will be able to take on the management of only a minority of cases, i.e. those with the most severe current problems or greatest risk of postnatal breakdown. In a case-register survey by Nott (1982) only 0.39% of a consecutive series of childbearing women made any sort of contact with psychiatric services up to 1 year postpartum. Depending on circumstances, the psychiatrist may also be able to attend clinics in health centres in the community and, in conjunction with the GP and health visitor, provide some domiciliary care for women who cannot, or do not, regularly attend antenatal clinics. Planning for labour, delivery and postnatal care for individual subjects with the patient's obstetrician and midwife is another important task. Finally, close links with social worker colleagues will ensure that cases are 'allocated' in time, that planning meetings take place, and that delays do not occur postnatally in calling child protection meetings.

(c) Postnatally, the psychiatrist should be available to deal rapidly with acute crises, to follow through 'cases' referred antenatally or postnatally either personally or through the community team, and to alert them of possible impending problems – e.g. the likely occurrence of postnatal depression in a mother whose marriage is breaking down, whose pregnancy was unwanted and who has severe housing and financial problems.

In-patient mother-and-baby service for assessing risk to the infant

The main function of psychiatric services for mentally ill mothers and their babies is effective treatment and rehabilitation of the mother while sustaining and facilitating her relationship with her infant. Since the Children Act 1989 came into effect, there seems to have been an increase in the demand for another kind of specialised service: the expert assessment of a mother's competence and motivation to rear her infant in the context of a severe mental illness or personality disorder. As the emphasis on parental responsibility has been increased, so it has become necessary for far more detailed and systematic evidence to be laid before the courts if it is being argued that a child will be better raised apart from its biological parents or parent.

There is a surprisingly small amount of literature published either before or after the implementation of the Children Act 1989 on this most important subject (see Stewart & Gangbar, 1984; Appleby & Dickens, 1993). It is a matter for the courts to reach decisions about the future welfare of infants whose mothers suffer from severe mental illnesses, but there is no published information about criteria upon which experts base judgements about maternal competency to care for babies, nor is it known what information they must have before they can make sound recommendations to courts. How long are mother and child to be observed together and in what kind of setting before reliable conclusions can be reached? Who is qualified to pass judgements on a mother's competence and safety and motivation to care for her child now and in the future? (See discussion by Black *et al*, 1991.) There does not seem to be available a published series of cases which has come before the High Courts in England and Wales where one major concern has been the presence of mental illness in the mother. There are very few reports of cases where experts have systematically evaluated the factors associated with decisions to remove from a mother the care and control of her child. Potentially relevant factors are the nature and severity of the mother's illness, the degree of impairment of her social functioning, the supports available to her in the form of her spouse, her family and others. Similarly there does not seem to have been any published report of a series of cases where mentally ill mothers were given care and control or extensive access to their children within a defined setting, to see what was the outcome for the child. What kinds of maternal illness carry a 'good' prognosis in this respect? It is a remarkable fact that the answers to all these questions still remain to be found.

In the past few years, the clinical team of the Mother and Baby Unit, Bethlem Royal Hospital, has begun systematically to address the problem of assessment of risk to the infant in the context of severe maternal mental illness, in particular schizophrenia. Such an assessment procedure has been firmly linked with the parallel developments of the consultation and liaison service in order to try to make the whole process anticipatory and systematic. The presence of severe mental illness in the expectant mother is usually well known to those looking after her and to social services, yet it is surprising how often a referral is made from a postnatal ward as if it had just been realised that the mother might be incompetent to care for herself, let alone a new baby.

The assessment procedure ideally begins during pregnancy by means of a referral to the consultation clinic when the suitability of the proposed referral can be discussed and preliminary information gathering begun. Such initial data collection includes access to previous psychiatric, social work and forensic reports, case notes (medical, psychiatric, obstetric, etc.) and knowledge of any restrictions under the Mental Health Act. Ideally, all such admissions should be planned and a decision to undertake an assessment of a mother and baby made only after the relevant clinical and social data have been reviewed and referrers have made concrete plans to take the patient back with or without the baby. Options such as supervised accommodation, family aids, day nurseries, mother and baby hostels and foster parents should have been explored before the referral is made. Finally, in the current market of the NHS, the referrers must be able to pay for the costs of the admission and for the expert reports arising out of the assessment. The duration of any such assessment must also be negotiated and, in their turn, the clinical team must undertake to provide rapid feedback in the form of case conferences as well as formal, written reports for submission to courts. It is possible in most cases to complete such assessments over two to four weeks, and, if it is felt that mother and baby can safely remain together, the report must contain practical recommendations for the next steps for rehabilitation and supervision.

The assessment is multidisciplinary, comprising a medical and psychiatric 'work-up' with conclusions reached about the diagnosis, severity and nature of the illness and consequent disability and indications of response to treatment and prognosis. The social work input consists of evaluation of the patient's current circumstances and needs and a review, in liaison with area social workers, of what is available in the community. The social worker plays a key role in organising conferences and in linking with the legal department of area social services. The nursing team is able to provide systematic measures of the mother's condition on a day-to-day basis, her competence and safety, and her motivation in her maternal role. These observations are fundamental to the assessment and may be supplemented by analogous observations in less structured circumstances such as 'home visits' and by measures made by other professionals with specialist expertise – such as developmental psychologists with skills in observing the mother's responsiveness to her infant and her ability to learn new and adaptive behaviours. Psychometry of the mother may be very valuable because the presence of significant mental impairment may be a cause for concern in that it may indicate future problems in adapting to the growing needs of the developing child. Paediatric and developmental assessments of the infant are also important because infants who fail to thrive or who are 'difficult' or non-responsive may be so because of some inherent problem rather than as a consequence of maternal illness. In terms of prognosis, another vital set of observations comes from occupational therapy, where it is possible to assess the daily living skills of the mother and to form an accurate picture of how she will cope outside hospital with her infant.

Each discipline aims to arrive at a set of recommendations before the end of the 2–4-week period and individual written reports are prepared and discussed in a conference with relevant staff from the community, mainly social workers. There may also be the GP, the health visitor, the police and members of voluntary agencies such as the NSPCC. Finally a consensus report is synthesised and submitted for use in any court proceedings and the aim is to have this done within a week of the end of the assessment period.

The procedure outlined above is in the early stages of its evolution and development and it is hoped that it will become more systematic as experience grows. A follow-up is essential to validate the assessments but this is complicated by the fact that the recommendations which emanate from the assessments are intended to determine outcome.

References

APPLEBY, L. & DICKENS, C. (1993) Mothering skills of women with mental illness. *British Medical Journal*, **306**, 348–349.
———, FOX, H., SHAW, M., *et al* (1989) The psychiatrist in the obstetric unit. Establishing a liaison service. *British Journal of Psychiatry*, **154**, 510–515.
BEBBINGTON, P., HARRY, J., TENNANT, C., *et al* (1981) Epidemiology of mental disorders in Camberwell. *Psychological Medicine*, **11**, 561–579.
BLACK, D., WOLKIND, S. & HARRIS, J. H. (eds) (1991) Assessing parenting capacity. In *Child Psychiatry and the Law* (2nd edn), Chapter 6, pp. 31–35. London: Gaskell.
COX, J., KUMAR, R., OATES, M., *et al* (1992) Report of the General Psychiatry Section Working Party on Postnatal Mental Illness. *Psychiatric Bulletin*, **16**, 519–522.
DALTON, K. (1989) *Depression after Childbirth* (2nd edn). Oxford: Oxford University Press.
DEAN, C., WILLIAMS, J. R. & BROCKINGTON, I. F. (1989) Is puerperal psychosis the same as bipolar manic depressive disorder? A family study. *Psychological Medicine*, **19**, 637–647.
ELLIOTT, S. A. (1988) Psychological strategies in the prevention and treatment of postnatal depression. In *Clinics in Obstetrics and Gynaecology*, vol. 3, no. 4 (ed. M. Oates), pp. 879–903. London: Baillière Tindall.
HAMILTON, J. A. & SICHEL, D. A. (1992) Prophylactic measures. In *Postpartum Psychiatric Illness: a Picture Puzzle* (eds J. A. Hamilton & P. N. Harberger), pp. 219–234. Philadelphia: University of Pennsylvania Press.
HANNAH, P., CODY, D., GLOVER, V., *et al* (1993) The tyramine test is not a marker for postnatal depression: early postnatal euphoria may be. *Journal of Psychosomatic Obstetrics and Gynaecology*, **14**, 295–304.
HENDERSON, A. F., GREGOIRE, A. J. P., KUMAR, R., *et al* (1991) Treatment of severe postnatal depression with oestradiol skin patches. *Lancet*, **338**, 816–817.
HOLDEN, J. M., SAGOVSKY, R. & COX, J. L. (1989) Counselling in a general practice setting: controlled study of health visitors' intervention in treatment of postnatal depression. *British Medical Journal*, **298**, 223–226.
JERMAIN, D. M. (1992) Psychopharmacologic approach to postpartum depression. *Journal of Women's Health*, **1**, 47–52.
KENDELL, R. E., WAINWRIGHT, S., HAILEY, A., *et al* (1976) The influence of childbirth on psychiatric morbidity. *Psychological Medicine*, **6**, 297–307.
KUMAR, R. (1982) Neurotic disorders in childbearing women. In *Motherhood and Mental Illness* (eds I. F. Brockington & R. Kumar), pp. 71–118. London: Academic Press.

—— (1985) Pregnancy, childbirth and mental illness. In *Progress in Obstetrics and Gynaecology*, vol. 5 (ed. J. Studd), pp. 146–159. Edinburgh: Churchill Livingstone.

MARKS, M. N., WIECK, A., CHECKLEY, S. A., *et al* (1992) Contribution of psychological and social factors to psychotic and non-psychotic relapse after childbirth in women with previous histories of affective disorder. *Journal of Affective Disorders*, **29**, 253–264.

NOTT, P. (1982) Psychiatric illness following childbirth in Southampton: a case register study. *Psychological Medicine*, **12**, 557–561.

OATES, M. (1988) The development of an integrated community oriented service for severe postnatal mental illness. In *Motherhood and Mental Illness 2* (eds R. Kumar & I. F. Brockington), pp. 133–158. London: Wright.

—— (1989) Normal emotional changes in pregnancy and the puerperium. In *Baillière's Clinical Obstetrics and Gynaecology*, vol. 3, no. 4, pp. 791–804. London: Baillière Tindall.

O'HARA, M. W. & ZEKOSKI, E. M. (1988) Postpartum depression: a comprehensive review. In *Motherhood and Mental Illness 2* (eds R. Kumar & I. F. Brockington), pp. 17–63. London: Wright.

PUGH, T. F., JERATH, B. K., SCHMIDT, W. M., *et al* (1963) Rates of mental disease related to childbearing. *New England Journal of Medicine*, **268**, 1224–1228.

REGIER, D. A., BOYD, J. H. & BURKE, J. D., *et al* (1988) One month prevalence of mental disorders in the United States. *Archives of General Psychiatry*, **45**, 977–986.

RILEY, D. (1986) An audit of obstetric liaison in psychiatry in 1984. *Journal of Reproductive and Infant Psychology*, **4**, 99–115.

SCHOPF, J., BRYOIS, C., JONQUIERE, M., *et al* (1984) On the nosology of severe postpartum disorders. *European Archives of Psychiatry & Neurological Sciences (Berlin)*, **234**, 54–63.

SHEPHERD, M., COOPER, B., BROWN, A. C., *et al* (1966) *Psychiatric Illness in General Practice*. London: Oxford University Press.

STEWART, D. E. & GANGBAR, R. (1984) Psychiatric assessment of competency to care for a new-born. *Canadian Journal of Psychiatry*, **29**, 583–589.

——, KLOMPENHOUWER, J. L., KENDELL, R. E., *et al* (1991) Prophylactic lithium in puerperal psychosis, the experience of three centres. *British Journal of Psychiatry*, **158**, 393–397.

SURTEES, P. G., DEAN, C., INGHAM, J. G., *et al* (1983) Psychiatric disorder in women from an Edinburgh community: associations with demographic factors. *British Journal of Psychiatry*, **142**, 238–246.

5 Can non-psychotic depression be prevented?

JENI HOLDEN

"My husband wants another baby. The idea is quite nice, but it really frightens me to think that after having the baby I would be like this again. I wouldn't mind the morning sickness, or the actual birth. It is the postnatal depression that really frightens me, I don't think I could face that again. It was horrific."

(Holden, 1989)

The unexpected distress suffered by at least one in ten women following the birth of a baby is a matter for deep concern. In this chapter we consider whether postnatal depression can be prevented, and if so, how this could be done. Women's contact with health professionals is at a peak around the time of childbirth, and in the changing climate of priorities surrounding the delivery of health care, we need to ensure that these contacts are used to respond with maximum efficiency to the needs of individual women. Developing and practising preventive measures is cost-effective as well as humane and the importance of allocating scarce resources to prevention strategies rather than treatment is increasingly acknowledged. As Reed (1992) points out, the prevention of mental illness is of importance not only for the people who suffer from mental illness, but also because of the very heavy burdens it imposes on their families.

On a personal level, the experience of postnatal depression can be devastating. Pitt (1968) noted that many of the women in his study "felt quite changed from their usual selves, and most had never been depressed like this before". Although recent research suggests that the symptoms and duration of postnatal depression are not noticeably different from that occurring at other times (Cooper *et al*, 1988) depression after having a baby is unarguably unusual in that its effects are experienced at a time when exceptional physical and emotional demands are being made on the mother in caring for her infant and family. Untreated depressions may persist for several years (Kumar *et al*, 1984; Watson *et al*, 1984) and may be the precursor of further depressive episodes.

Targets for prevention in mental health recently outlined in the White Paper *Health of the Nation* (1992) not only include improving the quality of life for people suffering from mental illness, but also emphasise the importance of significantly reducing the suicide rate. Although several researchers have reported that pregnancy and the postnatal year are a time of very low risk of suicide (Appleby, 1991) suicidal feelings were commonly reported by women with postnatal depression in an Edinburgh study (Holden, 1991). Early intervention in the form of extra contact and emotional support may help to counteract such despair.

Depression not only affects the quality of a woman's own life and her experience of mothering, but can cast a long shadow on the whole family. The depressed mother's reduced sensitivity may have adverse effects on her infant's emotional and cognitive development (Murray & Stein, 1989; Stein *et al*, 1989; Cogill *et al*, 1986). Other children may also be affected (Richman *et al*, 1982; Pound & Mills, 1985). For partnered women, increased irritability and lowered libido (Pitt, 1968), combined with a lack of knowledge of what is happening, may affect the couple's relationship or even lead to break-up of the family (Holden, 1991).

The implications of depression for the mother herself and the possible long-term harmful effects on the family as a whole show clearly that prevention, early diagnosis and active treatment of postnatal depression should be a matter of the highest priority.

Preventing postnatal depression

According to Caplan (1964), prevention can be divided into primary, secondary and tertiary activities, as follows:

(a) *Primary prevention:* prevents the *incidence* of mental disorder by counterbalancing adverse factors before they can cause a disorder.
(b) *Secondary prevention:* this refers to early diagnosis and interventions which shorten the length of episodes of the illness, minimise the chances of transmission, and limit the adverse consequences of the disorder. Secondary prevention aims to reduce the *prevalence* of the condition.
(c) *Tertiary prevention:* this refers to measures which limit disability and handicap caused by an illness which may not in itself be fully treatable.

   Primary prevention can be further categorised (as adapted from Jenkins, 1992) as follows:

(a) *Universal measures:* these are measures directed at the whole population.
(b) *Selective measures:* these are directed at relatively large subgroups whose risk of becoming unwell is higher than normal (for example, all pregnant women are potentially at risk of postnatal depression).

(c) *Indicated measures:* these include measures directed at relatively small subgroups who are at high risk of developing the condition (for example, pregnant women who have a number of vulnerability factors).

Primary prevention of postnatal depression – universal measures

Factors common to all mothers, for which society in general should take responsibility, include the relatively low status of motherhood and the lack of ritual markers of the transition to motherhood (Seel, 1986; Cox, 1988). Fifty years ago, it was common for women to have a 'lying-in' period of a month to get over the birth. Today they are expected to take childbirth in their stride and carry on with their normal lives. Apart from personal satisfaction, the new status does not confer many advantages. On the contrary, like the newly disabled, mothers are more likely to find that they have forfeited many rights they previously took for granted, for example, the right to access in public places; even the right to go to the lavatory may be restricted by having a baby in tow. For women wishing or needing to work, their choice may be limited by the availability of adequate childcare.

Media idealisations (and some antenatal classes) camouflage the sheer exhaustion and emotional adjustment faced by most parents. In the context of limited knowledge and information on the realities of parenting, such images can be subtly pervasive; women who do not achieve the ideal of a joyfully coping mother may believe themselves to be inadequate.

Embarking on parenthood is a stringent test for the most emancipated partnership, and sexual equality does not yet extend to equal shares in parenting (Beail, 1985; Moss *et al*, 1987). While maternity leave is short, paternity leave is virtually non-existent. The increasing numbers of women who are parenting single-handed, either by choice or because their partner has left, face even greater demands on their time and resources. Financial incentives for those who wish or need to stay at home with their infants would help to acknowledge the importance of the maternal role, and ideally, adequate nursery provision or other suitable childcare arrangements should be available to all women who wish or need to work or pursue a career.

Changing the social climate is not easy, but helping women to recognise their own needs, and to believe that these are valid, can empower them to lobby for change. Professionals and researchers, women themselves, and the media, all have a role to play in bringing about improvements in care and changes in attitudes.

The media

Media messages emphasising the realities of parenting rather than idealising motherhood would be helpful, as would raising consciousness about the need for improved access to public places and to transport, and improved childcare facilities.

Education

Education of schoolchildren

This is an important universal measure which could influence the whole population. Many children today grow up in small nuclear families with little experience of the impact a baby can have on day-to-day life, both on a practical and emotional level. 'Parentcraft' programmes for teenagers of both sexes, including the practicalities of childrearing and family life, would be a useful addition to the school curriculum.

Education of health professionals

Freeling (1992) argues that an understanding of the concepts of primary, secondary and tertiary prevention are an absolute requirement for all practising doctors and essential learning for all medical students. He suggests that in teaching undergraduates in general practice about anxiety and depression, students should be asked to record answers to the following three questions in all case reports:

  (a) Could this problem have been prevented?
  (b) Could intervention have been made earlier? If yes, where (and why) was there a delay?
  (c) What steps could be taken to avoid recurrence of the problem or any delay?

Education of health professionals can be viewed either as a 'universal' or a 'selective' preventive measure. Teaching interpersonal communication skills (see section on secondary prevention and early identification, p. 68) is likely to influence a larger population. In teaching specifically about postnatal depression, attention would be directed to the needs of a selected population, that is, pregnant women and their partners.

Selective prevention of postnatal depression

The important role of the primary care team in the prevention of depression and anxiety was examined in an HMSO report published in 1992. It is certainly appropriate that prevention of postnatal depression should be considered in this context. Although depression after childbirth may sometimes be severe enough to require specialist care, the majority of women with non-psychotic postnatal depression never reach the attention of the psychiatric services (if indeed they are identified at all; see Cox *et al*, 1982) and those who do may be dismissed by some psychiatrists as 'the worried well'. Most women who experience it are dealt with in a primary care setting. For those women whose depression does not respond to simple measures, primary care is not only the first point of contact, but "the central base from which other care is obtained" (Strathdee, 1992).

The primary care setting provides the greatest opportunities for both primary and secondary prevention of mental illness and it is here that recognition of risk factors and detection of illness usually occurs (Reed, 1992). It is also the ideal place to consider issues such as continuity of care, and to plan individualised and holistic care programmes, based on an intimate understanding and knowledge of all the aspects of a woman's life and circumstances. A sensitised approach to the varying needs of individual childbearing women by a primary care team armed with knowledge of how the condition may be identified and the circumstances which can contribute to its manifestation and persistence, may well be our best hope in preventing postnatal depression.

Training courses for practising health visitors

Training combined with a counselling intervention (Holden *et al*, 1989) and a trial of preventive measures (Elliott *et al*, 1988) was implemented in Edinburgh, Stoke-on-Trent and Lewisham, London. Prevention strategies included the setting up of information and support groups for antenatal and postnatal women, encouraging the use of local voluntary services and agencies. Using the Edinburgh Postnatal Depression Scale (EPDS) as baseline and outcome measure, the percentage of women scoring high at 6–9 months was significantly reduced after training and implementation of the programme (Gerrard *et al*, 1993). The health visitors were given information about the nature and effects of postnatal depression and its possible origins, and the value of preventive strategies, including:

(a) continuity of care
(b) an empathic, non-directive, empowering approach
(c) setting up information/support groups, bringing together new and experienced mothers
(d) early antenatal contact: establishing a trusting relationship; providing information about the realities of parenthood, including the possibility of low mood and where to get help; information about the role of the health visitor and other health professionals and about sources

of support in the area, e.g. mother and toddler groups, baby-sitting groups and leaflets about postnatal depression; encouragement to talk about self and feelings of pregnancy; introduction to other expectant mothers if wished; a telephone contact number and times available
(e) late antenatal contact: reassurance about postnatal visiting – i.e. supporting the woman, not just checking up on baby; encouragement to seek practical help and identify sources of support; stressing the value of talking about her feelings to partner, friend or professional; reassurance that each woman is seen as an individual and her wishes respected; listening and attending to any problems
(f) postnatal visit: encouragement to talk about her birth experience and early experience of mothering ('the baby's fine, but how are YOU?'); reassurance of availability; information about sources of support, including baby clinic; telephone contact number and times available.

Educating other health professionals

This training was supplemented with information given to other members of the primary care team, raising general awareness of the problem. However, prevention is not solely the prerogative of primary care. In order to be effective, preventive strategies will depend on close liaison with all other health professionals involved in the care of women at this time, and also on a shared understanding by other disciplines of the nature of postnatal depression and factors which are associated with the origins and maintenance of the condition. Informed obstetricians and midwives can do much to prevent emotional distress through their care and by recognising women in need of extra support. All health professionals involved in the care of childbearing women, including hospital staff (obstetricians and midwives), should be given specific training in the psychological needs of perinatal women. Psychiatrists, psychologists, psychiatric nurses and social workers may be less involved in prevention, but they are likely to receive referrals of depressed women from primary care. Primary care workers need to know not only where to refer patients who need more help, but that when they do refer, the woman will be met with perceptive, appropriate and non-stigmatising care. As perinatal mental illness has only recently been recognised in the *International Classification of Diseases*, these professionals are likely to need extra training. There is a growing body of pertinent reading material for health professionals, including a Marcé Society Distance Learning Package, but input from an educator with specialist knowledge is also important.

Prevention of depression should not be considered only as a medical prerogative. According to Jenkins (1992) 'good practice' in prevention should help people to find their own solutions and should also draw on and strengthen existing support systems.

Other agencies

Voluntary agencies, the woman's partner, friends, and her extended family may all have a role to play in the prevention of postnatal depression, and education should be extended as widely as possible to ensure that all women with small babies have a recognised status, support and the individualised care they deserve and need. Specialised study days, the media and an informed body of literature are all relevant sources of information.

Primary prevention: selective measures; education of parents

This category of preventive measures would be directed at pregnant women and their partners. Again, specific education is important. A common criticism by parents (Holden *et al*, 1989) was that antenatal preparation had concentrated on the practical aspects of pregnancy, delivery and basic infant care. Fathers complained of feeling 'left out', or that their own role was unclear, and both men and women wished they had been warned of the possibility of low mood. An empowering approach, which provides women and their partners with information and enables them to take control over their own lives, is likely to be the most helpful in preventing the long-term consequences of postnatal depression.

Gordon & Gordon (1960) reported that women who were encouraged during pregnancy to confide in their husbands and enlist his practical help not only got more help, but were less likely to become depressed. To traditional antenatal classes, they added two 40-minute sessions in which women and their partners were advised to seek information and practical help, to make friends with couples experienced in childcare, to avoid moving house, to get plenty of rest, to discuss plans and worries, to cut down unnecessary activities and arrange baby-sitters. Shereshefsky & Lockman (1973) showed that the marital relationships of women who received individual antenatal counselling about the possible effect of childbirth on their relationship remained stable whereas those in a control group had deteriorated by six-months postpartum.

Social support and information

The opportunity provided by antenatal education for women to form supportive relationships could be more fully exploited by health professionals. Formal hospital-based antenatal classes do not provide an ideal opportunity for women to get to know each other; meetings held near women's homes, which combine professional input with the opportunity for women to share experiences, are more likely to foster mutual postnatal support. Hillier & Slade (1989) reported that although both hospital- and community-based antenatal classes increased women's confidence in labour and care of their newborn infant, the latter had the advantage of promoting supportive social relationships. An added advantage is, of course, that women who live near each other and who have shared the experience of pregnancy will be likely to form a mutually supportive group after the child is born.

Elliott and her colleagues (1988) invited pregnant women to attend informal groups which met during pregnancy and for six months afterwards. Group facilitators provided information about the realities of parenthood and encouraged women to discuss their own agenda over a cup of tea, and the groups were gradually taken over and run by the women themselves. Similar groups could be set up by midwives and health visitors either as an adjunct to existing classes or as support groups in their own right, with information sessions provided by various members of hospital and primary care professionals as appropriate.

Discussion topics for such groups could include:

(a) the realities of parenting: a lot of joy and a lot of hard work
(b) possible effects of parenting on the couple's relationship and sex life
(c) the importance of asking for specific help from partner, relatives, friends
(d) encouraging visitors to wait on the new mother, rather than the opposite
(e) the advantages of confiding in partner, mother, or a close friend
(f) how to cut out all unnecessary work outside and inside the home – simplify routines, don't move house or take on new commitments
(g) planning extra rest and relaxation, including time away from baby to maintain own identity
(h) choice and implications of feeding method
(i) possible problems, such as obstetric intervention, baby needing special care, postnatal depression, sibling rivalry.

(From Elliott *et al*, 1988)

Education and social support in primary care

Routine contacts in health centre settings can be maximised to provide opportunistic teaching and support sessions. Primary care workers are ideally placed to put women in touch with others in a similar situation and to encourage 'befriending' of newcomers or women who have been at work and do not know their neighbours. Information exchange and supportive groups can be facilitated in antenatal clinic waiting-rooms by the provision of a friendly atmosphere and cups of tea. For example, a first-time mother, unsure whether to breastfeed, could be introduced to a woman who has breastfed a previous baby. The waiting-room should also be a place where first-time parents can find explanatory leaflets, for example, 'do's and 'dont's' to make life easier in pregnancy and around the time of birth. The primary care team could provide an updated list of information for pregnant women and their partners about facilities which are available in their area. Short informative videos could be shown, and a library of informative books could also be kept. Pace (1992) described a health education library in general practice where 400 books were freely available in the waiting-room for patients to 'dip into' or borrow. Books on mental health and child care proved the most popular!

Primary prevention: selective measures; the birth experience

Much preventive work can be carried out in the delivery room, where sensitive and individualised care may prevent adverse emotional sequelae, including postnatal depression. Odent (1984) found that women who were emotionally supported during delivery did not experience postpartum 'blues'. Although they did become emotionally labile in the few days after delivery, this was described as a pleasurable release of feelings. Sosa *et al* (1980) and Klaus *et al* (1986) employed non-professional women (extra to the normal staff on the delivery ward) who 'mothered' and supported women throughout the birth. The presence of a 'Doula' (as the women were known in the Guatemalan hospital where the studies took place) not only reduced the time of labour by half, but dramatically reduced complications for both mother and baby. These startling findings were recently confirmed in a randomised controlled trial by Kennell *et al* (1991) in the United States. Emotionally supported women had significantly lower rates of Caesarean section, forceps deliveries, use of oxytocin and epidural anaesthesia.

It may be supposed that the presence of the woman's partner during labour would serve a similar function to that of a 'Doula', but it is not quite so straightforward. Men may not be able, however willing, to provide their partner with total emotional support; they may, indeed, need to be supported emotionally themselves. A Scottish study by Niven (1985) showed that the woman's perception of the quality of the support she receives from her partner, and whether or not she actually desired her partner to be present at the birth affect the experience of pain. Niven observed that women who said that their partner's presence enhanced their experience of labour reported less pain than women who had no companion or those who found their partner's presence unhelpful. It is important to check with the woman whether her partner actually is her preferred companion, and if at all possible, to ensure that another person who could emotionally support the couple be present. (See Niven, 1992, for a fuller discussion of this and other aspects of psychological care.)

As I have already mentioned, another important issue is the provision of ongoing information as the birth progresses. Green and her colleagues (1992) showed that women's satisfaction with labour and their subsequent emotional well-being are strongly influenced by the degree to which they feel they have been kept informed and involved in decisions about labour.

Important elements in providing emotional support during labour

(a) Provide continuity of *empathic* care throughout labour and birth.
(b) Give parents 'centre-stage' – this is *their* day (but don't assume the father is providing emotional support – he may also *need* support).
(c) Be sensitively aware of the woman's ongoing emotional state.
(d) Listen to the woman's stated needs, keep her fully informed, and involve her in all decisions.
(e) Remember that women in childbirth have heightened perceptions and may remember casual remarks made by carers; it is important (and should be a matter of courtesy) not to talk to colleagues about the woman (or about anything else) as if she wasn't there.
(f) If the woman seems to be losing control, help her to regain her sense of self.
(g) Help the woman to deal with pain by recognising and validating her pain (something often underestimated by midwives and obstetricians), providing information about methods of pain relief, respecting her choice of strategies, but helping decide on alternatives if necessary, and by knowing the value of the emotional support you can provide.
(h) Don't intrude at the moment of creation – allow the parents time to be with each other and their infant.

(Adapted from the Marcé Society Distance Learning Package.)

Primary prevention in the postnatal ward

Ball (1987) and Niven (1992) have emphasised the need for ensuring that women have sufficient support, rest and peace in which to recover from the stress and excitement of delivery. They also need time and privacy in which to get to know their infant (Klaus & Kennell, 1978) and to feel confident in handling and feeding. Giving women the opportunity to talk about their feelings after delivery is psychologically strengthening in allowing them to integrate and make sense of their birth experience. Staffing levels should be sufficient to allow midwives to spend up to half an hour of 'quality listening time' with each mother every day, ensuring that she is given explicit encouragement to talk fully about her feelings and her early responses to mothering (Holden, 1990). Empathic listening is not only therapeutic in itself, but can facilitate the early recognition of women with problems in relating to their infants. Encouragement to talk about their feelings in the early postnatal period may help to prevent later emotional problems from developing. Women who experience severe blues symptoms or who seem to be in need of extra support for any other reason should be closely monitored while in hospital, and followed up after returning home.

64 *Perinatal psychiatry*

Primary prevention: indicated measures

These are preventive measures which can be applied to relatively small subgroups with high risk of developing the condition (e.g. pregnant women with a number of vulnerability factors). Newton (1988) emphasised the importance of targeting preventive strategies on high-risk groups; according to Brown (1992) it is now possible to identify with reasonable accuracy those at high risk of depression and opportunities for preventive action are appropriate at key transitional stages such as pregnancy.

Primary care teams now take increased responsibility for antenatal care, providing the ideal opportunity for identifying vulnerable women in pregnancy. The continuing relationship also means that family doctors, midwives and health visitors are well placed to provide follow-up care and support. In a recent study by Sharp (1992), 200 women were observed from early pregnancy until the end of the first postnatal year, using Goldberg's Clinical Interview Schedule and self-report scales; the HAD (Snaith *et al*, 1976) which measures anxiety and depression, Barnett *et al*'s (1983) scale for measuring obstetric life events, and Kumar & Robson's maternal adjustment scale (1984). Factors which were predictive of psychiatric problems during pregnancy and after delivery were identified as: poor social support, adverse life events, an unplanned pregnancy, a poor relationship with partner, financial difficulties and a psychiatric history. At one year, being at home but wanting to work and problems with the baby were also relevant. According to Sharp, predictive vulnerability factors can be detected readily during pregnancy and the puerperium by family doctors and other members of the primary care team, and suitable follow-up care provided.

Women with vulnerability factors may also be detected at hospital-based antenatal clinics, although care should then be taken to ensure that a suitable liaison scheme is in operation to alert members of the primary care team to high-risk women. Leverton & Elliott (1989) devised a questionnaire which was used in this setting to identify vulnerable women for inclusion in the parents' groups described by Elliott *et al* (1988).

Defining the target group

In *Preventing Mental Illness*, Newton (1988) stresses the importance of targeting prevention on at-risk groups. Much research has been directed towards identifying factors associated with depression after childbirth. These findings not only help in understanding the aetiology of the condition but also provide clues about specific areas of vulnerability.

Summary of 'vulnerability' factors associated with postnatal depression

(a) *Biological factors*

    (i) Previous family or personal history of depression; this could be due to genetic vulnerability, but family dynamics are also relevant (Nilsson & Almgren, 1970; Zajicek & Wolkind, 1978; Paykel *et al*, 1980; Cox *et al*, 1982; O'Hara *et al*, 1983; Watson *et al*, 1984; Sharp, 1992).

    (ii) Previous postnatal depression (Uddenberg & Englesson, 1978; Wrate *et al*, 1985).

    (iii) Lowered progesterone in women who are fully breastfeeding and not taking oral contraceptives (Alder & Cox, 1983; Harris *et al*, 1989*a,b*).

(b) *Obstetric factors*

    (i) No direct relationship has been shown between type of delivery and depression. However, emotional support and feelings of being in control during labour are associated with postnatal emotional well-being (Sosa *et al*, 1980; Klaus *et al*, 1986; Kennell *et al*, 1991; Niven, 1985).

(c) *'Baby-related' factors*

    (i) Ambivalence about the pregnancy or 'lack of commitment' to the infant (Kumar & Robson, 1984; Murray, 1989)

    (ii) Previous stillbirth, miscarriage or termination (Cox *et al*, 1982; Watson *et al*, 1984; Kumar & Robson, 1984).

    (iii) Realistic worries about the baby's health (Sharp, 1992)

(d) *Psychosocial factors*

    (i) *External factors:* for example, housing or financial problems or having several small children to care for; a recent adverse life event which threatens the sense of self, e.g. bereavement, relationship crisis or loss of employment (Brown & Harris, 1978; Paykel *et al*, 1980; Watson *et al*, 1984; Kumar & Robson, 1984; Stein *et al*, 1989).

    (ii) *Internal factors:* external factors are more likely to lead to depression in women with low self-esteem or 'heightened interpersonal sensitivity'. Often this can be traced to the lack of a satisfying experience of being nurtured in their own childhood. The woman may have lost one or both parents; she may have been in care or otherwise separated from her parents; her parents may have been overcontrolling and lacking affection; or she may have suffered actual neglect or abuse (Frommer & O'Shea, 1973; Uddenberg, 1974; Boyce *et al*, 1991; Brown, 1992).

(e) *Relationships*

    (i) Having an unsupportive relationship with the woman's own mother (Nilsson & Almgren, 1970; Murray, 1989).

   (ii) Having an ongoing unsatisfying or unsupportive relationship with her partner (Paykel *et al*, 1980; Campbell *et al*, 1983; Robinson *et al*, 1989).

  (iii) Poor relationship with partner predating the birth (Whiffen, 1988).

(f) *Lack of support*

    (i) Emotional support, e.g. lack of any close relationship and having no one in whom to confide (Brown, 1992).

   (ii) Lack of practical help, e.g. with chores and childcare (Paykel *et al*, 1980).

(g) *Personal belief system, feelings of control*

    (i) The belief that events, circumstances or other people, rather than personal decisions, direct one's life (O'Hara *et al*, 1982; Boyce, see Chapter 6, this volume).

   (ii) Being in circumstances where actual control is difficult to achieve.

  (iii) Feeling that there is no escape from difficult circumstances (Brown, 1989).

(h) *Lack of employment* (or suitable childcare facilities) for women who wish to return to work (Sharp, 1992).

(i) *Not having time* (and little money) to spend on oneself.

Secondary prevention of depression in pregnant women identified as vulnerable

Having identified vulnerable women, what then? Can we actually prevent them from developing postnatal depression? Using Jenkins' (1992) categorisation, it is useful to look at possible preventive strategies in three categories: biological, social and psychological.

Biological prevention for women in high-risk groups

Physical treatments
Pregnant women may suffer from a deficit of vitamin B6. Riley (1986) found less depression at one month and one year following delivery in high-risk women treated with pyridoxine.

Progesterone

Intensive progesterone treatment is claimed by some to prevent recurrence of depression in high-risk women. This treatment has not yet been tested in a double-blind placebo trial, however. As previously mentioned, Harris and his colleagues (1989*a*,*b*) suggest that progesterone therapy may help to prevent depression in women who are fully breastfeeding and not taking oral contraceptives. (For a fuller description of the role of hormones in perinatal mental illness, see Chapter 7.)

Thyroid function tests

Harris *et al* (1989*b*) suggest that the thyroid function level of depressed postnatal women should be checked.

Psychosocial strategies

Psychosocial consequences of breastfeeding could explain the association with low mood. Low oestrogen is associated with loss of libido (and vaginal dryness), and the mother is more likely to be exhausted than if she were bottle-feeding. Total breast-feeders have little chance of time off from their baby, and may find it more difficult to resume their social life. While some women find the baby's dependence fulfilling, others may find it hard to cope with the baby's control of their life.

Women choosing to breast-feed should not only be given extra information and continuing support but encouraged to seek help with routine household tasks, and to care for themselves as well as the infant. Family, friends and especially partners may all need to be educated into the need to provide extra help.

Psychosocial factors: life events and chronic difficulties

Hobfoll & Lerman (1988) found that high self-esteem is influential in limiting postnatal depression. Self-esteem is largely dependent on the extent to which we feel valued; according to Cohen & Wills (1985) a single close and confiding relationship may be enough to mitigate the effects of stress. Cutrona & Troutman (1986) reported that at three months postnatal, social support exerted a protective function against depression.

Brown (1992) describes three essential elements of effective 'crisis support' from a partner or friend which may enable vulnerable women to survive a severe event without succumbing to depression. Considering birth as a severe event for women identified as vulnerable in pregnancy, these criteria seem appropriate in this context:

(a) the presence of someone close in whom the person 'at risk' may confide about the severe event

(b) receipt of active ongoing support from that person
(c) the avoidance by the person giving the support of making any negative comments about the person seeking support (i.e. to her or himself personally) during the required period of support.

From a study of vulnerable women in Islington Brown (1992) reported that only 4% of married women who expected and received such support from their partner became depressed. On the other hand, 26% of those who did not confide and did not receive crisis support became depressed, while those who confided, expected support but did not get it, were the most likely to become depressed.

Interestingly, those who did not expect and did not get crisis support from their partner but did get support from someone else close to them (usually a woman) were least likely to become depressed. For women who do not already have a confiding relationship or someone they can count on, pregnancy would seem to be a good time to encourage them to make a confidant either of their partner or another woman. Asking women if they have anyone they can trust in this way may be an indicator of vulnerability, and the possible need for extra support.

Sharp (1992) believes that support from relevant professional colleagues and services, the woman's family and friends, and local self-help groups, together with early intervention, can prevent or modify the effects of postnatal depression.

Secondary prevention: early identification and treatment

This refers to measures which shorten the length of episodes of the illness. The importance of identification cannot be overemphasised. The typically gradual onset of postnatal depression means that it is not easily distinguishable from the fatigue and emotional lability experienced by most mothers as they recover from delivery and adjust to the demands of the new baby. Early contacts with mothers are still more commonly oriented towards physical rather than emotional well-being, and some clinicians may still believe that emotional disturbance at this time is predictable and self-limiting. Also, depressed women may find it difficult to confide.

Goldberg (1992) describes the collusion which can occur between doctor and patient: "to keep the consultation as non-psychological as possible". According to Goldberg: "patients whose distress is not detected by their doctor are usually complaining of somatic symptoms and may have real physical illnesses which do not account for their present symptoms". Collusion may result from the fear that if they admit to how they are really feeling that they will be referred. For many people there is a stigma attached to psychiatric referral (Langer & Abelson, 1974; Doherty, 1975), and women with small babies run the added risk that they may be perceived as inadequate mothers.

Some professionals hold the view that if you tell a patient that they are depressed, this may add to their depressed feelings (see Elliott's excellent discussion in Chapter 14). Goldberg (1992), however, mentions two naturalistic studies which both showed that depression which has been recognised by the family doctor has a better outcome than depression which is missed. Freeling (1992) showed that unrecognised depression lasts longer than recognised depression, whereas Ormel and colleagues (1990) showed that this finding is not due to any particular treatment. These results substantiate an earlier finding by Malan and his colleagues (1975). In a review of 24 studies of the outcome of psychotherapy for depression in an attempt to discover why many clients appear to recover while on the waiting-list for treatment, they found that a "respectable number of clients feel helped by a single assessment interview". Having their feelings validated by a diagnosis of clinical depression appears to make patients feel better. Goldberg's opinion is that improvement may be due to the fact that the distress has been shared with another person. So detection in itself appears to be beneficial to the patient and can therefore be seen as secondary prevention.

Some doctors are, according to Goldberg, naturally better at detecting signs of emotional distress than others. Linda Gask, who has been involved for several years in teaching psychiatric interviewing skills to general practitioners, agrees but further believes that these skills can easily be learned using video and audio feedback of their own consultations with patients. In her teaching programme, a problem-based approach is used to enable doctors to help patients to discern and clarify their problems (Gask, 1992). The four main steps involve the following:

(a) accuracy in sensing and detecting patients' problems
(b) concise, complete description of elicited problems
(c) determination of patients' motivation and ability to change
(d) a mutually agreed plan for solving or improving the problems.

Sensitivity to the patient's tone of voice, posture, general appearance and demeanour are all important diagnostic aids, as are the doctor's own emotional responses to the patient. Gask explains that if the doctor feels anger or dislike for the patient, the patient may have the same effect on their relatives and friends, leaving them with no one to tell their problems to, which, as already discussed, is a key factor in depression.

As an adjunct to these sensitivity skills, the identification of postnatal depression can be simplified by screening all postnatal women using the Edinburgh Postnatal Depression Scale. (For information on using the EPDS in clinical practice, see Chapter 9.) Using the EPDS routinely can raise professional alertness to women's feelings and can facilitate a cooperative approach to postnatal depression as all members of the primary care team become involved. Women quickly learn from others that the EPDS is being used, and the resulting climate of increased openness may in itself be preventive.

Wright (1992) believes that the judicious use of computers could help to overcome problems with communication which are often present in the early stages of professional consultation. A computerised version of the EPDS by Glaze & Cox (1991) compared favourably with pencil-and-paper testing, and was found to be acceptable to patients. Although this approach should not be thought of as having the ability to replace doctor/patient contact, it could provide a useful adjunct.

Tertiary prevention

Tertiary prevention refers to measures which limit disability and handicap caused by an illness which might not in itself be fully treatable (Caplan, 1964). According to Jenkins (1992) "it is often not so much the disease *per se*, but how the health care system responds, which determines the extent of a person's disability". Rutter & Madge (1976) point out that early detection and treatment may disrupt the 'cycle of disadvantage', the predisposition to mental illness in adult life which can result from having had parents who suffer from mental illness, and this may also apply to postnatal depression.

Medication

Early treatment with antidepressants prescribed in appropriate dosage may limit the disabling effects of postnatal depression. However, as Cox (1989) points out, compliance can be extremely poor. Explanation of the rationale behind the treatment and reassurance that the side-effects will diminish and the depression will start to improve are needed to persuade women of the value of persisting with treatment. It should also be explained that antidepressants, unlike tranquillisers, are not addictive. Taken in sufficient dosage, antidepressants can lift a woman's mood sufficiently for her to be able to start to think about and deal with her situation, especially if this is combined with counselling.

Empowering women: psychological strategies

This category of tertiary prevention is likely to be the most effective in the long-term, because it aims to help the individual to live her life more effectively, increasing her feelings of personal worth and self-esteem. It includes schemes which would help the woman to alter what may be long-standing self-defeating beliefs (for example, that she is helpless or is always controlled by events or other people) to a recognition of her ability to take charge of her own life.

Counselling

Counselling may be the ideal first line of treatment for women who are experiencing emotional problems after childbirth. In an Edinburgh trial, health visitors were given a brief training in the principles of non-directive counselling and were asked to pay eight regular weekly 'listening' visits to women with postnatal depression. Of a group of 24 depressed mothers who received the extra visits from their health visitor, 69% had recovered from their depression after three months, compared with only 35% of 26 controls. Recovery was evaluated by a psychiatrist using Goldberg's Standardised Psychiatric Interview. The difference in recovery rate between the groups was 31.7% (95% confidence interval 5–58, $\chi^2 = 5.06$, d.f. = 1, $P = 0.03$) (Holden *et al*, 1989). Other researchers have had similar results, for example, Ring & McLean (1993) reported that giving non-directive counselling to 20 women with EPDS scores of 14 or over, as well as advice and support from their GP, resulted in 'complete recovery' for 80% of the women, measured by EPDS scores and by the women's own reports in a clinical interview. Cullinan (1991) offered counselling to 60 depressed women, leading to the reported improvement of 87% of this sample, measured by lowered EPDS scores and clinical opinion.

A counsellor is a professional confidant, who can provide social and emotional support. Counselling means empathic listening without giving opinions or advice. Depressed mothers are particularly vulnerable to feelings of inadequacy, which can be confirmed by the willingness of experts to give advice. For example, a mother who does not feel confident in her own judgement about whether to bottle or breast-feed her baby may ask the nurse or health visitor to make the decision for her. While this may seem easier in the short term, what she really needs is encouragement to make her own decisions and the confidence to believe that these are valid.

Health professionals often have a pre-set agenda, and a mental checklist of questions about the welfare of the mother and infant. Although they may also be sensitively aware of the mother's ongoing emotional state, this may not be apparent to the mother. They may inadvertently ask questions which make the mother feel inadequate, and it may be evident that they are working under time pressure. Depressed women need specific permission and encouragement to take up the time of a busy professional by talking about their feelings; however, our health visitor intervention study (outlined below) showed that, given the opportunity, they will do so. Non-recovered counselled women also benefited from this intervention, as demonstrated by their subsequent help-seeking behaviour. When their doctors were asked about their further progress a year later, 75% of non-recovered counselled women had sought medical help, compared with only 13% of non-recovered controls. The attention of their health visitor may have encouraged counselled women to view their depression as a legitimate reason to consult, and may also have increased compliance with further treatment.

Counselled women were also significantly more likely to have an altered perception of the health visitor's role. Of those counselled 85% said they thought the health visitor was there for them as well as the baby, compared with only 21% of controls. Many had been surprised by the realisation that the health visitor was prepared to discuss feelings.

Important elements of a health visitor intervention study

- (a) The health visitors provided an explicitly 'mother-oriented' rather than a 'baby-oriented' service, so the mother knew the extra attention was for her, rather than imagining that the health visitor was concerned about her ability to care for the baby.
- (b) The health visitors set up a 'contract' with women to visit for a set number of weeks at a pre-arranged time.
- (c) Having a regular weekly appointment meant that the mother knew when her health visitor was coming, and could prepare for the visit with things she wanted to talk about.
- (d) Asking the woman to arrange for her baby and/or children to be cared for during this time not only assured the mother that she was being taken seriously, but gave her 'permission' to ask for help from other people.
- (e) The woman was reassured by knowing she had support, that someone understood, and that other people go through similar experiences.
- (f) The woman was encouraged to talk about her experiences in her own way, without having to answer questions relating to an 'interviewer's agenda'. (Any questions asked were open-ended 'encouragers'.)
- (g) Talking about her feelings helped the woman to think more clearly about her situation and decide what she could do.
- (h) Not being given advice gave the woman confidence in her ability to make her own decisions.

Health professionals who wish to add non-directive counselling to their repertoire of helping skills may need extra training. The important message is to concentrate on the mother rather than the baby, to encourage her to talk about her feelings, to listen empathically, not to make judgements, offer gratuitous advice or 'bandaid' (the 'there-there' response).

Depressed women should be encouraged to cry if they need to. A further description of this counselling can be found in John Cox's book, *Postnatal Depression: A Guide for Health Professionals* (1986).

Counselling health visitors need the informed acknowledgement of managers that this extra service needs extra time. They may also need support for themselves: sharing another person's pain is personally demanding. All health visitors may not wish to become personally involved in counselling depresed women, especially if they are already stretched to their limits. Doctors may also find counselling too time-consuming. Many primary care teams now have specialist counsellors working in the practice, and this would seem to be a valid alternative and a worthwhile allocation of funds. Alternatively, one doctor, health visitor, midwife or community psychiatric nurse in the team could become a specialist in postnatal depression counselling, and either counsel all depressed women or provide support for colleagues. Community psychiatric nurses are an invaluable resource, especially if they know about the special emotional needs of postnatal women. In the three-centre health visitor programme for prevention and intervention in postnatal depression described on page 71, community psychiatric nurses provided added back-up to health visitors by taking referrals or assessing women and offering advice and support.

Befriending

Befriending groups such as Newpin and Homestart, or a supportive midwife or health visitor who acts in a way that empowers the woman and helps her to gain a sense of her own competence, can change women's lives. Newpin was started by Anne Jenkins, a former health visitor with marriage guidance training. Jenkins believes that health professionals have lost their ability to see people as unique, which leads to underestimation of their individual needs. Newpin offers an emotionally secure environment in which isolated women can make friends and gain support, while gradually taking control of their own lives. Newpin operates in comfortable homelike premises with a living room, playroom and kitchen, open all week so that women can drop in at any time. Mothers are referred to the centre by health visitors, social workers and family doctors, or by other mothers. The only criteria for involvement with Newpin is that people are mothers or the main carers of children.

Women who come with needs to be met gradually assume responsibility for befriending others. Training for supporting is provided, which in itself leads to a change in how the women see their status and their own potential. Women who become involved in the training programme are also encouraged to explore their own feelings with a trained counsellor, and receive ongoing support. Help is given in supporting the mother to recognise her own competence in dealing with agencies such as social security or the housing department. In their evaluation of Newpin, Pound & Mills (1985) noted that a third of women who were depressed recovered completely, and all but one of the others became less depressed. The scheme also has beneficial effects on relationships with partners due to more open communications, and helps the women to relate more lovingly and happily with their children. The scheme is based on respect for the individual woman, the establishment of trust, and the development of self-esteem and self-confidence.

Another empowering scheme is Homestart, a voluntary home visiting programme with over 100 branches operating all over the UK. Homestart works closely with both statutory and voluntary agencies in the community, has paid organisers and secretaries, and teams of volunteers who have been "realistically recruited, carefully prepared, sensitively matched with only one or two families at a time, and meticulously supported" (Harrison, 1992). Homestart offers friendship, support and practical help to young families experiencing difficulties. Volunteers visit young families on a regular basis for up to two years, helping with the problems and worries of everyday life, acting as a friend and confidant, and helping to build self-confidence in using other services. As with Newpin, many women go on to become volunteers themselves. Harrison (1992) who has been involved in the Homestart project for 17 years, says: "people who have been on the receiving end of welfare services, sometimes for quite a long time, often need to come out and volunteer themselves. They gain enormous benefit from that experience".

Self-help groups can also help to increase self-confidence by giving women the opportunity to discuss shared experiences. MAMA, the Meet-a-Mum Association, offers informal home-based groups for mothers who feel isolated after the birth. Cry-sis is a rather specialised association for parents whose babies cry excessively, with groups and telephone contacts throughout the country. The Association for Postnatal Illness has had an important role in helping individual women and in publicising postnatal depression.

The Stoke-on-Trent Parent-and-Baby Day Unit

Most empowering initiatives are found within the voluntary sector. North Staffordshire, however, is uniquely favoured by having the facility of a psychiatric day unit for parents and their babies. The atmosphere is informal and welcoming, and the philosophy of the unit is that many cases of postnatal depression are likely to have psychosocial origins. The multi-disciplinary team are trained in Rogerian non-directive counselling, and are also familiar with the range of antidepressant medication, including indications for electroconvulsive therapy. Cognitive therapy is carried out by a clinical psychologist. Other psychosocial treatments include yoga, meditation, individual and group therapy, relaxation, a stress management group, assertiveness training and creative therapy (which involves art and role play). There is also a parents-and-older-children group (inspired by the Newpin project) which facilitates parent–child interactions (Cox *et al*, 1993).

Links with other health professionals

Primary care staff need the reassurance that referral of resistant cases will result in prompt and effective help. As Elliott (1989) points out, in theory, Health Service departments have always been able to cross-refer; in practice, communications are enhanced and the speed and quality of referral improved when formal links are established. The parent-and-baby day unit was a distinct advantage in the instigation of the health visitor intervention training programme in North Staffordshire; health visitors had the security of knowing that expert advice, domiciliary assessment and/or treatment for women with special problems was readily available, giving them additional confidence in their ability to help depressed women. The parent-and-baby psychiatric day unit acts as the 'hub of the wheel' for postnatal services in North Staffordshire, receiving referrals from family doctors, midwives, consultants and social workers as well as health visitors. There is also a proportion of self-referrals. For regions lacking such a specialised facility Cox (1989) recommends that within each health district at least two community psychiatric nurses should be identified who have a particular concern for the prevention and treatment of postpartum mood disorder and can provide essential back-up to other health professionals. A specialist consultant psychiatrist would also be an appropriate use of resources; Oates (1988) has demonstrated that in a health district of 500 000, seeing all referred women with children under one year would justify a full-time consultant appointment.

Postnatal depression groups

Many health visitors have set up support groups for postnatal women, and there is a smattering of specialist therapy groups around the country. Care and sensitivity must be employed in extending invitations to such groups; in the early stages of depression, women are likely to need the nurture provided by a one-to-one relationship and may find it threatening to attend a group. They may also have difficulty organising themselves to get out of the house to attend a group, which could intensify their feelings of failure if this was the only resource offered. Professionals may be able to put women with low mood in touch with others who have had similar experiences. Or they could refer them to the Association for Postnatal Illness, an influential self-help organisation in which women who have themselves experienced postnatal depression 'befriend' women who are currently suffering, offering them a telephone 'hotline'. Depressed women find it both comforting and helpful to talk about their day-to-day experiences and problems to someone who has the been through the experience and recovered. Group support or group therapy are likely to be helpful as the woman starts to recover.

Conclusions

The reasons why women become depressed vary with each individual, and it is unlikely that we will ever be able to prevent all postnatal depressions. Responding to women's individual needs and responses, involving them in decisions about their care and creating a climate in which women, their partners, and caregivers feel free to discuss the emotional impact as well as the practical implications of parenthood, are, however, important steps towards promoting the psychological well-being of women and their families. Education of the public, health professionals and the women and their partners, will all help to bring about change. Most importantly, we need to ensure that resources, both in terms of specialist personnel and suitable venues, are available to help depressed women to help themselves. The extent to which these aims can be accomplished is largely dependent on recognition by the government and purchasers and providers of health care that the prevention of postnatal depression deserves adequate allocation of funding and resources.

Acknowledgements

The EPDS validation and counselling intervention study was supported by the Scottish Home and Health Department, and the three-centre training trial was supported by a grant from the Gatsby Charitable Foundation. I would like to express my thanks to Ruth Sagovsky, without whose untiring work in conducting the psychiatric interviews neither the EPDS study nor the counselling intervention trial would have been possible. Thanks also to Marjorie Dodd, John Cox's secretary at the Royal Edinburgh Hospital, who taught me to use a word processor, read all that I wrote, and made herself indispensable in so many ways, including taking responsibility for the random allocation of women to groups in the intervention trial and typing the audiotaped interviews with women – a mammoth task. Thanks to Sandra Elliott, for sharing her ideas and directing the 3-centre study, to Janice Gerrard, who trained the Stoke-on-Trent health visitors, contributing her own expertise as counsellor and nurse manager of the Charles Street Parent-and-Baby Day Unit, to Richard Bambridge for his support and especially to John Cox, without whom nothing would have happened.

References

ALDER, E. M. (1989) Sexual behaviour in pregnancy, after childbirth and during breastfeeding. In *Psychosocial Aspects of Obstetrics and Gynaecology* (ed. M. R. Oates). Clinical Obstetrics and Gynaecology, Vol. 3, No. 4. London: Baillière-Tindall.
—— & COX, J. L. (1983) Breast-feeding and postnatal depression. *Journal of Psychosomatic Research*, **27**, 139–144.
APPLEBY, L. (1991) Suicide during pregnancy and in the first postnatal year. *British Journal of Psychiatry*, **302**, 137–140.
BALL, J. (1987) *Reactions to Motherhood*. Cambridge: Cambridge University Press.

BARNETT, B. & PARKER, G. (1986) Possible determinates, correlates and consequences of high levels of anxiety in primiparous mothers. *Psychological Medicine*, **16**, 177–185.

BEAIL, N. (1985) Fathers and infant caretaking. *Journal of Reproductive and Infant Psychology*, **3**, 54–64.

BOYCE, P., PARKER, G., BARNETT, B., *et al* (1991) Personality as a vulnerability factor to depression. *British Journal of Psychiatry*, **159**, 106–114.

BROWN, G. (1992) Life events and social support: possibilities for primary prevention. In *The Prevention of Depression and Anxiety: the Role of the Primary Care Team* (eds R. Jenkins, J. Newton & R. Young). London: HMSO.

—— (1989) Discussant. In *Childbirth as a Life Event* (eds J. L. Cox, E. S. Paykel & M. L. Page), pp. 94–103. Southampton: Duphar Medical Publications.

—— & HARRIS, T. (1978) *Social Origins of Depression*. London: Tavistock Publications.

CAMPBELL, E., COPE, S. J. & TEASDALE, J. D. (1983) Social factors and affective disorder: an investigation of the Brown and Harris model. *British Journal of Psychiatry*, **143**, 548–553.

CAPLAN, G. (1964) *Principles of Preventive Psychiatry*. New York: Basic Books.

COGILL, S. R., CAPLAN, H. L., ALEXANDRA, H., *et al* (1986) Impact of maternal postnatal depression on cognitive development of young children. *British Medical Journal*, **292**, 1165–1167.

COHEN, S. & WILLS, T. A. (1985) Stress, social support and the buffering hypothesis. *Psychological Bulletin*, **98**, 310–357.

COOPER, P. J., CAMPBELL, E. A., DAY, A., *et al* (1988) Non-psychotic disorder after childbirth: a prospective study of prevalence, incidence, course and nature. *British Journal of Psychiatry*, **152**, 799–806.

COX, J. L. (1986) *Postnatal Depression: A Guide for Health Professionals*. Edinburgh: Churchill Livingstone.

—— (1988) The life event of childbirth: sociocultural aspects of postnatal depression. In *Motherhood and Mental Illness, Vol. 2. Causes and Consequences* (eds R. Kumar & I. F. Brockington), pp. 64–75. London: Wright.

—— (1989) Postnatal depression: a serious and neglected postpartum complication. In *Psychosocial Aspects of Obstetrics and Gynaecology* (ed. M. R. Oates), Clinical Obstetrics and Gynaecology, vol. 3, no. 4, pp. 839–857. London: Baillière Tindall.

——, CONNOR, Y. & KENDELL, R. E. (1982) Prospective study of the psychiatric disorders of childbirth. *British Journal of Psychiatry*, **140**, 111–117.

——, HOLDEN, J. M. & SAGOVSKY, R. (1987) Detection of postnatal depression: development of the Edinburgh Postnatal Depression Scale. *British Journal of Psychiatry*, **150**, 782–786.

——, GERARD, J., COOKSON, D., *et al* (1993) Development and audit of Charles Street Parent and Baby Day Unit, Stoke-on-Trent. *Psychiatric Bulletin*, **17**, 711–712.

CULLINAN, R. (1991) Health visitor intervention in postnatal depression. *Health Visitor*, **64**, 412–414.

CUTRONA, C. E. & TROUTMAN, B. R. (1986) Social support, infant temperament and parenting self-efficacy: a mediational model of postpartum depression. *Child Development*, **57**, 1507–1518.

DOHERTY, E. G. (1975) Labelling effects. *Archives of General Psychiatry*, **32**, 562–568.

ELLIOTT, S. A. (1989) Psychological strategies in the prevention and treatment of postnatal depression. In *Psychological Aspects of Obstetrics and Gynaecology* (ed. M. R. Oates), Clinical Obstetrics and Gynaecology, vol. 3, no. 4, pp. 879–905. London: Baillière-Tindall.

——, SANJAK, M., LEVERTON, T. (1988) Parents groups in pregnancy; a preventive intervention for postnatal depression? In *Marshalling Social Support. Formats, Processes and Effects* (ed. B. H. Gottlieb). California: Sage Publications.

FREELING, P. (1992) Implications for general practice training and education. In *The Prevention of Depression and Anxiety: the Role of the Primary Care Team* (eds R. Jenkins, J. Newton & R. Young), pp. 57–68. London: HMSO.

FROMMER, E. A. & O'SHEA, G. (1973) Antenatal identification of women liable to have problems in managing their infants. *British Journal of Psychiatry*, **123**, 149–156.

GASK, L. (1992) Teaching psychiatric interview skills to general practitioners. In *Prevention of Depression and Anxiety: the Role of the Primary Care Team* (eds R. Jenkins, J. Newton & R. Young). London: HMSO.

GERRARD. J., HOLDEN, J. M., ELLIOTT, S. A., *et al* (1994) A trainer's perspective of an innovative training programme to teach health visitors about the detection, treatment and prevention of postnatal depression. *Journal of Advanced Nursing* (in press).

GLAZE, R. & COX, J. L. (1991) Validation of a computerised version of the 10-item (self-rating) Edinburgh Postnatal Depression Scale. *Journal of Affective Disorders*, **22**, 73–77.

GOLDBERG, D. (1992) Early diagnosis and secondary prevention. In *Prevention of Depression and Anxiety in General Practice* (eds R. Jenkins, J. Newton & R. Young), pp. 33–39. London: HMSO.

GORDON, R. E. & GORDON, K. K. (1960) Social factors in prevention of postpartum emotional adjustment. *Obstetrics & Gynecology*, **15**, 433–438.

GREEN, J. M., COUPLAND, V. A. & KITZINGER, J. V. (1992) Expectations, experiences and psychological outcomes of childbirth: A prospective study of 825 women. *Birth*, **17**, 15–24.

HARRIS, B., JOHNS, S., FUNG, H., *et al* (1989) The hormonal environment of postnatal depression. *British Journal of Psychiatry*, **154**, 660–667.

——, FUNG, H., JOHNS, S., *et al* (1989) Transient postpartum thyroid dysfunction and postnatal depression. *Journal of Affective Disorders*, **17**, 243–249.

HARRISON, M. (1992) Linking with voluntary and community resources: Homestart consultancy. In *Prevention of Depression and Anxiety in General Practice* (eds R. Jenkins, J. Newton & R. Young), pp. 140–144. London: HMSO.

HILLIER, C. A. & SLADE, P. (1989) The impact of antenatal classes on knowledge, anxiety and confidence in primiparous women. *Journal of Reproductive and Infant Psychology*, **7**, 3–15.

HMSO (1992) *The Prevention of Depression and Anxiety: The Role of the Primary Care Team*. London: HMSO.

HOBFOLL, S. E. & LIEBERMAN, M. (1988) Personal relationships, personal attributes and stress resistance: mother's reactions to their child's illness. *American Journal of Community Psychology*, **16**, 565–589.

HOLDEN, J. M. (1986) Counselling for health visitors. In *Postnatal Depression – a Guide for Health Professionals* (ed. J. L. Cox). Edinburgh: Churchill Livingstone.

—— (1989) A randomised controlled trial of counselling by health visitors in the treatment of postnatal depression. MPhil thesis, Faculty of Medicine, University of Edinburgh.

—— (1990) Emotional problems relating to childbirth. In *Midwifery Practice: Postnatal Care* (eds J. Alexander, V. Levy & S. Roch). Basingstoke: McMillan Publications.

—— (1991) Postnatal depression: its nature, effects and identification using the Edinburgh Postnatal Depression Scale. *Birth*, **18**, 211–221.

——, SAGOVSKY, R. & COX, J. L. (1989) Counselling in general practice setting: a controlled study of health visitor intervention in treatment of postnatal depression. *British Medical Journal*, **298**, 223–226.

JENKINS, R. (1992) Depression and anxiety: an overview of preventive strategies. In *The Prevention of Depression and Anxiety: the Role of the Primary Care Team*. London: HMSO.

KENNELL, J., KLAUS, M., McGRATH, S., *et al* (1991) Continuous emotional support during labour in a US hospital: a randomised controlled trial. *Journal of the American Medical Association*, **265**, 2197–2201.

KLAUS, M. H. & KENNELL, J. H. (1978) Future care of parents. *Birth and Family Journal*, **5**, 246–248.

——, KENNEL, J. H., ROBERTSON, S. S., *et al* (1986) Effects of social support during parturition on maternal and infant morbidity. *British Medical Journal*, 585–587.

KRUK, S. & WOLKIND, S. N. (1983) A longitudinal study of single mothers and their children. In *Families at Risk* (ed. N. Madge). London: Heinemann.

KUMAR, R. & ROBSON, K. M. (1984) A prospective study of emotional disorders in child-bearing women. *British Journal of Psychiatry*, **144**, 35–47.

LANGER, E. J. & ABELSON, R. P. (1974) A patient by any other name. *Journal of Consulting and Clinical Psychology*, **42**, 4–9.

LEVERTON, T. J. & ELLIOTT, S. A. (1989) Transition to parenthood groups; a preventive intervention for postnatal depression? In *The Free Woman. Women's Health in the 1990s* (eds E. V. van Hall & W. Everaerd), pp. 479–486. Amsterdam: Parthenon.

MALAN, D. H., HEATH, E. S., BACAL, H. A., *et al* (1975) Psychodynamic changes in untreated neurotic patients – II. Apparently genuine improvements. *Archives of General Psychiatry*, **32**, 110–126.

MOSS, P., BOLLAND, G., FOXMAN, R., *et al* (1987) The division of household work during the transition to parenthood. *Journal of Reproductive and Infant Psychology*, **5**, 71–87.

MURRAY, L. (1988) Effects of postnatal depression on infant development: the contribution of direct studies of early mother–infant interactions. In *Motherhood and Mental Illness* (eds R. Kumar & I. Brockington), vol. 2. London: John Wright.

—— (1989) The Cambridge Study of Postnatal Depression and Infant Development. In *Childbirth as a Life Event* (eds J. L. Cox, E. S. Paykel & M. L. Page), pp. 23–38. Southampton: Duphar Medical Publications.

—— & STEIN, A. (1989) The effects of postnatal depression on the infant. In *Psychological Aspects of Obstetrics and Gynaecology* (ed. M. R. Oates), Clinical Obstetrics and Gynaecology, vol. 3, no. 4, pp. 921–935. London: Baillière-Tindall.

NEWTON, J. (1988) *Preventing Mental Illness*. London: Routledge.

—— (1992) Crisis support: utilising resources. In *The Prevention of Depression and Anxiety: the Role of the Primary Care Team* (eds R. Jenkins, J. Newton & R. Young), pp. 68–77. London: HMSO.

NILSSON, A. & ALMGREN, P. E. (1970) Paranatal emotional adjustment. A prospective investigation of 165 women. *Acta Scandinavica* (suppl. 220), 9–41.

NIVEN, C. A. (1985) How helpful is the presence of the husband at childbirth? *Journal of Reproductive and Infant Psychology*, **3**, 45–53.

—— (1992) *Psychological Care for Families Before, During and After Birth*. Oxford: Butterworth-Heinemann.

NOTT, P. (1989) The Southampton Study. In *Childbirth as a Life Event* (eds J. L. Cox, E. S. Paykel & M. L. Page), pp. 57–62. Southampton: Duphar Medical Publications.

O'HARA, M. W. (1985) Depression and marital adjustment during pregnancy and after delivery. *American Journal of Family Therapy*, **4**, 49–55.

—— (1986) Social support, life events and depression during pregnancy and the puerperium. *Archives of General Psychiatry*, **43**, 569–573.

——, REHM, L. P., & CAMPBELL, S. B. (1982) Predicting depressive symptomatology; cognitive–behavioural models and postpartum depression. *Journal of Abnormal Psychology*, **91**, 457–461.

——, —— & —— (1983) Postpartum depression: A role for social network and life stress variables. *Journal of Nervous and Mental Disorders*, **171**, 336–341.

——, ZEKOSKI, E. M., PHILIPPS, L. H., *et al* (1990) Controlled prospective study of postpartum mood disorders; comparison of childbearing and non-childbearing women. *Journal of Abnormal Psychology*, **99**, 3–15.

OATES, M. (1988) The development of an integrated community-oriented service for severe postnatal illness. In *Motherhood and Mental Illness, vol. 2, Causes and Consequences* (eds R. Kumar & I. F. Brockington). London: John Wright.

—— (1989) Normal emotional changes in pregnancy and the puerperium. In *Psychological Aspects of Obstetrics and Gynaecology* (ed. M. R. Oates), Clinical Obstetrics and Gynaecology, vol. 3, no. 4, London: Baillière-Tindall.

ODENT, M. (1984) *Birth Reborn*. London: Souvenir Press.

ORMEL, H., KOESTER, M., VAN DER BRINK, W., *et al* (1990) The extent of non-recognition of mental problems in primary care and its effect on management and outcome. In *The Public Health Impact of Mental Disorder* (eds D. Goldberg & D. Tantum). Bern: Hogrefe and Huber.

PACE, C. (1992) A health education library in general practice. In *The Prevention of Depression and Anxiety: the Role of the Primary Care Team* (eds R. Jenkins, J. Newton & R. Young), pp. 131–135. London: HMSO.

PAYKEL, E. S., EMMS, E., FLETCHER, J., *et al* (1980) Life events and social support in puerperal depression. *British Journal of Psychiatry*, **136**, 339–346.

PITT, B. (1968) Atypical depression following childbirth. *British Journal of Psychiatry*, **114**, 1325–1335.

POUND, A. & MILLS, M. (1985) A pilot evaluation of Newpin: home visiting and befriending scheme in South London. *Association of Child Psychiatry and Psychology Newsletter*, 7, 13–15.

REED, J. (1992) Foreword. In *The Prevention of Depression and Anxiety: the Role of the Primary Care Team* (eds R. Jenkins, J. Newton & R. Young), pp. xiii–xiv. London: HMSO.

RICHMAN, N., STEVENSON, J. & GRAHAM, P. (1982) *Preschool to School: A Behavioural Study*. London: Academic Press.

RILEY, D. (1986) An audit of obstetric liaison psychiatry in 1984. *Journal of Reproductive and Infant Psychology*, 4, 99–115.

RING, N. & McLEAN, T. M. (1994) Routine postnatal depression screening and the effects on health visitor practice. *Journal of Advanced Nursing* (in press).

ROBINSON, G. E., OLMSTED, M. P. & GARNER, D. M. (1989) Predictors of postpartum adjustment. *Acta Psychiatrica Scandinavica*, 80, 561–565.

ROBSON, K. M. & KUMAR, R. (1980) Delayed onset of maternal affection after childbirth. *British Journal of Psychiatry*, 136, 347–353.

RUTTER, M. L. & MADGE, N. (1976) *Cycles of Disadvantage*. London: Heinemann.

SEEL, R. M. (1986) Birth rite. *Health Visitor*, 59, 182–184.

SHARP, D. (1992) Liaison between providers of primary care: early detection of difficulties: Predicting postnatal depression. In *Prevention of Depression and Anxiety: the Role of the Primary Care Team* (eds R. Jenkins, J. Newton & R. Young), pp. 101–113. London: HMSO.

SHERESHEFSKY, P. M. & LOCKMAN, R. F. (1973) Comparison of counselled and non-counselled groups. In *Psychological Aspects of a First Pregnancy* (eds P. M. Shereshefsky & L. J. Yarrow), pp. 151–163. New York: Raven Press.

SOSA, R., KENNEL, J. R., KLAUS, M., *et al* (1980) The effect of a supportive companion on perinatal problems, length of labour and mother–infant interaction. *New England Journal of Medicine*, 303, 597–600.

STEIN, A., COOPER, P., CAMPBELL, E. A., *et al* (1989) Social adversity and perinatal complications: their relation to postnatal depression. *British Medical Journal*, 298, 1073–1074.

——, GATH, D. H., BUCHER, J., *et al*, (1991) The relationship between postnatal depression and mother–child interaction. *British Journal of Psychiatry*, 158, 46–52.

STRATHDEE, G. (1992) Liaison between primary and secondary care teams towards early intervention; a general approach. In *The Prevention of Depression and Anxiety: the Role of the Primary Care Team* (eds R. Jenkins, J. Newton & R. Young), pp. 113–124. London: HMSO.

THOME, M. (1991) Emotional distress during the postpartum period, from the second to the sixth month, assessed by community nurses. *Nordic Midwives and Research Oslo*, 9, 25–27.

UDDENBERG, N. (1974) Reproductive adaptation in mother and daughter: a study of personality development and adaptation to motherhood. *Acta Psychiatrica Scandinavica* (suppl. 254), 1–115.

—— & ENGLESSON, I. (1978) Prognosis of postpartum mental disturbance: prospective study of primiparous women and their four-and-a-half-year-old children. *Acta Psychiatrica Scandinavica*, 58, 201–212.

WATSON, J. P., ELLIOTT, S. A., RUGG, A. J., *et al* (1984) Psychiatric disorder in pregnancy and the first postnatal year. *British Journal of Psychiatry*, 144, 453–462.

WHIFFEN, V. E. (1988) Vulnerability to postnatal depression: a prospective multivariate study. *Journal of Abnormal Psychology*, 97, 467–474.

WOLKIND, S. N. & DE SALIS, W. (1982) Infant temperament, maternal depression and child behaviour problems. In *Temperamental Differences in Infants and Young Children* (ed. M. Rutter).

WRATE, R. M., ROONEY, A. C., THOMAS, P. F., *et al* (1985) Postnatal depression and child development: a 3-year follow-up study. *British Journal of Psychiatry*, 146, 622–627.

WRIGHT, A. (1992) The computer will see you now: meeting the challenge of hidden psychiatric morbidity in general practice. In *Prevention of Depression and Anxiety: the Role of the Primary Care Team* (eds R. Jenkins, J. Newton & R. Young), pp. 101–113. London: HMSO.

ZAJICEK, E. & WOLKIND, S. (1978) Emotional difficulties in married women during and after the first pregnancy. *British Journal of Medical Psychology*, 51, 379–385.

Further reading

BALL, J. (1987) *Reactions to Motherhood*. Cambridge University Press.

BROCKINGTON, I. F. & KUMAR, R. (eds) (1982) *Motherhood and Mental Illness*. London: Academic Press.

COMPORT, M. (1987) *Towards Happy Motherhood: Understanding Postnatal Depression*. Guernsey: Corgi.

COX, J. L. (1986) *Postnatal Depression: A Guide for Health Professionals*. Edinburgh: Churchill Livingstone.

DAINOW, S. & BAILEY, C. (1988) *Developing Skills with People: Training for Person to Person Client Contact*. Chichester: John Wiley.

DIX, C. (1986) *The New Mother Syndrome. Coping With Postnatal Depression*. London: Allen & Unwin.

ELLIOTT, S. A. (1989) Psychological strategies in the prevention and treatment of postnatal depression. In *Psychological Aspects of Obstetrics and Gynaecology* (ed. M. R. Oates). Clinical Obstetrics and Gynaecology, vol. 3, no. 4. London: Baillière-Tindall.

JENKINS, R., NEWTON, J. & YOUNG, R. (eds) (1992) *The Prevention of Depression and Anxiety: the Role of the Primary Care Team*. London: HMSO.

NEWTON, J. (1988) *Preventing Mental Illness*. London: Routledge.

NIVEN, C. A. (1992) *Psychological Care for Families Before, During and After Birth*. Oxford: Butterworth-Heinemann.

RAPHAEL-LEFF, J. (1991) *Psychological Processes of Childbirth*. London: Chapman & Hall.

SAPSTED, A. M. (1990) *Banish Post-baby Blues*. Wellingborough: Thorson's Publishing Group.

WELBURN, V. (1980) *Postnatal Depression*. Glasgow: Fontana.

6 Personality dysfunction, marital problems and postnatal depression

PHILIP BOYCE

Postnatal depression is a common disorder, affecting about 10% of women in the first six months postpartum. While its prevalence is high, the rate of depression among women at other times of the life cycle is similar (Kumar, 1982; Cooper *et al*, 1988; O'Hara *et al*, 1990). Further, the symptoms of postnatal depression are essentially the same as neurotic depression (Kumar, 1982; Cooper *et al*, 1988), although some symptoms such as fatigue and irritability may be over-represented (Pitt, 1968; Snaith & Taylor, 1985). Postnatal depression is, in essence, no different from neurotic depression. However, it is important to consider it to be a specific 'type' of depression for three reasons. First, it has a predictable time of onset and association with childbirth. Second, it causes considerable distress at a critical time in a woman's life and may impede successful adaptation to this life transition. It may also have a profound long-term effect on the woman and her long-term relationships (Cox, 1989). Finally, the affected woman may be unresponsive to her infant, which may have a detrimental effect on the infant's development (Murray *et al*, 1991). Infants raised by women suffering from postnatal depression may have cognitive impairment (Cogill *et al*, 1986) and attachment difficulties (Murray & Stein, 1989; Stein *et al*, 1991).

Postnatal depression needs to be distinguished from two other types of mood disorder occurring postnatally. Firstly, there is the transient 'blues' affecting up to 70% of women. It is most likely that hormonal and biological factors are the major contributors to this mood disturbance (Pitt, 1973; Stein, 1982; Kennerley & Gath, 1986; Campbell, 1992), and psychosocial factors such as personality are unlikely to be involved (Pitt, 1973; Nott *et al*, 1976). Secondly, there is puerperal psychosis, a severe psychiatric illness related to manic–depressive illness. Puerperal psychosis arises within the first two to three weeks after childbirth and has an incidence of between one and two per thousand deliveries (Brockington *et al*, 1981; Kendell, 1985; Kendell *et al*, 1987). The disorder is biologically mediated, with one possible mechanism being dopamine supersensitivity induced by the rapid fall in oestrogen (Weick *et al*, 1991). Psychosocial stresses, such as being unmarried or having a caesarean section or a stillbirth, appear to contribute to the disorder. However, an excess of life events (Martin *et al*, 1989; Marks *et al*, 1991), deficient social support (Martin *et al*, 1989) or an overly critical partner (Marks *et al*, 1992) do not appear to increase the risk of developing puerperal psychosis (Martin *et al*, 1989; Brockington *et al*, 1990).

Postnatal depression, in contrast to the blues and puerperal psychosis, arises principally as a result of psychosocial variables (Kumar, 1982), similar to those associated with depression at other times (O'Hara & Zekoski, 1988). While the predominant causal influences are psychosocial, the role of hormonal factors such as thyroid dysfunction (e.g. Harris *et al*, 1992) cannot be discounted. It is most likely that postnatal depression has a multifactorial causality, being determined by an interaction between social, psychological, interpersonal and hormonal or biological factors (Cox, 1986; O'Hara & Zekoski, 1988; Gotlib *et al*, 1989). Brown & Harris (1978) have described a psychosocial model for depression. This model proposes that, following adversity, vulnerable women have an increased risk of becoming depressed. They identified four vulnerability factors: loss of one's mother before the age of 11; having three or more young children at home; no confiding relationship; and no outside employment. In a later study, this model was expanded to include 'negative evaluation of the self' as a vulnerability factor (Brown *et al*, 1990*a,b*). The role of these and other vulnerability factors, such as having experienced dysfunctional parenting (Boyce *et al*, 1988; Gotlib *et al*, 1988), have been the focus of many studies of postnatal depression. Two psychosocial variables stand out as being particularly relevant to the genesis of postnatal depression: being in a dysfunctional relationship and having a vulnerable personality style. While these are considered to contribute to vulnerability, both could also be a consequence of postnatal depression. This chapter will focus on these factors as possible risk factors to postnatal depression.

Personality style as a risk factor

The experience of pregnancy, childbirth and looking after a newborn infant is an important event in a woman's life. For many women this is a positive and enriching transition to a new phase in the life cycle. However, as with all life transitions, it is stressful; Brown & Harris (1978, p. 141) have stated, "pregnancy and birth, like other crises, can bring home to a woman the disappointment and hopelessness of her position – her aspirations are made more distant as she becomes even more dependent on an uncertain relationship". The stresses, which may have an impact on women with a vulnerable personality style, include body image and role changes, changes in social relationships and the demands of having to nurture a dependent infant. In addition to the physical symptoms and discomfort of pregnancy, a woman has to cope with her changing body image as the foetus develops. This may have an impact on her self-esteem. At the same time she has to contend with a number of significant role changes, particularly taking on the role of 'mother'. A woman's social support network will also change over this period. She may lose some of her familiar support group (single women and those with no children) and need to replace them by finding new sources of support. If she gained role satisfaction through work and her self-esteem was invested in this, she may lose, temporarily or permanently, an important part of her self-concept. Finally, she has to cope with looking after and nurturing her dependent infant. This may be particularly stressful for a woman who has difficulty in giving to others, especially when she may not have experienced good-enough mothering herself (Boyce *et al*, 1991).

Personality and postnatal depression

A number of vulnerable personality styles have been proposed for depression in general which could, theoretically, also predispose women to postnatal depression. These include dependency (Hirschfeld *et al*, 1976; Birtchnell, 1984), orality (Chodoff, 1972), neuroticism (Coppen & Metcalf, 1965; Hirschfeld *et al*, 1989), obsessionality (Abraham, 1911; Klein & Depue, 1985), a dysfunctional cognitive style (Abrahamson *et al*, 1978), and a personality style characterised by high interpersonal sensitivity (Boyce & Parker, 1989). A number of these traits have been examined as possible risk factors to postnatal depression, especially neuroticism, a dysfunctional cognitive style, external locus of control and interpersonal sensitivity. Studies examining these traits are summarised in Table 6.1. Although it is closely aligned with neuroticism, the role of anxiety as a risk factor has not been included since it is a symptom (albeit an important predictor of postnatal depression) rather than an enduring personality trait (Meares *et al*, 1976; Barnett & Parker, 1986; O'Hara & Zekoski, 1988).

Investigation of these personality traits as vulnerability factors have not yielded clear answers for four principal reasons. First, there is probably no unique personality style which renders women vulnerable to postnatal depression. More likely there are a number of traits, either alone or in conjunction with others, which render women vulnerable. Second, the time at which postnatal depression is assessed will influence findings (Boyce *et al*, 1990). Some studies have sought to determine personality vulnerability close to childbirth (e.g. Manly *et al*, 1982) when any depression would be more likely to reflect the 'blues'. As previously mentioned, this depression

TABLE 6.1
Studies of personality and postnatal depression

Authors	Sample size	Personality measures	Relevant findings
Tod, 1964	322	Interview	Depressed women had previous 'inadequate' personality
Pitt, 1968	62	MPI	Women with postnatal depression: high neuroticism and low extraversion
Hayworth et al, 1980	166	HDHQ Locus of control	High hostility and external locus of control associated with postnatal depression
O'Hara et al, 1982	170	SCQ ASQ DAS	Depressive symptoms predicted by dysfunctional attributional style after prepartum depression controlled for Dysfunctional attributional style predicted depressive symptoms
Manly et al, 1982	50	ASQ	Attributional style *did not* predict depressive symptoms
Cutrona, 1983	85	ASQ	Dysfunctional attributions predicted depressed symptoms at 2 and 8 weeks postpartum
O'Hara et al, 1984	99	SCQ ASQ	Attributional style *did not* predict depressive symptoms Dysfunctional self-control attitude predicted depressive symptoms
Watson et al, 1984	128	EPQ	Women with postnatal depression: high neuroticism, low extraversion and high psychoticism
Whiffen, 1988	115	Attributional style	Attributional style *did not* predict postnatal depression
Robinson et al, 1989	89	Sociotropy– autonomy scale	High symptom women scored higher on 'freedom from others control' scale
Kumar & Robson, 1984	119	EPI	No personality differences detected
Boyce et al, 1990	164	EPI IPSM	No differences detected at 1 and 3 months postpartum. Women depressed at 6 months postpartum: high inter-personal sensitivity and high neuroticism
Gotlib et al, 1991	730	DAS Ways of coping	Women with postnatal depression: increased escape *No increase* in dysfunctional attitudes

ASQ: Attributional Style Questionnaire (Peterson *et al*, 1982)
DAS: Dysfunctional Attitudes Scale (Weissman, 1980)
EPI: Eysenck Personality Interview (Eysenck & Eysenck, 1975)
HDHQ: Hostility and Direction of Hostility Questionnaire (Caine *et al*, 1967).
IPSM: Interpersonal Sensitivity Measure (Boyce & Parker, 1989)
MPI: Maudsley Personality Interview (Eysenck, 1959)
SCQ: Self-Control Questionnaire (Rhem *et al*, 1981)
Ways of Coping (Folkman & Lazarus, 1985)

is likely to be determined by hormonal or biological factors and not by personality factors. Furthermore, if depression is assessed early in the postpartum period the full impact of the stress of being a new mother may not have hit, particularly as support systems are more likely to be available at this period.

Ann B coped well initially after delivery and only became depressed in the second month postpartum. It was clear from her history that she had a vulnerable personality style – she had a history of coping poorly with life stresses. It transpired that for the first six weeks postpartum her mother had come to stay to help her look after the baby. Ann only became depressed when her mother had to return home and she was left to cope on her own.

Third, some of the personality measures, particularly those measuring negative cognitive style, may not be sufficiently sensitive to identify 'latent' or dormant personality traits (Boyce & Mason, 1994) when the assessment is made prior to childbirth. Finally, there is the contribution of methodological problems to add to the confusion. These problems include insufficient statistical power to detect differences when relatively small samples are used. The use of several personality measures mean that the results are hampered because of the issue of multiple inference (O'Hara & Zekoski, 1988); there is also the fact that, compared with when they are well, depressed individuals tend to describe their personality as more deviant (Kendell & DiScipio, 1968; Hirschfeld *et al*, 1989; Boyce *et al*, 1990). Consequently, personality questionnaire scores obtained while a person is depressed are not a true reflection of their premorbid personality. The postnatal assessment of a woman's personality when she is depressed will suggest that she has a dysfunctional personality whereas, when she is well, no such dysfunction is evident.

Neuroticism

Neuroticism is one of the most widely studied personality traits. The concept of neuroticism refers to a tendency to decompensate under stress. Persons with high trait neuroticism are easily aroused and tend to overreact to stresses. Pitt (1968) was the first to report high levels of neuroticism among postnatally depressed women. However, in that study, neuroticism was measured when the women were depressed, so the high scores could have been the result of their depressed state. High levels of neuroticism were found to predict depression by Watson *et al* (1984), and to some extent by Boyce *et al* (1990) but not by Kumar & Robson (1984). While research evidence regarding the role of neuroticism as a risk factor is equivocal there is ample clinical support for the fact that women with high levels of neuroticism do appear to be at risk for developing postnatal depression.

Karen M was a 28-year-old married school teacher who first sought treatment for depression prior to the birth of her first child. She had become depressed following a series of life events; she had to have a termination of pregnancy because of hyperemesis gravidarum, her mother had been sick and she was experiencing considerable work stress. Karen was always anxious and had a lifelong history of not coping well with life stresses. She worried about everything and was hypochondriacal. She was fussy and perfectionistic – which contributed to her finding difficulties in teaching.

Karen fell pregnant just as she recovered from her depression. Her hypochondriasis became a major problem during the pregnancy as she agonised over every symptom and movement of the foetus, and demanded constant reassurance.

She delivered a healthy baby and initially appeared to cope well. However, at about two months postpartum Karen became increasingly depressed. She was anxious, worrying about everything, overly concerned about how the baby was and constantly demanded reassurance from her husband and others. Her husband was extremely supportive of her, providing considerable instrumental and emotional support. It was clear that her high neuroticism was a major factor contributing to her postnatal depression.

Cognitive style

When people are depressed they tend to see themselves, the world and the future in a negative way, such that they feel hopeless and helpless (Kovacs & Beck, 1978). A woman with postnatal depression sees herself as deficient, inadequate and worthless. According to Beck's model (Beck *et al*, 1979) she will tend to distort the way she views the world, a result of faulty information processing. Beck *et al* (1979) have described a number of such distortions: selective abstraction, arbitrary inference, overgeneralisation, magnification and all-or-nothing thinking. These distortions in thinking mean that events are interpreted in a negative way, in spite of evidence to the contrary. In particular, cognitive distortions will relate to a woman's competence and ability to cope as a mother. For example, in selective abstraction a single negative event such as the baby crying may be focused on by the depressed mother exclusively, while positive events such as the baby being contented at other times are ignored.

The most important component of Beck's model with reference to vulnerability to postnatal depression is what he described as a schema. A schema is an individual's assumption about the world, determined by early life experiences. Thus, when an individual appraises a situation, his or her perception of the situation is determined by the schema. Beck (1964) proposed that schemas are "relatively stable cognitive structures which channel thought processes, irrespective of whether or not these are stimulated by the immediate environmental situation". Beck has proposed that the schema is a latent structure which comes into play under adverse circumstances. In this model, women prone to developing postnatal depression have a dysfunctional schema. A problem with the concept of the schema is its 'latent' quality. It is presumed to be part of an aspect of the personality, but, because it is latent it cannot, by definition, be readily identified. This has contributed to methodological problems in identifying women at risk prior to their onset of depression.

A second cognitive model looks at the way depressed people explain events. Abrahamson *et al* (1978) suggested that depressed people explain negative events as being caused by themselves, applicable to all situations and stable over time. Specifically they proposed that attributions for negative events are internal, global and stable. A woman with postnatal depression will interpret negative events, such as the baby not sleeping, as arising because of her failure as a mother (an internal attribution) and not because the baby is teething. She may go on to believe that she is a failure in all things (a global attribution) and that she will never succeed (a stable attribution).

A number of studies have been conducted to determine whether a dysfunctional cognitive style predicts postnatal depression. Dysfunctional attitudes, measured using the Dysfunctional Attitudes Scale (Weissman, 1980), were found by O'Hara *et al* (1982) to predict depressive symptoms postnatally. However, it was likely that these findings were the result of prepartum depressive symptoms. Dysfunctional attitudes did not predict postnatal depression in the study by Gotlib *et al* (1991). A dysfunctional attributional style predicted postnatal depression in two studies (O'Hara *et al*, 1982; Cutrona, 1983) but failed to do so in other studies (O'Hara *et al*, 1984; Whiffen, 1988). Other studies have focused on the extent to which individuals regard behaviour as under their control, another aspect of cognitive style. Women with an external locus of control or those who believe events to be out of their control have been found to be at risk of developing depression in two studies (Hayworth *et al*, 1980; O'Hara *et al*, 1984) but, in another (O'Hara *et al*, 1982), self-control was associated with prepartum and not postnatal depression.

While the research findings are equivocal, we often see women with a dysfunctional cognitive style who are suffering from postnatal depression.

Mary D was referred for treatment of postnatal depression when her infant was nine months old. She had been depressed for about six months. She felt worthless and considered herself to be a bad mother, despite the evidence that she cared well for her daughter. She was overly critical of herself, and if things weren't going well blamed herself. She also had sleep and appetite disturbance, and a lack of interest and enjoyment in activities.

Prominent among her depressive symptoms was the way she construed the world. If she had not achieved anything perfectly or if her baby was crying Mary would explain this as resulting from her being a bad mother. If her husband was annoyed, she would believe it was because of her, not that he had had a bad time at work. She lacked motivation to change things because she felt that if she did she would fail in her task.

In reviewing her history it became clear that Mary had a life-long pattern of thinking negatively. Her self-esteem had always been low and she had always been self-critical. If she did not succeed in a task she believed it was because of her worthlessness. Any success she achieved was 'luck'. It transpired, during the course of treatment, that as a child she had been sexually abused, a major contributor to her low self-esteem. Mary explained the sexual abuse as evidence that she was 'bad' and that she had deserved it. She had been married previously and, during the relationship, her husband had abused her when drunk. This was also explained as being her 'fault', a characteristic of her personality style.

Obsessionality

An obsessional or perfectionistic personality style has often been reported to be associated with depression. This association is most frequently seen among persons with endogenous depression or manic–depressive illness (Abraham, 1911; Klein & Depue, 1985; Kendell & DiScipio, 1970). Obsessional women could easily become overwhelmed when having to cope with the demands of a dependent baby. Babies tend not to keep to routines and are inclined to be messy. Such behaviours will be stressful for the houseproud, orderly, obsessional woman. As her routine becomes disrupted she may become depressed. While a number of women with such a personality style do become depressed it is not always the case. An association between an obsessional personality style and puerperal psychosis has been noted (Hemphil, 1952; Pitt, 1982). There have been no studies addressing the question of an association between obsessionality and postnatal depression.

Interpersonal sensitivity

Overly sensitive women are also likely to become depressed postpartum with the emotional and physical demands of having to care for their infant. Boyce *et al* (1990) found that high interpersonal sensitivity, measured antenatally, increased a woman's risk of becoming depressed at six months, but not three months postpartum. Interpersonal sensitivity is an umbrella term that covers a constellation of traits concerned with a person's sensitivity to the behaviour and feelings of others (Boyce & Parker, 1989). The Interpersonal Sensitivity Measure (IPSM), an instrument developed to measure this trait, consists of five subscales defining the underlying traits of interpersonal sensitivity (Boyce & Parker, 1989). These traits are 'interpersonal awareness', 'need for approval', 'separation anxiety', 'timidity' and 'fragile inner self'. Women who scored high on the 'interpersonal awareness' and 'timidity' subscales of the IPSM were at risk of developing postnatal depression. Those who scored more than one standard deviation above the mean on the whole scale were ten times more likely to be depressed six months postpartum than the remaining women. Interpersonal awareness refers to sensitivity to interpersonal interactions, particularly to the way an individual appraises interpersonal interactions. Women high on this trait were overly sensitive to interpersonal events, including those that might be expected to accompany the life changes and role transitions following parenthood. Timidity refers to a more behavioural aspect of interpersonal sensitivity, particularly the inability to assert oneself. Women high on this trait would have difficulty coping with the increased demands placed upon them in their mothering role, when they might find the demands of the baby, their spouse and their own needs difficult to reconcile. As they are unable to assert themselves, they receive little positive reinforcement from the environment, which contributes to their becoming depressed.

Alison H was referred for treatment of postnatal depression when she was five months postpartum. She had a lifelong pattern of being overly sensitive. As a child she was shy, but craved for affection and would do what she could to please her parents in order to gain their approval. She would become mortified if she was criticised. She still recalled, with a sense of humiliation, being told off while at primary school by her teacher for spilling some paint on her desk while doing some painting. As an adult, Alison worried about what other people thought about her, and was constantly vigilant in case they might be critical. She was unable to assert herself, preferring to do what others demanded. She would become upset if her intimates were unhappy or angry.

She had difficulty coping with her baby. She constantly worried about him, and was overly anxious to ensure that he was happy. She would become devastated when he cried and she was unable to settle him. She was unable to ask her husband's assistance with the baby. For example, Alison could not ask him to get up at night to the baby as she felt he needed his sleep so he would be able to function at work.

Personality dysfunction as a consequence of postnatal depression

Postnatal depression may affect a woman's personality in two ways. First, when people are depressed their personality changes, such that they appear to be dysfunctional (Boyce *et al*, 1990). Women with postnatal depression may appear to have a dysfunctional personality style when, in fact, their personality functioning is the result of their depression. Most notably they appear overly dependent, as shown by their need for reassurance and their lack of confidence.

Sue N, a 28-year-old woman, was referred for treatment of postnatal depression after the birth of her first child. She and her husband had been running a newsagency business prior to the birth of the child. The pregnancy was planned and they both anticipated with pleasure the birth of their child. Sue took great care of herself while pregnant; she avoided being around people who smoked, consumed no alcohol and was careful about her diet to ensure a healthy baby was born. Towards the latter stage of the pregnancy her father became ill and required chemotherapy, although he denied to her that he was suffering from cancer. Her sister-in-law had a miscarriage, something which upset Sue.

The labour and delivery were normal; however, the baby was born with a cleft palate and hare lip. Sue found that nursing the baby was very difficult because of his disability, which stressed her considerably. Her husband had to work long hours to maintain their family business, leaving home at 4.00 a.m. and returning late at night. Sue's father was unable to provide the support he would normally provide because of his declining health. In these circumstances Sue became profoundly depressed.

During her depression, her personality was that of an anxious worrier, lacking resilience and overly dependent. However, in reviewing her history carefully, it became clear that Sue's personality was functional and adaptive before she had the baby. She had shown that she could cope with stressors and, although she was sensitive to other people's needs, this previously had not caused her undue distress. She had a close and very supportive relationship with her family and was very distressed by her father's illness.

When Sue recovered from her depression she demonstrated that her resilience had returned. She coped well with stressors, particularly after her father died of cancer. She organised the funeral and was able to look after and support her mother. She was also able to plan effectively to deal with the major surgery involved with her son's hare lip and cleft palate. It was clear that the depression in this case contributed to dysfunction in her personality.

Secondly, postnatal depression may affect personality because some symptoms of postnatal depression overlap with the area of personality functioning. Postnatally depressed women are often irritable and, as noted earlier, will have a negative cognitive style. These symptoms could easily be considered to be aspects of the woman's habitual personality style yet may often be the result of the postnatal depression. Similarly, there is the appearance of being overly sensitive, tearful and overly concerned about separations. These personality attributes arise as a consequence of the depression and are not necessarily antecedents to the depression. Similarly, the cognitive dysfunction noted among many women with postnatal depression, particularly the negative view of themselves, of themselves as mothers and of the future, will be due to the depression.

Postnatal depression, if untreated, tends to be a chronic condition (Nott *et al*, 1987). It is likely that experiencing such a chronic depression will have an effect on subsequent personality functioning. A woman may have a marked loss of self-esteem and develop a pervasive sense of hopelessness and helplessness. The depression will contribute to her withdrawing from her social network, so that she will become more isolated and have increasing difficulty in dealing with others.

Marital dysfunction and postnatal depression

Childbirth is clearly an important event in a relationship (*de facto* or marital), marking a major life-cycle transition. This relationship will change over this transitional phase, requiring adaptation by both partners (Hopkins *et al*, 1984). For some couples the associated stresses may lead to a decline in the quality of their relationship (Miller & Sollie, 1980; Belsky *et al*, 1985). Adaptation to the new baby can be particularly difficult for the male partner during the first few months postpartum as the new mother may only wish to be involved with the baby. In the early postpartum weeks she may focus all of her attention and affection on the new baby. Winnicott (1956) labelled this state 'primary maternal preoccupation'. He considered that this state was

TABLE 6.2
Studies of marital interaction and postnatal depression

Authors	Sample size	Marital measure	Relevant findings
Tod, 1964	322	Interview*	Depressed women more likely to report 'abnormal marital conditions'
Nilsson & Amgren, 1970	165	Interview	Women reporting an unsatisfactory relationship had more symptoms
Uddenberg, 1974	112	Semi-structured interview	Quality of relationship antenatally did not predict postpartum symptoms. Symptomatic postpartum women reported a poor relationship
Martin, 1977	401	Interview*	Postnatally depressed women reported an unhappy relationship
Braverman & Roux, 1978	120	Questionnaire (2-item)	Postnatal depression predicted by marital problems and feeling unloved
Paykel et al, 1980	120	Interview*	Poor communication with husband. Inadequate instrumental support
Cox et al, 1982	105	Interview – any change in marital relationship	Deterioration in marital relationship
O'Hara et al, 1983	30	1. Semi-structured interview to assess marital happiness (7-point scale) 2. Postnatal interview of stressful circumstances and assessment of emotional and instrumental support	No differences on the prenatal assessment of marital satisfaction. Depressed women reported less marital satisfaction, lower instrumental and emotional support than non-depressed women at the postnatal assessment
Watson et al, 1984	128	Interview with husband and wife	Association between postnatal depression and marital dissatisfaction
Kumar & Robson, 1984	119	Semi-structured interview	Postnatally depressed women reported more marital conflict. A history of emotional instability in spouses related to postnatal depression
O'Hara, 1986	99	Social support interview DYAS	Depressed women reported deficient instrumental and emotional support and less marital satisfaction
Whiffen, 1988	115	MAT	Low marital satisfaction predicted depressive symptoms postnatally

(Continued)

TABLE 6.2 *(Continued)*

Authors	Sample size	Marital measure	Relevant findings
Robinson *et al*, 1989	89	SIS	Women with high symptom scores reported low intimacy and less marital satisfaction
O'Hara *et al*, 1990	182 (189 controls)	DYAS Marital adjustment scale of SAS–SR	Childbearing women reported greater marital satisfaction during pregnancy than controls Childbearing women showed a decline in marital adjustment postpartum Depressed childbearing women reported marital maladjustment
Boyce *et al*, 1991	150	IBM	Postnatal depression predicted by spouses perceived as being uncaring and overcontrolling
Gotlib *et al*, 1991	730	DYAS	Depressed women reported lower marital satisfaction antenatally

*Marital relationship was rated postpartum
DYAS: Dyadic Adjustment Scale (Spanier, 1976)
IBM: Intimate Bond Measure (Wilhelm & Parker, 1988)
MAT: Marital Adjustment Test (Locke & Wallace, 1959)
SAS–SR: Social Adjustment Scale–Self-Report (Weissman & Boswell, 1976)
SIS: Social Intimacy Scale (Miller & Lefcourt, 1982)

required for a mother to enable her "to adapt delicately and sensitively to the infant's need at the very beginning". While she is 'preoccupied' with the baby her partner may feel excluded. This may contribute to marital difficulty, especially if the relationship was not secure beforehand. Not only may the partner feel excluded, but he still needs to provide support to the mother over this critical time. In order to make the task of mothering easier, and more rewarding, a woman will benefit from being in a secure, intimate and caring relationship. She will also benefit from having both practical help and emotional support. She will look principally, but not exclusively, to her husband for this support, and if it is deficient this may contribute to her becoming depressed. In summary, for a successful transition, the relationship will need to maintain intimacy with a sense of collaboration between the parental dyad in caring for the new baby.

Marital dissatisfaction

It is hardly surprising that new mothers who have to cope with the additional stress of a dysfunctional relationship often experience postnatal depression. A number of studies have reported that marital dysfunction, present prior to the birth of the baby, predicts postnatal depression (Table 6.2). Women suffering from postnatal depression are more likely than their non-depressed counterparts to have described their marriage antenatally as being characterised by marital conflict or problems (Kumar & Robson, 1984) or general dissatisfaction (Watson *et al*, 1984; O'Hara, 1986; Whiffen, 1988; O'Hara *et al*, 1990; Gotlib *et al*, 1991). Postnatally depressed women are more likely to report that their relationship lacks intimacy (Robson *et al*, 1989), or that their partners are perceived as uncaring or overcontrolling (Boyce *et al*, 1991) or that they feel unloved (Braverman & Roux, 1978).

> Annette T, a 26-year-old professional woman, became depressed six weeks postpartum. Annette's marriage had been difficult prior to her falling pregnant. She and her husband would argue over trivial matters, and had difficulties with intimacy, yet they both felt committed to the relationship. Annette thought that having a child would improve their relationship.
> Initially everything went well postpartum, but as time went on she began to resent the amount of time her husband had to put in at work, even though he did help with looking after the baby when he was at home. When he was at home he felt tired from work and helping with household matters and disgruntled by his wife's resentment. As a consequence, he withdrew affection from Annette so that she felt rejected and became depressed.

Instrumental support

Instrumental support refers to the necessary practical support new mothers require. It includes such things as helping with household chores, changing nappies, bathing the baby, nursing the baby, getting up at night, and taking care of the baby during the day so that the mother can have some 'time out'. Postnatally depressed women report a deficiency in the amount of instrumental support they receive (Paykel *et al*, 1980; O'Hara *et al*, 1983; O'Hara, 1986).

Jane C, a 24-year-old weight loss counsellor, became depressed and anxious when her first daughter was 10 weeks old. Although she had planned to return to work Jane only managed to work for one day as she became disabled by overwhelming depression and anxiety. She had been apprehensive about getting back to her paid job and was particularly worried about how she would manage the schedule working and looking after her daughter.

Jane had been married for two years and the pregnancy was planned. Initially, she reported that her relationship with her husband was good; however, on closer review it appeared there were some problems. He worked long hours as a salesman. Outside of his work his major interest was playing football. He trained two evenings a week and had a match every weekend. He also spent considerable time with his 'mates' at the football club. When at home he protested that he was exhausted and was unable to help with household chores and he had little contact with the baby. He did not help with the baby – he had not changed a nappy, bathed her, or got up at night to her when she was crying. Jane didn't feel she could ask him to do more around the house because he was so tired from his work.

Emotional support

Emotional support refers to the extent to which the woman's partner listens to her, discusses with her the events of the day and acknowledges the importance of her role in looking after the baby. He needs to be sensitive to her needs and not overly demanding of her attention. He will also need to be sympathetic to her reduced libido (Alder & Bancroft, 1988; Robson & Kumar, 1981) and not construe it as a rejection, or be excessively demanding. Emotional support embraces the concept of a confiding relationship as described by Brown & Harris (1978). A supportive relationship at this time is particularly important as the new mother may be housebound and overwhelmed by the demands of the baby. Furthermore, she may have difficulty obtaining support from other network members or may even have had to find a new social network. Women with postnatal depression have reported low emotional support (Paykel *et al*, 1980; O'Hara *et al*, 1983; O'Hara, 1983), a lack of intimacy in the relationship (Gotlib *et al*, 1991) and perceiving their partner as being uncaring (Boyce *et al*, 1991).

Denise N and her husband both worked as veterinary surgeons until Denise fell pregnant. The pregnancy had been planned and they both looked forward to having a child. Denise planned to stop working for three years to look after the baby. The labour and delivery were normal and the first few weeks postpartum went well. Denise became increasingly depressed over the next few months, her self-esteem fell and she experienced difficulty coping with the baby. Her husband helped around the house, yet didn't appreciate what she was experiencing. She felt unable to talk to him about her activities during the day and, when she did, he appeared bored. He would however delight in telling her what an interesting day he had had. After he returned from work, he would say to his wife, "What useful things have you done today?" She felt devastated by this lack of emotional support from him and became increasingly depressed.

Marital dysfunction as a result of postnatal depression

Marital satisfaction generally tends to decrease over the postpartum period (Miller & Sollie, 1980; Belsky *et al*, 1985), which may contribute to the relationship deteriorating further for postnatally depressed women. This may be particularly so if the husband has his own psychological problems (Kumar & Robson, 1984) and is jealous of the attention given to the baby. Symptoms of postnatal depression such as irritability, fatigue, loss of interest and withdrawing from social contact, may also contribute to increased marital dissatisfaction. Cox *et al* (1982) and O'Hara *et al* (1990) found a deterioration in the marital relationship of postnatally depressed women. O'Hara *et al* suggested that this may be because the necessary marital adjustment following childbirth may be too difficult for depressed women to cope with. In an earlier study, O'Hara *et al* (1983) found that prenatal assessment of marital satisfaction did not discriminate between women who did or did not become depressed postnatally. However, at the postpartum assessment the postnatally depressed women reported less marital satisfaction than the non-depressed women, supporting the view that the depression contributed to marital discord. Other studies of postnatally depressed women have reported similar results to the prospective studies, with the postnatally depressed women reporting more marital discord than their non-depressed counterparts (Martin, 1977) or that their spouses did not provide sufficient emotional or instrumental support (Paykel *et al*, 1980). While there has not been a larger number of studies examining whether postnatal depression actually causes marital problems, it would be hard to imagine that such an illness would not put a strain on even the best marital relationship. Clinically, we frequently see marital relationships becoming dysfunctional as a result of postnatal depression.

> Karen D became depressed when her baby was about six weeks old. Prominent among her symptoms was fatigue. She lacked confidence, had poor concentration, felt miserable and irritable. In spite of being fatigued she had difficulty sleeping, and was continually worrying about the baby.
>   Her husband found it difficult to understand what Karen was experiencing. He would return home after long hours at work to find nothing had been done around the house and his wife had spent the day watching TV. He was

critical of her for not looking after the house properly. She became increasingly irritable in response to his criticism, which led to increasing disharmony. It appeared as if the disharmony was the cause of her depression, but they both reported that the relationship had been good antenatally. Upon remission of her depression their marital satisfaction improved and the relationship resumed functioning well.

Treatment implications

In this chapter two risk factors to postnatal depression have been described. In the general psychiatric literature, both marital and personality dysfunction have been reported to contribute to chronicity, or poor response to treatment. For example, Weissman *et al* (1978), Hirschfeld *et al* (1986) and Boyce *et al* (1992) have all shown that people with dysfunctional personality style such as high neuroticism, being 'thin skinned' or overly sensitive, have a poorer prognosis than people who have a healthy personality. Similarly, the outcome of a depressive episode is worse if the depressed subject is in a dysfunctional relationship (Rounsaville *et al*, 1979; Hooley *et al*, 1986; Hickie & Parker, 1992). Clearly, women suffering from postnatal depression caused by, or contributing to, these risk factors will require therapy aimed at ameliorating them.

The assessment of a woman with postnatal depression should include an assessment of the marital relationship and personality functioning. Assessment of the marriage will involve a thorough review of the quality of the marital relationship, with particular emphasis on how much support her partner is providing for her. Instrumental support may be assessed by asking whether her spouse helps her look after the baby and with household chores. Specifically, she can be asked whether he changes the nappies, feeds or baths the baby or gets up at night to settle the baby. She can also be asked whether he helps with cooking or housework. Emotional support can be assessed by asking whether he is prepared to pay attention to her, listen to her needs and appear accepting of them. The amount of intimacy, care, and affection between the couple should also be assessed. Ideally, the woman's partner should also be interviewed so that his perceptions about the relationship can be explored.

Personality can be assessed by asking the woman what type of person she considers herself to be. Specifically she can be asked if she was always a worrier and how she had coped in the past with stressful events. Her cognitive style can be assessed by asking her if she has a tendency to view things in a pessimistic and negative way. She can also be asked about how she understands negative events: are they generally her fault or are there other explanations? The extent to which she perceives her life to be under her control can also be assessed. The woman's ability to assert herself and her sensitivity to other people should be explored.

If marital difficulties are identified, it will be necessary to clarify the specific problems and whether they contributed to, or were a consequence of, the postnatal depression. Involving the spouse at this stage is important as he may be unaware of the specific problems, or, in many cases, unaware that she is suffering from postnatal depression. I have found that many partners do not appreciate either how demanding it is to look after a child, or that they need to be actively involved. In such instances, educating the husband about postnatal depression and the role he should take in providing support may lead to an improvement in both the relationship and the depression. If the marital problem is the consequence of postnatal depression both partners will require support and reassurance that the relationship will improve when the depression lifts. Should marital problems still persist after this educational approach then more intensive marital therapy is indicated.

If the woman is found to have a dysfunctional personality style, supportive therapy aimed at bolstering her coping style and problem solving will be helpful. More specific treatment aimed at overcoming particular personality dysfunction can also be implemented. For example, cognitive behavioural therapy can be used to modify her cognitive style, and assertiveness training can be used to help her cope better with interpersonal relationships. If personality problems are more deep seated then a course of psychotherapy may be indicated.

Summary and conclusions

In this chapter I have reviewed the role of personality dysfunction and marital problems as risk factors to postnatal depression. A number of vulnerable personality styles, such as having high levels of neuroticism, a negative cognitive set or being overly sensitive have been discussed. Marital problems, specifically being in a relationship characterised by insufficient support or lacking in intimacy, put women at risk of developing postnatal depression. Postnatal depression may contribute to marital difficulties and lead one to consider that a postnatally depressed woman has a dysfunctional personality. The amelioration of these risk factors therefore needs to be addressed as part of the treatment of women suffering from postnatal depression.

References

ABRAHAM, K. (1911) Notes on the psychoanalytical investigation and treatment of manic-depressive insanity and allied conditions. In *Selected Papers on Psychoanalysis* (ed. K. Abraham), pp. 137–147. London: Hogarth Press.
ABRAHAMSON, L. Y., SELIGMAN, M. E. P. & TEASDALE, J. D. (1978) Learned helplessness in humans: critique and reformulation. *Journal of Abnormal Psychology*, **87**, 49–74.

ALDER, E. & BANCROFT, J. (1988) The relationship between breast feeding persistence, sexuality and mood in postpartum women. *Psychological Medicine*, **18**, 389–396.

BARNETT, B. & PARKER, G. (1986) Possible determinants, correlates and consequences of high levels of anxiety in primiparous mothers. *Psychological Medicine*, **16**, 1–9.

BECK, A. T. (1964) Thinking and depression: 2 theory and therapy. *Archives of General Psychiatry*, **10**, 561–571.

——, RUSH, A. J., SHAW, B. F., *et al* (1979) *Cognitive Therapy for Depression*. New York: Guilford.

——, EPSTEIN, N., HARRISON, R. P., *et al* (1983) Development of the sociotropy–autonomy scale: a measure of personality factors in psychopathology. Unpublished manuscript, University of Pennsylvania.

BELSKY, J., LANG, E. & ROVINE, M. (1985) Stability and change in marriage across the transition to parenthood: a second study. *Journal of Marriage and the Family*, 855–865.

BIRTCHNELL, J. (1984) Dependence and its relationship to depression. *British Journal of Medical Psychology*, **57**, 215–225.

BOYCE, P. & PARKER, G. (1989) Development of a scale to measure interpersonal sensitivity. *Australian and New Zealand Journal of Psychiatry*, **23**, 341–351.

——, HADZI-PAVLOVIC, D., PARKER, G., *et al* (1990) Depressive type and state effects on personality measures. *Acta Psychiatrica Scandinavica*, **81**, 197–200.

——, HICKIE, I. & PARKER, G. (1991*a*) Parents, partners or personality? risk factors for post-natal depression. *Journal of Affective Disorders*, **24**, 245–255.

——, PARKER. G., BARNETT, B., *et al* (1991*b*) Personality as a vulnerability factor to depression. *British Journal of Psychiatry*, **159**, 106–114.

——, ——, ——, *et al* (1992) Interpersonal sensitivity and the one-year outcome of a depressive episode. *Australian and New Zealand Journal of Psychiatry*, **26**, 156–161.

—— & MASON, C. (1994) An overview of depression-prone personality traits and the role of interpersonal sensitivity. *Australian and New Zealand Journal of Psychiatry* (in press).

BRAVERMAN, J. & ROUX, J. F. (1978) Screening for the patient at risk for postpartum depression. *Obstetrics and Gynecology*, **52**, 731–736.

BROCKINGTON, I. F., CERNIK, K. F., SCHOFIELD, E. M., *et al* (1981) Puerperal psychosis: phenomena and diagnosis. *Archives of General Psychiatry*, **38**, 929–933.

——, MARTIN, C., BROWN, G. W., *et al* (1990) Stress and puerperal psychosis. *British Journal of Psychiatry*, **157**, 331–334.

BROWN, G. W. & HARRIS, T. (1978) *Social Origins of Depression: a Study of Psychiatric Disorders in Women*. London: Tavistock.

——, ANDREWS, B., BIFULCO, A., *et al* (1990*a*) Self-esteem and depression. *Social Psychiatry and Psychiatric Epidemiology*, **25**, 200–209.

——, BIFULCO, A. & ANDREWS, B. (1990*b*) Self-esteem and depression. *Social Psychiatry*, **25**, 235–243.

CAMPBELL, J. (1992) Maternity blues: a model for biological research. In *Postpartum Psychiatric Illness: A Picture Puzzle* (eds J. A. Hamilton & P. N. Harberger). Philadelphia: University of Pennsylvania Press.

CAINE, T. M. (1970) Personality and illness. In *The Psychological Assessment of Mental and Physical Handicap* (ed. P. Mittler), pp. 781–817. London: Methuen.

——, FOULDS, G. A. & HOPE, K. (1967) *Manual of the Hostility and Direction of Hostility Questionnaire (HDHQ)*. London: University of London Press.

CHODOFF, P. (1972) The depressive personality: a critical review. *Archives of General Psychiatry*, **27**, 666–673.

COGILL, S. R., CAPLAN, H. L., ALEXANDRA, H., *et al* (1986) Impact of maternal postnatal depression on cognitive development of young children. *British Medical Journal*, **292**, 1165–1167.

COOPER, P. J., CAMPBELL, E. A., DAY, A., *et al* (1988) Non-psychotic psychiatric disorder after childbirth: a prospective study of prevalence, incidence, course and nature. *British Journal of Psychiatry*, **152**, 799–806.

COPPEN, A. & METCALF, M. (1965) Effect of a depressive illness on M.P.I. scores. *British Journal of Psychiatry*, **111**, 236–239.

Cox, J. L. (1986) *Postnatal Depression. A Guide for Health Professionals.* Edinburgh: Churchill Livingstone.

—— (1989) Depression in the puerperium: a conceptual controversy. In *Depression: An Integrative Approach* (eds K. Herbst & E. Paykel), pp. 125–139. Oxford: Heinemann Medical Books.

——, Connor, Y. & Kendell, R. E. (1982) Prospective study of the psychiatric disorders of childbirth. *British Journal of Psychiatry*, **140**, 111–117.

Cutrona, C. E. (1983) Causal attributions and perinatal depression. *Journal of Abnormal Psychology*, **92**, 161–172.

Eysenck, H. J. (1959) *Manual of the M.P.I.* London: London University Press.

—— & Eysenck, S. G. B. (1975) *Manual of the Eysenck Personality Questionnaire.* London: Hodder and Stoughton.

Folkman, S. & Lazarus, R. S. (1985) If it changes it must be a process: a study of emotion and coping during three stages of a college examination. *Journal of Personality and Social Psychology*, **48**, 150–170.

Gotlib, I. H., Mount, J. H., Cordy, N. I., *et al* (1988) Depression and perceptions of early parenting: a longitudinal investigation. *British Journal of Psychiatry*, **152**, 24–27.

——, Whiffen, V. E., Mount, J. H., *et al* (1989) Prevalence rates and demographic characteristics associated with depression in pregnancy and the postpartum. *Journal of Consulting and Clinical Psychology*, **57**, 269–274.

——, ——, Wallace, P. M., *et al* (1991) Prospective investigation of postpartum depression: factors involved in onset and recovery. *Journal of Abnormal Psychology*, **100**, 122–132.

Harris, B., Othman, S., Davies, J. A., *et al* (1992) Association between postpartum thyroid dysfunction and thyroid antibodies and depression. *British Medical Journal*, **305**, 152–156.

Hayworth, J., Little, B. C., Carter, S. B., *et al* (1980) A predictive study of post-partum depression: some predisposing characteristics. *British Journal of Medical Psychology*, **53**, 161–167.

Hemphil, R. E. (1952) The incidence and nature of puerperal mental illness. *British Medical Journal*, ii, 1232.

Hickie, I. & Parker, G. (1992) The impact of an uncaring partner on the course of non-melancholic depression. *Journal of Affective Disorders*, **25**, 147–160.

Hirschfeld, R. M. A., Klerman, G. L., Korchin, S., *et al* (1976) Dependency–self-esteem—clinical depression. *Journal of the American Academy of Psychoanalysis*, **4**, 373–388.

——, Clayton, P. J., *et al* (1983) Assessing personality: effects of the depressive state on trait measurement. *American Journal of Psychiatry*, **140**, 695–699.

——, ——, Andreasen, N. C., *et al* (1986) Psycho-social predictors of chronicity in depressed patients. *British Journal of Psychiatry*, **148**, 648–654.

——, ——, Lavori, P., *et al* (1989) Premorbid personality assessments of first onset major depression. *Archives of General Psychiatry*, **46**, 345–350.

Hooley, J. M., Orley, J. & Teasedale, J. D. (1986) Levels of expressed emotion and relapse in depressed patients. *British Journal of Psychiatry*, **148**, 642–647.

Hopkins, J., Marcus, M. & Campbell, S. B. (1984) Postpartum depression: a critical review. *Psychological Bulletin*, **95**, 498–515.

Jansson, B. (1964) Psychic insufficiencies associated with childbirth. *Acta Psychiatrica Scandinavica* (suppl. 172).

Kendell, R. E. (1985) Emotional and physical factors in the genesis of puerperal mental disorders. *Journal of Psychosomatic Research*, **29**, 3–11.

—— & DiScipio, W. J. (1968) Eysenck Personality Inventory scores of patients with depressive illness. *British Journal of Psychiatry*, **114**, 767–770.

—— & —— (1970) Obsessional symptoms and obsessional personality traits in patients with depressive illnesses. *Psychological Medicine*, **1**, 65–72.

——, Chalmers, J. C. & Platz, C. (1987) Epidemiology of puerperal psychoses. *British Journal of Psychiatry*, **150**, 662–673.

Kennerley, H. & Gath, D. (1986) Maternity blues reassessed. *Psychiatry Developments*, **1**, 1–17.

Klein, D. N. & Depue, R. A. (1985) Obsessional personality traits and risk for bipolar affective disorder: an offspring study. *Journal of Abnormal Psychology*, **94**, 291–297.

KOVACS, M. & BECK, A. T. (1978) Maladaptive cognitive structures in depression. *American Journal of Psychiatry*, **135**, 525–533.

KUMAR, R. (1982) Neurotic disorders in childbearing women. In *Motherhood and Mental Illness* (eds I. F. Brockington & R. Kumar), pp. 71–118. London: Academic Press.

—— & ROBSON, K. M. (1984) A prospective study of emotional disorders in childbearing women. *British Journal of Psychiatry*, **144**, 35–47.

LOCKE, H. J. & WALLACE, K. M. (1959) Short marital adjustment and predictions tests: their reliability and validity. *Journal of Marriage and Family Living*, **21**, 251–255.

MANLY, P. C., MCMAHON, R. J., BRADLEY, C. F., DAVIDSON, P. O. (1982) Depressive attributional style and depression following childbirth. *Journal of Abnormal Psychology*, **91**, 245–254.

MARKS, M. N., WIECK, A., CHECKLEY, S. A., et al (1991) Life stress and post-partum psychosis: a preliminary report. *British Journal of Psychiatry*, **158**, 45–49.

——, ——, SEYMOUR, A., et al (1992) Women whose mental illness recur after childbirth and partners' levels of expressed emotion during late pregnancy. *British Journal of Psychiatry*, **161**, 211–216.

MARTIN, C. J., BROWN, G. W., GOLDBERG, D. P., et al (1989) Psycho-social stress and puerperal depression. *Journal of Affective Disorders*, **16**, 283–293.

MARTIN, M. (1977) A maternity hospital study of psychiatric illness associated with childbirth. *Irish Journal of Medical Science*, **146**, 239–244.

MEARES, R., GRIMWADE, J. & WOOD, C. (1976) A possible relationship between anxiety in pregnancy and puerperal depression. *Journal of Psychosomatic Research*, **20**, 605–610.

MILLER, B. C. & SOLLIE, D. L. (1980) Normal stresses during the transition to parenthood. *Family Relationships*, 459–465.

—— & LEFCOURT, H. M. (1982) The assessment of social intimacy. *Journal of Personality Assessment*, **28**, 79–82.

MURRAY, R. M. & STEIN, A. (1989) The effects of postnatal depression on the infant. *Baillière's Clinical Obstetrics and Gynaecology*, **3**, 921–933.

——, COOPER, P. J. & STEIN, A. (1991) Postnatal depression and infant development. *British Medical Journal*, **302**, 978–979.

NILSSON, A. & ALMGREN, P. (1970) Para-natal emotional adjustment: a prospective investigation of 165 women. Part II. The influence of background factors, psychiatric history, parental relations, and personality characteristics. *Acta Psychiatrica Scandanavica*, **220**, 62–141.

NOTT, P. N. (1987) Extent, timing and persistence of emotional disorders following childbirth. *British Journal of Psychiatry*, **151**, 523–527.

——, FRANKLIN, M., ARMITAGE, C., et al (1976) Hormonal changes and mood in the puerperium. *British Journal of Psychiatry*, **128**, 379–383.

O'HARA, M. W. (1986) Social support, life events, and depression during pregnancy and the puerperium. *Archives of General Psychiatry*, **43**, 569–573.

——, REHM, L. P. & CAMPBELL, S. B. (1982) Predicting depressive symptomatology: cognitive–behavioral models and postpartum depression. *Journal of Abnormal Psychology*, **91**, 457–461.

——, —— & —— (1983) Postpartum depression: a role for social network and life stress variables. *Journal of Nervous and Mental Disease*, **171**, 336–341.

——, NEUNABER, J. & ZEKOSKI, E. M. (1984) Prospective study of postpartum depression: prevalence, course and predictive factors. *Journal of Abnormal Psychology*, **93**, 158–171.

—— & ZEKOSKI, E. M. (1988) Postpartum depression: a comprehensive review. In *Motherhood and Mental Illness 2: Causes and Consequences* (eds R. Kumar & I. F. Brockington), pp. 17–63. London: Wright.

——, ——, PHILIPPS, et al (1990) Controlled prospective study of postpartum mood disorders: comparison of childbearing and nonchildbearing women. *Journal of Abnormal Psychology*, **99**, 3–15.

PAYKEL, E. S., EMMS, E. M., FLETCHER, J., et al. (1980) Life events and social support in puerperal depression. *British Journal of Psychiatry*, **136**, 339–346.

PETERSON, C., SEMMEL, A., VON BAYER, C., et al (1982) The attributional style questionnaire. *Cognitive Therapy and Research*, **6**, 287–300.

PITT, B. (1968) 'Atypical' depression following childbirth. *British Journal of Psychiatry*, **114**, 1325–1335.

—— (1973) Maternity blues. *British Journal of Psychiatry*, **122**, 431–433.

—— (1982) Depression and childbirth. In *Handbook of Affective Disorders* (ed. E. S. Paykel), pp. 361–378. London: Churchill Livingstone.

REHM, L., KORNBLITH, S. J., O'HARA, M. W., *et al* (1981) An evaluation of the major elements in a self-control therapy program for depression. *Behavior Modification*, **5**, 459–489.

ROBINSON, G. E., OLMSTED, M. P. & GARNER, D. M. (1989) Predictors of postpartum adjustment. *Acta Psychiatrica Scandinavica*, **80**, 561–565.

ROBSON, K. M. & KUMAR, R. (1981) Maternal sexuality during first pregnancy and after childbirth. *British Journal of Obstetrics and Gynaecology*, **88**, 882–889.

ROTTER, J. B. (1966) Generalised expectancies for internal versus external control of reinforcement. *Psychological Monographs: General and Applied*, **80**, 1–28.

ROUNSAVILLE, B. J., WEISSMAN, M. M., PRUSOFF, B., *et al* (1979) Marital disputes and treatment outcome in depressed women. *Comprehensive Psychiatry*, **20**, 483–490.

SNAITH, R. P. & TAYLOR, C. M. (1985) Irritability: definition, assessment and associated factors. *British Journal of Psychiatry*, **147**, 127–136.

SPANIER, G. B. (1976) Measuring dyadic adjustment: new scales for assessing the quality of marriage and similar dyads. *Journal of Marriage and the Family*, **38**, 15–28.

STEIN, G. (1982) The maternity blues. In *Motherhood and Mental Illness* (eds I. F. Brockington & R. Kumar), pp. 119–154. London: Academic Press.

——, GATH, D. H., BUCHER, J., *et al* (1991) The relationship between post-natal depression and mother–child interaction. *British Journal of Psychiatry*, **158**, 46–52.

TOD, E. D. M. (1964) Puerperal depression. *Lancet*, 1264–1266.

UDDENBERG, N. (1974) Reproductive adaptation in mother and daughter. A study of personality development and adaptation to motherhood. *Acta Psychiatrica Scandinavica* (suppl. 254).

WATSON, J. P., ELLIOTT, S. A., RUGG, A. J., *et al* (1984) Psychiatric disorder in pregnancy and the first postnatal year. *British Journal of Psychiatry*, **144**, 453–462.

WEISSMAN, A. W. (1980) Assessing depressogenic attitudes: a validation study. *51st Annual Meeting of the Eastern Psychological Association*, Hartford, CT.

—— & BOTHWELL, S. (1976) Assessment of social adjustment by patient self-report. *Archives of General Psychiatry*, **33**, 1111–1115.

——, PRUSOFF, B. A. & KLERMAN, G. L. (1978) Personality and the prediction of long-term outcome of depression. *American Journal of Psychiatry*, **135**, 797–800.

WHIFFEN, V. (1988) Vulnerability to postpartum depression: a prospective multivariate study. *Journal of Abnormal Psychology*, **97**, 467–474.

WIECK, A., KUMAR, R., HIRST, A. D., *et al* (1991) Increased sensitivity of dopamine receptors and recurrence of affective psychosis after childbirth. *British Medical Journal*, **303**, 613–616.

WILHELM, K. & PARKER, G. (1988) The development of a measure of intimate bonds. *Psychological Medicine*, **18**, 225–234.

WINNICOTT, D. W. (1956) Primary maternal preoccupation. In *Through Paediatrics to Psychoanalysis*, pp. 300–305. London: Hogarth Press.

7 Hormonal theories and therapy for postnatal depression

SHAUGHN O'BRIEN and BRICE PITT

Postnatal depression (PND), together with premenstrual syndrome (PMS) and menopausal disorders, are probably determined by several factors, among which hormonal change and neuroendocrine sensitivity to such change are likely to be prominent. While there is little doubt about the relationship between hypo-oestrogen status and menopausal symptoms, in both PMS and postnatal depression there is a shortage of facts to support theories of lack or excess of particular hormones: it is probably the normal hormone change of these physiological events which is important. Thus the search for aetiology should be aimed less at differences in hormonal activity than at neuroendocrine differences. Treatment might then be directed: (a) to eliminate or modulate the hormonal 'trigger'; or (b) to modulate the neuroendocrine response.

Possible hormonal mechanisms of postnatal depression

The endocrine changes following childbirth are unmatched by any other biological event in terms of rapidity and magnitude. Endocrine changes through pregnancy are, in the main, the direct or indirect consequence of placental activity. At the end of pregnancy oestrogen levels are many times those of non-pregnant women, and rapidly return to normal postpartum.

Gelder (1978) acknowledged that the precipitous fall in circulating total oestrogen and in progesterone over the first few days of the puerperium suggests that mental disturbance might result from a failure of adjustment to these changes. Endocrine differences between women who are depressed or not would be evidence for an endocrine cause, but failure to show such a difference, or even failure to respond to hormonal therapy, would not rule it out: psychosis related to disorders of thyroid or adrenal function, for example, often persists after endocrine balance has been restored.

103

Oestrogen and progesterone changes are the best known, but there are also marked changes in the components of the renin–angiotensin system, aldosterone, corticosteroids and prolactin, as well as in many other non-hormonal substances which markedly diminish from the moment that the placenta separates.

Just before delivery morning levels of free cortisol double. There are some similarities, according to Hamilton (1962), between early puerperal syndromes and cortisone-induced psychoses, with their tendency to acute onset, euphoria, insomnia, restlessness, excitement and "a major departure of thought content from reality".

Bower & Altschule (1956) advanced the theory that high levels of placental progesterone depress anterior pituitary activity, and thus the adrenal cortex, while placental ACTH directly stimulates the adrenal cortex. The loss of the latter stimulus postpartum might explain the 'blues', while the loss of progesterone might lead to a rebound anterior pituitary activity and stimulation of the adrenal cortex which, if excessive, could cause psychosis. These workers therefore gave progesterone (after other somatic treatments) to 16 of 39 postpartum psychotics: all but one had lasting remissions compared with often temporary remission in the controls. In another approach, steroid-suppressing drugs (aminoglutethimide, ketoconazole, metyrapone) were used for two months in the treatment of treatment-resistant major (not puerperal) depression in an open trial with benefit to 60% (Murphy *et al*, 1991).

Railton (1961) on the other hand regarded the postpartum drop in the level of circulating corticoids as the cause of the 'blues' and possibly of the more serious PND. She gave prednisolone 5–10 mg b.d. for 3–4 weeks postpartum to 8 depressed women and 8 with a history of PND. None of the latter relapsed, while the depressed women took an average of only two months to recover; a control group of 16 with 'postpartum psychological difficulties' treated with psychotherapy took an average of 8 months to recover.

'Blues' symptoms cluster round the third postpartum day and the frequency with which they appear has led to much speculation about hormonal causes. Some features – irritability, lability, sleep disturbance, subjective 'confusion' – are consistent with an 'organic' cause. Nott *et al* (1976) found no difference between 'blues' and 'no blues' sufferers in progesterone, oestrogen, the ratio of one to the other, LH, FSH or prolactin before and after delivery. Feksi *et al* (1984), however, found significantly higher salivary oestradiol and progesterone in 'blues' sufferers on the day when their symptoms occurred than in matched, symptom-free controls. 'Blues' subjects more often reported PMS (see also Yalom *et al*, 1968) which could indicate particular susceptibility to hormonal change, or a lower threshold for minor discomfort.

Psychoses in the puerperium usually begin between the third day postpartum and the end of the second week, but after only 1 in every

500–1000 births and in women with a family and personal psychiatric history similar to that of non-puerperal psychotic women. The occurrence of post-operative psychoses (Stengel *et al*, 1958), which have in common with puerperal psychoses a two-day latency period, early confusion, and a mixture of schizophrenic and affective symptoms at a time of readjustments in cortisol production, excretion and in binding globulins, supports the notion of a trait susceptibility to any normal hormonal change.

Blumberg & Billig (1942) suggested a disturbed progesterone balance in a woman with postpartum schizophrenia and exacerbations in the proliferative phase of menstruation and claimed that the administration of progesterone completed the recovery induced by insulin therapy.

An important breakthrough in the identification of susceptibility to affective psychosis has been the discovery that 8 out of 15 women with a history of bipolar or schizoaffective psychosis who relapsed postpartum had increased sensitivity of dopamine receptors in the hypothalamus (and possibly elsewhere in the brain) (Wieck *et al*, 1991); such changes might be triggered by the sharp fall in circulating oestrogens after delivery.

Gelder (1978) states that postnatal depression is very imprecisely defined, in terms of time of onset, duration and severity, for the purpose of hormone studies. The typical picture, though, is that of 'neurotic' depression, and tiredness; anxiety and irritability may be more prominent than depression. Pitt (1968) suggested the criteria that subjects should spontaneously admit to depression arising in or worsening since childbirth, and that this should be unusual in their experience, at least partly disabling (with unexpected difficulty in coping with the baby, housework and shopping) and of more than two weeks' duration.

Harris *et al* (1989*a*) measured salivary progesterone six to eight weeks postpartum. In bottle-feeding women the levels correlated positively, and in breast-feeding mothers negatively, with a number of indices of depression; if replicated this would suggest that both too little and too much progesterone could increase susceptibility to PND. In a prospective study of 97 primiparous Australian women (Smith *et al*, 1990), those whose mood deteriorated from 38 weeks' gestation to postnatal day 2 had larger falls in plasma beta-endorphin after delivery than those whose mood improved or stayed constant. They also had significantly higher MADRS (Montgomery–Åsberg Depression Rating Scale; Montgomery & Åsberg, 1979) depression scores at three months postpartum.

Prolonged thyroid disorder has been suggested as a cause of asthenic forms of depression. Danowski *et al* (1953) showed that pregnancy was often accompanied by raised serum protein-bound iodine (PBI), that after delivery the PBI decreased rapidly and that unduly low levels might persist for as long as a year. Hamilton and 13 co-workers (Ballachey *et al*, 1958) tried L-triiodothyronine followed after two weeks by thyroid in 12 postpartum patients, mostly suffering from depression, and reported favourable results, including a placebo-controlled double-blind cross-over trial on two subjects. Parry (1989) suggests that alterations in thyroid function may be a feature both of rapid cycling and of postpartum affective disorder in women. Dussault & Rousseau (1987) state that 'postpartum thyroiditis' (probably a special form of silent lymphocytic thyroiditis) prevails in 5–10% of pregnant women and may be responsible for a substantial proportion of cases of postpartum depression; thyroid hormone replacement therapy is recommended for persistent disease. Okano & Nomura (1989) found lower T3 levels in four women who developed major depression at one month postpartum than in 38 controls, while Harris *et al* (1989*b*) recruited 65 women seropositive for thyroid microsomal or thyroglobulin antibodies at delivery and found that at 6–8 weeks postpartum 8 showed thyroid dysfunction, of whom 3 were depressed.

Though the balance of evidence may point to social and psychological causes, the dramatic changes in endocrine status in late pregnancy and the puerperium make theories linking major placental/ovarian flux and postnatal depression very attractive. Gard *et al* (1986) found no clear relationship between levels of progesterone, oestrogen and PND developing between two weeks and nine months after delivery, so again the hypothesis of an enhanced central response to normal endocrine events seems the more likely.

Hormonal treatment and prophylaxis in postnatal depression

The most likely agents for the neuroendocrine dysfunction triggered by normal hormonal change relate to noradrenaline, dopamine, serotonin or possibly neurotransmitter precursors such as tryptophan. Despite this likely scenario there has been great enthusiasm for replacing the now 'missing' hormone. Oestrogen and progesterone have, not surprisingly, received the most attention.

It is probably true to say that obstetricians virtually never prescribe antidepressants, or for that matter psychoactive drugs in general. It is also true to say that psychiatrists rarely prescribe hormones. As PND develops some three weeks or more after delivery, the obstetrician is not usually involved, and hence treatment with antidepressants is far more likely than hormonal therapy. Prophylactic treatment, also, has rarely been instigated by the obstetrician. However, in recent years, mainly in the context of research, both oestrogen and progesterone have been evaluated in PND – mainly to prevent rather than treat the disorder.

Progesterone

Progesterone was used for postpartum psychosis over 50 years ago (Schmidt, 1943) and for postnatal depression by several other workers (Billig

& Bradley, 1942; Dalton, 1984, 1985, 1989). It is surprising that in a disorder where a high placebo effect could be expected that in none of these studies was the hormone compared to placebo.

Dalton has long been an exponent of progesterone therapy for PND, the 'blues', PMS and even during pregnancy to improve the offspring's IQ! In her first study (1985) she looked at a series of 221 women with a history of PND and found a relapse rate of 68%. She claims in a second study (1985), of 94 women, that a regime of 100 mg progesterone intramuscularly from the completion of labour daily for seven days followed by progesterone suppositories for two months or until the return of menstruation reduced the relapse rate to 10%. The subjects were highly self-selected, the study was uncontrolled and it was largely conducted by post.

The 1989 study involved 242 women who had written to her requesting progesterone prophylaxis because of previous PND. These were sent a letter asking the general practitioner to prescribe the following: 100 mg by intramuscular injection from the completion of labour daily for a week, then 400 mg suppositories twice daily for the next two months or until menstruation. Patients could increase their medication by going back to the GP.

At six months after the expected date of delivery questionnaires were sent to the subjects, their GPs and obstetricians. A control group comprised 21 women who were not treated with progesterone, who were compared with the 181 women who received progesterone according to the protocol. Severe PND occurred in 12 (7%) of the treated and 14 (67%) of the untreated women – a difference said to be significant ($P < 0.001$). There were few adverse side-effects. These optimistic results warrant further research in properly controlled trials.

Oestrogen

Postnatal oestrogen levels fall dramatically following delivery and remain low until the menstrual cycles return, or longer during the course of breast-feeding. It has been postulated that just as hypo-oestrogenism at the menopause is associated with many symptoms, including depression in some women, postnatal depression might be prevented or treated by the administration of oestrogen.

It has been suggested that oestrogen withdrawal provokes affective psychotic disorder through complex interaction with dopamine synthesis or activity (Wieck *et al*, 1991). Henderson *et al* (1991) reported preliminary data on the treatment of PND with oestrogen in a letter to the *Lancet*. A double-blind, placebo-controlled trial was used to evaluate transdermal oestrogen patches in severe non-psychotic PND. The dose was 200 μg, presumably every third day (a high dosage). Randomisation was made either to this regime or identical placebo patches. Because prolonged stimulation of the endometrium with unopposed oestrogen may give rise to endometrial hyperplasia (or even cancer), dihydrogesterone 10 mg daily was given for 12 days. Endometrial sampling with curettage showed no histological changes.

Recruitment was made on the basis of an Edinburgh Postnatal Depression Scale (EPDS) score of 14 or more, the diagnosis of a major depressive disorder was then made using Research Diagnostic Criteria (RDC) and the Schedule for Affective Disorders and Schizophrenia (SADS; Endicott & Spitzer, 1978).

Because of a high drop-out rate an interim analysis was made. Of 35 recruits, 7 of the placebo group dropped out because of social and financial reasons and 3 of the treatment group because they felt better. This left 25 subjects for analysis, 18 in the active group, 7 on placebo. The active subjects showed a significant, persistent improvement in their EPDS scores while the controls showed only minor improvement over the first three months. The oestrogen levels in the treated group – in the region of 680 pmol/l – were significantly greater than those of controls.

There are some deficiencies in this study. More precise data are needed, for example of the RDC diagnoses. No reference is made to the presence or absence of menstruation, nor of the timing of the EPDS within the menstrual cycle. Had the placebo group been measured during the premenstrual phase in women with significant PMS, a major error might have been introduced into the evaluation. Indeed, it is likely that the active group were amenorrhoeic while the controls were not. The symptoms of PMS are not unlike those of PND as recorded by the EPDS, women who suffer PND may well also suffer from PMS, and the same group (Watson *et al*, 1989) has reported that similar doses of oestradiol can treat PMS: hence the importance of taking both the menstrual cycle and PMS into account.

Antidepressant therapy

Postnatal depression cannot, of course, be diagnosed by the EPDS. The EPDS is a screening instrument, indicating women who might be suffering from PND. To make the diagnosis a clinical assessment is required, usually by the general practitioner, often involving an interview with the baby's father as well as the mother.

Most cases of PND meet DSM–III–R criteria (American Psychiatric Association, 1987) for major depression. The syndrome is very similar to that of depression occurring at other times, in either sex, except that the baby looms large both in the mother's preoccupations and in the things she has to do. Consequently, although we are unaware of controlled trials of the efficacy of antidepressant therapy in the postpartum period, there is no reason to doubt that antidepressants appropriately prescribed at this time are as effective as at any other. Part of their action at this time may be by modulating neuroendocrine sensitivity to hormonal changes. If the depression is trivial or transitory, or if the mother is much opposed to medication, the drugs should be withheld. On the other hand, if depression is moderately severe or, worse, distressing, disabling and persistent, treatment with the usual repertoire of antidepressants should be offered.

Among the tricyclics dothiepin 75–150 mg, or lofepramine 70–210 mg (less sedative than dothiepin) are suitable, while the newer serotonin-specific reuptake inhibitors (SSRIs) such as fluoxetine or paroxetine, 20 mg daily (as effective as the older drugs and sometimes better tolerated), are becoming very popular. Monoamine oxidase inhibitors (MAOIs, e.g. phenelzine, 15 mg three times daily) are useful for the 'neurotic' depression most typical in the puerperium, but because of dietary precautions are a second choice and perhaps best left to psychiatrists to prescribe. Breast feeding may be continued despite the use of these drugs because they enter breast milk only in very tiny quantities (Loudun, 1987).

The prophylactic use of antidepressants where there is a history of severe PND has, again, not been subject to a controlled trial, although the practice does make sense. Depending on the previous time of onset they could be given early in the puerperium or even in late pregnancy.

Conclusions

Progesterone has psychoactive as well as endocrine effects. In high doses it is sedative and anaesthetic. It may well account for the relative euphoria of pregnancy. Premenstrual syndrome disappears during pregnancy (though this is more likely due to the elimination of menstruation than to the psychotropic effects of progesterone). It would not be surprising if withdrawal of this euphoric effect was associated with depression. If high dose progesterone is effective against PND (which has not yet been demonstrated by a satisfactory double-blind placebo-controlled study), then it may be due to a sedative effect on the central nervous system.

If oestrogen is effective against PND, again the mechanism must be explained. Theoretical parallels can be drawn between the menopause and the relatively enormous deficiency postpartum compared with the levels to which mothers are exposed in pregnancy; so profound an 'instant menopause' might be plausibly associated with severe depression. Breast feeding, by preventing ovulation and the return of oestrogenic activity, may exaggerate the effect by prolonging the oestrogen deficient phase. This mechanism would support a role for oestrogen prophylaxis, the worth of which, however, has yet to be proved.

However, all women experience these profound postpartum changes in endocrine function, probably to much the same degree, yet only a minority suffer PND. Other differences, therefore, must be present – in psychosocial background, underlying depression, and sensitivity to endocrine changes possibly secondary to abnormalities in neurotransmitter status (these making antidepressant therapy logical).

Thus there is a place for psychological and psychiatric treatments in prophylaxis and treatment although the choice and balance between psychodynamic or cognitive interventions or psychoactive drugs is not yet clear. It does seem as if the role of hormonal therapy will remain limited. It is certainly unproven.

References

AMERICAN PSYCHIATRIC ASSOCIATION (1987) *Diagnostic and Statistical Manual of Mental Disorders* (3rd edn, revised) (DSM–III–R). Washington, DC: American Psychiatric Press.

BALLACHEY, E. L., CAMPBELL, D. G., CLAFFEY, B., et al (1958) Response of post-partum psychiatric problems to L-triiodothyronine. *Journal of Clinical and Experimental Psychopathology*, **19**, 170.

BILLIG, O. & BRADELY, J. D. (1942) Hormonal influence upon 'puerperal psychosis' and neurotic conditions. *Psychiatric Quarterly*, **15**, 454–462.

BLUMBERG, M. A. & BILLIG, O. (1942) Hormonal influence upon 'puerperal psychosis' and neurotic conditions. *Psychiatric Quarterly*, **16**, 454.

BOWER, W. H. & ALTSCHULE, M. D. (1956) Use of progesterone in the treatment of post-partum psychosis. *New England Journal of Medicine*, **254**, 157.

COX, J. L., HOLDEN, J. M. & SAGOVSKY, R. (1987) Detection of postnatal depression: development of a 10-item Edinburgh Postnatal Depression Scale. *British Journal of Psychiatry*, **150**, 782–786.

DALTON, K. (1984) *The Premenstrual Syndrome and Progesterone Therapy*, pp. 203–205. London: Heinemann.

—— (1985) Progesterone prophylaxis used successfully in postnatal depression. *Practitioner*, **229**, 507–508.

—— (1989) Successful prophylactic progesterone for idiopathic postnatal depression. *International Journal of Uterine Prenatal and Perinatal Studies*, **1**, 323–327.

DANOWSKI, T. S., HUFF, S. J., MRVOS, D., et al (1953) Is pregnancy followed by relative hypothyroidism? *American Journal of Obstetrics and Gynecology*, **65**, 77.

DUSSAULT, J. H. & ROUSSEAU, F. (1987) Immunologically mediated hypothyroidism. *Endocrinology and Metabolism Clinics of North America*, **16**, 417–429.

ENDICOTT, J. & SPITZER, R. L. (1978) A diagnostic schedule for affective disorders and schizophrenia. *Archives of General Psychiatry*, **35**, 837–844.

FEKSI, A., HARRIS, B., WALKER, R. F., et al (1984) Maternity blues and hormones in saliva. *Journal of Affective Disorders*, **6**, 351–355.

GARD, P. R., HANDLEY, S. L., PARSONS, A. D., et al (1986) A multivariate investigation of postpartum mood disturbance. *British Journal of Psychiatry*, **148**, 567–575.

GELDER, M. (1978) Hormones and post-partum depression. In *Mental Illness in Pregnancy and the Puerperium* (ed. M. Sandler). Oxford: Medical Publications, Oxford University Press.

HAMILTON, J. A. (1962) *Post Partum Psychiatric Problems*. St Louis: C. V. Mosby.

HARRIS, B., JOHNS, S., FUNG, H., et al (1989a) The hormonal environment of post natal depression. *British Journal of Psychiatry*, **154**, 660–667.

——, FUNG, H., JOHNS, S., et al (1989b) Transient post-partum thyroid dysfunction and postnatal depression. *Journal of Affective Disorders*, **17**, 243–249.

HENDERSON, A., GREGOIRE, A., KUMAR, R. C., et al (1991) Treatment of severe postnatal depression with oestrogen skin patches. *Lancet*, **338**, 816–817.

LOUDUN, J. B. (1987) Prescribing in pregnancy: psychotropic drugs. *British Medical Journal*, **294**, 167–169.

MONTGOMERY, S. A. & ÅSBERG, M. (1979) A new depression scale designed to be sensitive to change. *British Journal of Psychiatry*, **134**, 382–389.

MURPHY, B. E., DHAR, V., GHADIRIAN, A. M., *et al* (1991) Response to steroid suppression in major depression resistant to antidepressant therapy. *Journal of Clinical Psychopharmacology*, **11**, 121–126.

NOTT, P. N., FRANKLIN, M., ARMITAGE, C., *et al* (1976) Hormonal changes and mood in the puerperium. *British Journal of Psychiatry*, **128**, 379–383.

OKANO, T. & NOMURA, J. (1989) Maternity blues and postnatal depressive disorders – with special reference to clinical statistics and endocrinologic studies. *Seistin Shinkeigaku Zassti*, **91**, 628–633.

PARRY, B. L. (1989) Reproductive factors affecting the course of affective illness in women. *Psychiatric Clinics of North America*, **12**, 207–220.

PITT, B. (1968) 'Atypical' depression following childbirth. *British Journal of Psychiatry*, **114**, 1325–1335.

RAILTON, I. E. (1961) The use of corticoids in postpartum depression. *Journal of the American Women's Association*, **16**, 450.

SCHMIDT, H. J. (1943) The use of progesterone in the treatment of postpartum psychosis. *Journal of the American Medical Association*, **190**, 2.

SMITH, R., CUBIS, J., BRINSMEAD, M., *et al* (1990) Mood changes, obstetric experience and alterations in plasma cortisol, beta-endorphin and corticotrophin-releasing hormone during pregnancy and the puerperium. *Journal of Psychosomatic Research*, **34**, 53–69.

STENGEL, E., ZEITLYN, B. B. & RAYNER, E. H. (1958) Post-operative psychoses. *Journal of Mental Science*, **104**, 389.

WATSON, N. R., STUDD, J. W. W. & SAVVAS, M. (1989) Treatment of severe premenstrual syndrome with oestradiol patches and cyclical norethisterone. *Lancet*, i, 730–732.

WIECK, A., KUMAR, R., HIRST, A. D., *et al* (1991) Increased sensitivity of dopamine receptors and recurrence of affective psychosis after childbirth. *British Medical Journal*, **303**, 613–616.

YALOM, I. D., LUNDE, D. T., MOOS, R. H., *et al* (1968) "Post partum blues" syndrome. *Archives of General Psychiatry*, **18**, 16–27.

Part II. The Edinburgh Postnatal Depression Scale

8 Origins and development of the 10-item Edinburgh Postnatal Depression Scale

JOHN COX

Introduction: the social context to the research

In this chapter the origins and development of the Edinburgh Postnatal Depression Scale are described; I shall also recall as clearly as possible the clinical observations and research findings which led in 1980 to the successful grant application to the Scottish Home and Health Department. The professional and personal circumstances which underpinned the development of this questionnaire were fortuitous as well as planned – and linked to my work sojourns in London, Kampala and Edinburgh. By working across these cultures I was first sensitised to consider particularly the socio-cultural aspects of postnatal mental illness; Brice Pitt (1968) had already published his study of depression following childbirth in women in East London and developed a self-report scale to measure changes in depression from before to after delivery.

I was especially interested to carry out a somewhat similar prospective study in Uganda; in this study 10% of Ugandan women were found to be suffering from clinical depression 3–5 months after delivery (Cox, 1983), a similar proportion to that found by Pitt in London. Such depression markedly interfered with their ability to grow and prepare food. Although a Ugandan mental illness 'Amakiro' had symptoms similar to those found in the puerperal psychoses (Cox, 1979) the non-psychotic depression did not have a local African equivalent. Such depressed women, as in the West, were mostly unrecognised and rarely treated by either Western or traditional healers, yet most were regarded by the African health visitor as distressed and socially disabled.

It was already evident therefore that there was an urgent need to develop methods to identify such depression for use in primary care settings whether in a developed or a developing country.

A meeting with Channi Kumar, who was at that time planning a prospective study of postnatal depression, was particularly helpful because

115

he intended to use the Clinical Interview Schedule (Goldberg *et al*, 1970) which I had used in East Africa; we found we could therefore share research and clinical experience.

The later research collaboration with Robert Kendell in Edinburgh was of particular importance to the further development of our research strategies. With Yvonne Connor, we carried out a prospective study of postnatal depression on a fully representative sample of women attending antenatal clinics at the Simpson Memorial Maternity Pavilion (Cox *et al*, 1982). Kendell in an earlier study had found a 16-fold increased onset rate of severe postnatal mental disorders (mostly psychoses) within a month of childbearing, and at that time was planning a major study on a larger sample of women using Edinburgh Psychiatric and Obstetric Case Register data. However, this study was restricted to women who made contact with psychiatric services as in-patients or out-patients, and I was particularly interested to determine the rates of depression among a non-referred population and to compare the prevalence of postnatal depression in Scotland with that found in Africa.

Edinburgh prospective study

A study was carried out therefore to determine the frequency and onset rate of postnatal depression and to search for any association with obstetric factors, psychosocial variables, as well as the postnatal 'blues'. We also considered the possibility that such depression could adversely affect the temperament, feeding and development of the baby, although the number of completed health visitor reports was insufficient for any detailed analysis of these data. We were nevertheless alerted to the central role of health visitors in the provision of care to women with young infants.

It was during the course of this study that we first recognised the serious limitations of existing self-report scales to detect psychiatric disorder in childbearing women. Although this was partially overcome by conducting personal interviews on a subsample, the limitations of the Anxiety and Depression Self-report Scale (SAD) of Bedford & Foulds (1978) were abundantly apparent. We had used what was thought to be the best available depression questionnaire at that time, yet this scale failed to detect any increase in anxiety or depression associated with the postnatal blues which was readily detected by visual analogue scales. The validity of the SAD during pregnancy was most uncertain: of 13 women scoring above the threshold for personal illness (6 +) only three women when interviewed had any form of major psychiatric disorder whatsoever, 4 had minor symptoms only and in 6 there was no mental disorder at all.

We realised that these limitations of an established self-report scale when used with childbearing women may have major implications for interpreting studies which assumed a similar 'cut-off' score before and after delivery would delineate similar levels of psychiatric disorder.

The SAD scale also lacked 'face validity'; the 'depression' item was regarded by obstetricians as likely to upset a mother. 'User acceptability' is particularly important when a scale is administered to women attending an obstetric clinic. Further analysis of the SAD scale items as well as items from the Beck Depression Inventory (Beck *et al*, 1961) and the General Health Questionnaire (Goldberg, 1972) showed that somatic items were likely to be influenced by physiological changes of pregnancy (e.g. weight gain, breathlessness and tachycardia) and by the tendency for childbearing women to disclose normal worries.

The above items lacked their usual implication for the presence of an underlying psychiatric disorder; the item "recently I had gone to bed not caring if I never woke up", for example, was inappropriate because of the lack of a normal sleep routine after delivery. Likewise an item which linked sleep difficulties to a depressed mood was ambiguous and could not distinguish sleep difficulties associated with low mood from that caused by a crying baby, or a night feed. The SAD item which enquired about the presence of a depressed mood was given a morbid rating if there was no *explanation* for such depression; as some women regarded depression as an understandable consequence of childbirth, an appropriate rating of this item might not be given.

It was in the context of this work that we wrote (Cox *et al*, 1983):

> "If these difficulties with the SAD are replicated by others using different self-report questionnaires, then the implications for the reliable detection of neurosis in childbearing women are considerable. It might for example be necessary to redesign or revalidate self-report scales specifically for use during pregnancy and again for use in the puerperium. Furthermore, to assume that a similar point on these scales represents a similar degree of psychiatric morbidity before and after childbirth could also be misleading."

Kumar (1982) had also drawn attention to this important next step in postnatal depression research. It was in this way, therefore, and because of these methodological limitations, that the need for a depression scale specifically validated for use in the puerperium as well as pregnancy was more clearly recognised.

At that time I was aware that a research assistant who was a health visitor and trained psychologist would be an ideal colleague; a chance meeting with a Scottish psychologist (Kate Niven) at the Conference of the Society for Reproductive and Infant Psychology in York led to the suggestion that Jenifer Holden, who was completing a psychology degree and was an experienced health visitor, would have this expertise. Ruth Sagovsky, a part-time senior research registrar in Edinburgh also joined the team at that time, and carried out the psychiatric interviews in the validation study.

The Edinburgh Postnatal Depression Scale (EPDS)

At the outset of this research we recognised that a self-report scale could not fully measure the severity and personal impact of a depressive disorder which follows childbirth; the EPDS was designed as a screening questionnaire to identify possible depression in a clinical setting, and also for use in research. It was appreciated also that a complete understanding of postnatal depression was only possible if socio-cultural variables, relating to the attitudes towards childbirth and the processes of parenting, were fully understood.

With these limitations in mind, we decided to develop a screening scale for depression which would be acceptable to women who did not regard themselves as unwell, and was simple to complete. It should not require the health worker to have specialist knowledge of psychiatry and should have satisfactory validity and reliability as well as being sensitive to changes in the severity of depression over time.

We were encouraged in this task by Philip Snaith who had developed the Hospital Anxiety Depression Scale (HAD; Zigmund & Snaith, 1983), and recognised the need to modify existing self-report scales for use in specific clinical situations. Likewise Williams *et al* (1980) emphasised that questionnaires validated for use on hospital samples would need to be re-validated if used in the community.

With assistance from a general practitioner (Peter Holland) we set about our task by having detailed discussion about the suitability of depression items in existing questionnaires including the SAD (Bedford & Foulds, 1978), the HAD (Zigmond & Snaith, 1983) as well as the Beck Depression Inventory (Beck *et al*, 1961). We discarded items which lacked 'face validity' for postnatal depression and in particular many 'somatic' items which were misleading as indicators of depression in the puerperium.

Several Beck depression items were too detailed for use or too intrusive for screening a community sample of women. The Beck scale also contained several somatic items which were unsuitable for the reasons already mentioned. Other items lacked 'face validity' for women and health professionals as they did not take into account additional demands and the lack of leisure for new mothers: e.g. the HAD item for lack of interest (anhedonia), "I have enjoyed reading a book or watching television", was unsuitable because of reduced leisure at that time and two other HAD items "I have lost interest in my appearance" and "I feel as if I am slowed down" were rejected for similar reasons.

The clinical experience of the team in assessing and treating depressed women postpartum was used to identify suitable items which included several of our own construction. We tested the acceptability of these items by interviewing over 100 women attending local health centres, and by discussing the wording of items with health visitors. The only item which related to mothering "I have enjoyed my baby" was, surprisingly, not suitable; the depressed women were reluctant to admit not enjoying their baby. This item was therefore changed to "I have enjoyed being a mother" to emphasise mothering skills as we thought it unlikely that a depressed mother would not admit to being dissatisfied with motherhood, although reluctant to say she did not enjoy her infant.

After extensive discussion we agreed on 13 items which we thought would detect postnatal depression, and which proved satisfactory in the pilot interviews (Cox, 1986). These items were then re-written into the past tense, and each had four possible responses graded according to the severity and duration of the symptom during the previous seven days. The scoring method was simple: 0 for absence of the symptom; 3 for maximum severity and duration; 1 and 2 which were intermediate. The total score ranged from 0 to 30.

Validation study for the 13-item scale

The validation was carried out using the 13-item depression scale against the Research Diagnostic Criteria (Spitzer *et al*, 1978) derived from the Clinical Interview Schedule (Goldberg *et al*, 1970) administered by Ruth Sagovsky, who had no knowledge of the 13-item EPDS score, to a sample of women.

The women included in this study lived in Livingstone – a new town 15 miles from Edinburgh. If recently delivered, they were sent a letter inviting them to attend the health centre to complete a 'questionnaire' about postnatal depression, and to be interviewed by a member of the research team using the Clinical Interview Schedule. After our first letter 27 women attended the health centre, and a further 8 women after a follow-up letter. Of 9 women who were visited at home before a suitable appointment could be made, only 3 refused to participate at all. A total of 14 women were identified by their health visitor as having 'problems', and 2 were attending a psychiatric out-patient department. One mother recently had received psychiatric in-patient treatment and 2 others were referred from a postnatal depression support group.

The results of this validation study showed that this 13-item scale distinguished satisfactorily between the depressed and non-depressed women, but a factor analysis showed two separate factors: a 'depression' factor which explained 46% of the variance, and a second factor, which had its highest loadings on the 'mother' and two irritability items. It was therefore apparent that the 13-item scale could be shortened to 10 items without impairing its screening effectiveness for depression. We decided to carry out a validation of this shortened, 10-item scale to determine whether it would also have adequate psychometric properties. It was possible that a scale with 13 items might have been less acceptable than a 10-item scale; 13 is regarded by some as an unlucky number.

The 10-item Edinburgh Postnatal Depression Scale

The validation study of the 10-item EPDS was reported in the *British Journal of Psychiatry* (1987) by Cox, Holden and Sagovsky; this publication contained the scale items and scoring instructions, as well as guidance about the method of administration.

In this second validation study psychiatric interviews were again carried out by Ruth Sagovsky on 84 women in Livingstone. The women included in this study were taking part in a counselling intervention study (Holden *et al*, 1987) and were randomly allocated to an intervention and non-intervention group. Most women had been identified at six weeks after delivery by their health visitor as being 'possibly depressed'; the health visitor was instructed to record whether or not the mother was 'depressed' or had 'problems'.

As we envisaged that the optimum use of the questionnaire was to confirm clinical depression in women thought by health professionals to be possibly depressed, recruiting the sample in this way was appropriate. We nevertheless recognised that this sample was not representative and included a higher proportion of depressed women than would be found in the community.

We also wished to develop a scale that could be administered in a home setting because a home visit by a health visitor was important in linking a depressed woman to other primary care services. The women were interviewed at home by RS using Goldberg's Standardised Psychiatric Interview; the 10-item EPDS had been completed earlier and placed in a sealed envelope so that RS could again remain blind to the EPDS score. To prevent bias caused by RS knowing that a mother may be 'possibly depressed' or regarded as having 'problems', 12 non-depressed women were also included. A psychiatric diagnosis was made using the Research Diagnostic Criteria of Spitzer *et al* (1978). The women with a depressed mood but insufficient symptoms or abnormalities of the mental state to meet Research Diagnostic Criteria for depression, were separately identified.

Recruitment to this study was somewhat slower than we had anticipated and a further 12 women were interviewed by JLC at another health clinic. The validation of the 10-item EPDS was established by comparing the mean EPDS scores with RDC diagnosis at three months postpartum (Figure 8.1).

Figure 8.1 shows that above the threshold score 12/13, all women with a definite major depression and two of the three with a probable major depression were correctly identified. Of the 11 with a definite minor depression, only four had a 'false negative' score. There were 11 'false positives', although in 6 depressive symptoms were present but the full RDC criteria for depression were not met. The woman with the highest false positive score (21) had a personality disorder. There were three women with a psychiatric diagnosis other than depression who all scored below cut-off.

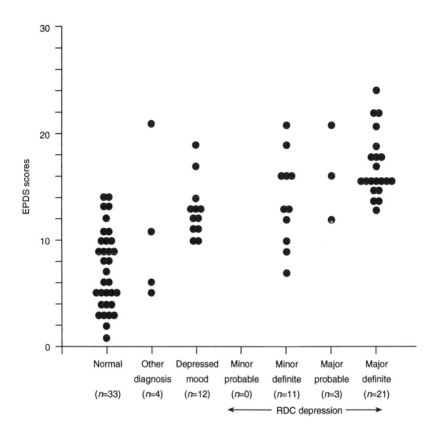

Fig. 8.1. Validation of Edinburgh Postnatal Depression Scale

The sensitivity of the EPDS (the proportion of RDC depressed women who were true positives) was 86%, and the specificity (proportion of non-depressed women who were true negatives) was 78%. The positive predictive value (the proportion of women above the threshold on the EPDS) ($n = 41$) who met RDC for depression ($n = 30$) was 73%. These findings suggested that the failed detection rate of cases could be reduced to under 10%, by using the lower cut-off 9/10; this is a cut-off we recommend if the EPDS is used in the first stage of screening in a community study.

Reliability

The split half reliability of the 10-item EPDS was 0.88 and the standardised alpha co-efficient 0.87. Sensitivity to change in severity of depression over time was established in a subsample by comparing EPDS scores obtained at the first interview when the depressed women were allocated to the counselling or routine treatment group, with that obtained after the counselled group had received eight weekly counselling visits. At this second follow-up interview the EPDS was again completed (EPDS-2) and a repeat CIS interview carried out (see Chapters 5 and 9).

The women found to be depressed at *both* interviews (i.e. who were still depressed at the follow-up interview) showed no significant difference between their mean EPDS-1 (16.5) and EPDS-2 (15.38) scores on these two occasions, whereas those women depressed at interview 1 but not at interview 2 ($n = 16$) showed a significant reduction in their mean EPDS score. The EPDS-2 score in all but one subject fell to below the threshold 12/13. The single subject whose EPDS-2 score increased but who was not depressed, had a probable carcinoma of the cervix, and suffered from an anxiety neurosis.

The three women with the highest EPDS score and three women with a 'false negative' score had other family members present when interviewed. We therefore advised that the EPDS is best completed when other family members are not present, because of the tendency for mothers to exaggerate, or minimise, psychiatric problems under these circumstances.

The 10-item EPDS was acceptable to women themselves and to their health visitors. A further advantage of the scale was its brevity; it took less than five minutes to complete, and was rapidly scored.

The EPDS, however, only screens for depression; subjects who score just below the cut-off (12/13) should not be assumed to have no psychiatric disorder. Our experience suggests that the cut-off 9/10 will detect almost all depressed women in a community sample. A high response rate (95%) is obtained when the EPDS is sent by post and a careful follow-up of non-responders carried out (Cox *et al*, 1993); this is a particular advantage if the scale is used to screen for depression in community studies.

Uses and misuses

The EPDS is particularly useful in the secondary prevention of postnatal depression by identifying the early onset of depressive symptoms, and can be administered at a postnatal or child health clinic. It is a useful first stage screening questionnaire as it is user and professional friendly, and has adequate psychometric properties – even when administered at six weeks (Murray & Carothers, 1990).

The instructions for using the EPDS and the scale items are included in the Appendix to Chapter 9. Users of the scale, however, are urged to read carefully Chapters 8–12 before embarking on a clinical investigation or research study. It is our belief that the scale is most optimally used by those health professionals who are familiar with the background research – much of which is included in this book. It is *not* recommended that the EPDS be used by women worried about their own mental state; it should be administered by a health professional. A woman with a high score, or an unexpectedly low score, should be interviewed by a health professional and/or referred to a general practitioner, community psychiatric nurse, psychologist or psychiatrist for a review. The EPDS can also be used to screen for depression during pregnancy (Chapter 12) and may even have wider uses, for example to screen for depression at other times, and to identify depressed fathers.

If this wider use becomes established and is fully supported by further validation studies then the scale may be renamed for this purpose the Edinburgh *Perinatal* Depression Scale (EPDS), or the Edinburgh Depression Scale (EDS).

In whatever setting the EPDS is used it is necessary to appreciate that it is not a measure of general psychiatric morbidity, and will not detect other common psychiatric disorders, such as phobias or anxiety states, or severe chronic mental illness such as schizophrenia. If it is necessary to screen for these disorders then the General Health Questionnaire (Goldberg, 1972) is an appropriate screening scale, and suitable personal interviews include the Present State Examination (Wing *et al*, 1974), the Schedule for Affective Disorders and Schizophrenia lifetime versions (Endicott & Spitzer, 1978) or the Clinical Interview Schedule (Goldberg *et al*, 1970).

References

BECK, A. T., WARD, C. H., MENDELSOHN, M., *et al* (1961) An inventory for measuring depression. *Archives of General Psychiatry*, **4**, 53–63.

BEDFORD, A. & FOULDS, G. (1978) *Delusions Symptoms States. State of Anxiety and Depression.* Windsor: National Foundation for Educational Research.

COX, J. L. (1979) Amakiro: a Ugandan puerperal psychosis? *Social Psychiatry*, **14**, 49–52.

—— (1983) Postnatal depression: a comparison of Scottish and African women. *Social Psychiatry*, **18**, 25–28.

—— (1986) *Postnatal Depression: a Guide for Health Professionals.* Edinburgh: Churchill Livingstone.

——, CONNOR, Y. & KENDELL, R. E. (1982) Prospective study of the psychiatric disorders of childbirth by personal interview. *British Journal of Psychiatry*, **140**, 111–117.

——, HENDERSON, I., McGUIRE, R. J., *et al* (1983) Prospective study of the psychiatric disorders of childbirth by self report questionnaire. *Journal of Affective Disorders*, **5**, 1–7.

——, HOLDEN, J. M. & SAGOVSKY, R. (1987) Detection of postnatal depression: development of the Edinburgh Postnatal Depression Scale. *British Journal of Psychiatry*, **150**, 782–786.

——, MURRAY, D. & CHAPMAN, G. (1993) A controlled study of the onset prevalence and duration of postnatal depression. *British Journal of Psychiatry*, **163**, 27–31.

ENDICOTT, J. & SPITZER, R. L. (1978) A diagnostic interview: the schedule for affective disorders and schizophrenia. *Archives of General Psychiatry*, **35**, 837–844.

GOLDBERG, D. P., COOPER, B., EASTWOOD, M. R., *et al* (1970) A standardised psychiatric interview for use in community studies. *British Journal of Preventive and Social Medicine*, **24**, 18–23.

—— (1972) *The Detection of Psychiatric Illness by Questionnaires.* Oxford: Oxford University Press.

HOLDEN, J., SAGOVSKY, R. & COX, J. L. (1987) Counselling in a general practice setting: a controlled study of health visitor intervention in the treatment of postnatal depression. *British Medical Journal*, **298**, 223–226.

KUMAR, R. (1982) Neurotic disorders in childbearing women. In *Motherhood and Mental Illness* (eds I. Brockington & R. Kumar). London: Academic Press.

MURRAY, L. & CAROTHERS, A. D. (1990) Validation of the Edinburgh Postnatal Depression Scale on a community sample. *British Journal of Psychiatry*, **157**, 288–290.

PITT, B. (1968) 'Atypical' depression following childbirth. *British Journal of Psychiatry*, **114**, 1325–1335.

SPITZER, R. L., ENDICOTT, J. & ROBINS, E. (1978) Research diagnostic criteria: rationale and reliability. *Archives of General Psychiatry*, **36**, 773–782.

WELBURN, V. (1980) *Postnatal Depression*. London: Fontana Books.

WILLIAMS, P., TARNOPOLSKY, A. & HAND, D. (1980) Case definition and case identification in psychiatric epidemiology. Review and Assessment. *Psychological Medicine*, **10**, 101–114.

WING, J. K., COOPER, J. E. & SARTORIUS, N. (1974) *The Measurement and Classification of Psychiatric Symptoms*. Cambridge: Cambridge University Press.

ZIGMOND, A. S. & SNAITH, R. P. (1983) The Hospital Anxiety and Depression Scale. *Acta Psychiatrica Scandinavica*, **67**, 361–370.

9 Using the Edinburgh Postnatal Depression Scale in clinical practice

JENI HOLDEN

This chapter is largely based on research experience of studies in which health visitors have tested the usefulness of the EPDS in routine clinical practice, both in our own work and in reports published by other health visitors. Much of the content is therefore biased towards this group of professionals, but could equally well apply to doctors or other health professionals who decide to become involved with administration of the EPDS. The reason health visitors were chosen in our own study is that they are already closely involved with mothers and their infants at this time and are ideally placed to form a trusting relationship with the mother. They can offer practical and emotional suport to the mother in her own home without fear of stigma, and can refer on to the family doctor or other agencies. Irrespective of who actually administers the scale, the importance of a team approach to intervention cannot be overemphasised.

Before advocating the use of the EPDS in clinical practice it is important to establish the following:

(a) the usefulness of the EPDS in identifying women with depression
(b) whether it is acceptable to the women who are asked to complete it
(c) whether it is practical and helpful for the health professionals who use it
(d) what problems may be encountered in administration.

Reliability of the EPDS in detecting depression

Let us first look at the usefulness of the scale in identifying depressed women. Our own validation data (Cox et al, 1987; see also Cox, Chapter 8, this volume) and that of other researchers (see Harris, Chapter 11) indicate that the scale is a reliable reflection of women's mood at the time of completion, and a useful indicator of those who may be suffering from depression.

As the EPDS is also quick to complete and does not require specialist knowledge to score, it is a useful screen for postnatal women in a general practice population.

Harris and his colleagues (1989) commented that although the EPDS is not a substitute for full psychiatric assessment, it clearly defines a population which needs further evaluation. This is a most important point; the EPDS should be used as an adjunct to, not a replacement for, clinical judgement.

In cases where reliance is being placed on the EPDS (i.e. in the absence of a psychiatrist to make a diagnosis, as would be the case in primary care) we advocate that a woman who scores high on the EPDS should be given the opportunity to discuss her feelings in more depth. She should also be asked to complete another EPDS after an interval of about two weeks, when a further high score is a reasonably accurate indication that she is depressed.

Acceptability of the EPDS to women

We first need to establish whether screening is acceptable to postnatal women, basically a healthy population who may not appreciate being asked to complete a depression questionnaire. It has even been suggested that giving the EPDS as a standardised screen to all postnatal women may have 'big brother' implications (see Comport, 1987, and Elliott, Chapter 14, this volume). Comport suggests that women may find the EPDS threatening, fearing that to fill in the form truthfully may result in their being labelled as a failure, 'ill', unsuited to care for their baby, or 'a suitable case for treatment'. Comport argues that a depressed woman may be uncooperative or even angry, feeling that she was being asked to pass one more test as a mother, or that her secrets were being 'winkled out of her' for her own good. She may also fear the risk of being labelled difficult if she refuses to cooperate.

Findings from studies in which the EPDS has been used to screen a postnatal population for depression seem to mitigate such criticisms. In their Cambridge study, Murray & Carothers (1990) mailed the EPDS to 702 women 6 weeks after birth, and concluded that a return rate of 97.3% indicated: ''impressive evidence of the scale's acceptability to postnatal women''. Certain factors in this study may, however, have helped to increase the acceptability of the EPDS. Firstly, all the women had been interviewed in hospital shortly after the birth. The aims of the research and the requirements of their involvement were explained to them, and therefore all the women who were sent an EPDS had already given their informed consent to participation in the study, and would have been expecting to fill in questionnaires. Secondly, the Cambridge population may be unusual; in this university city, women may have been more aware of the need for research and more prepared to cooperate. Thirdly, the fact that a stamped addressed envelope was enclosed for their reply may also have influenced this excellent return rate.

In other studies conducted in a range of different geographical and sociological areas, however, the EPDS has also proved its acceptability, even when given on several occasions to the same women. Ring & McLean (1994) carried out routine screening of 147 postnatal women in a general practice population in an urban/rural population in Central Scotland, consisting of two villages with higher than average unemployment. Taylor (1989) administered the scale to 150 women in two large housing suburbs in Aberdeen, and Stoke-on-Trent health visitors screened women in a mixed urban and rural population (Gerrard *et al*, 1993). The EPDS was also used by Cullinan (1991) in north-west Hertfordshire and by Angeli & Grahame (1990) in Walton-on-Thames. All authors reported that women voiced no objection to completing the scale.

Women who took part in the Edinburgh counselling intervention (Holden *et al*, 1989) were later asked about their response to being asked to complete the EPDS. Although this was a skewed sample in that all the women had been depressed, these are the very women who might be expected to feel threatened by: "having their secrets winkled out of them" (Comport, 1987). Most commented that it had been a relief to be asked about their feelings. For some, filling in the scale had clarified their knowledge that something was wrong, and seeing symptoms actually described made it easier to explain.

> "I was glad somebody had written something down, because it's hard to describe. It has to be written down to say what you are going through. I was glad to be able to just underline how I felt. It was much better than trying to describe it."

Some women saw the EPDS as a tangible 'permission to speak'. Others reported that filling in the scale had been therapeutic, regardless of whether or not it brought help. In contrast, one woman expressed frustration at being confronted with a form:

> "How can you tick a sentence on a bit of paper to say how you felt? If somebody had asked me, how did you feel last week, I could have told them. I wanted somebody to talk to."

This comment underlines the importance of using the EPDS as an adjunct to an interview in which the woman can then talk to a caring professional about how she feels, discussing responses to individual items on the EPDS.

Does the EPDS help professionals to detect depression?

It has been argued that health professionals do not need a piece of paper to determine whether someone is depressed. Does the EPDS actually increase recognition of depression? In our counselling intervention (Holden *et al*, 1989) health visitors were asked to indicate whether postnatal women in their caseload were, in their opinion, in need of extra help. They identified only 40% of women who obtained high scores at six weeks postnatal as having problems. In the three-centre trial described in Chapter 5 (pp. 58–59), many health visitors reported being surprised to learn that women they thought were coping, were actually very depressed (Gerrard *et al*, 1993).

These findings are echoed by other researchers; Thome (1991), who evaluated the EPDS with Icelandic women, found that nurses picked up 50% more cases of depression than they had done before using the scale. Angeli & Grahame (1990) found that health visitors had been unaware of 57% of the women identified as depressed using the EPDS. Cullinan (1991) also found that the EPDS identified a larger number of depressed women than would normally have been picked up. Ring & McLean (1993) reported:

> "At the outset of the study, we believed we had been adequately identifying and managing postnatal depression in our caseloads without using the EPDS. Routine screening identified the full extent of the problem and made us recognise that our previous approach had been patchy and therefore inadequate in meeting the needs of all postnatally depressed women."

It would seem that routine use of the EPDS can indeed help professionals to identify women with emotional problems.

Ways of using the EPDS

(a) To check whether an individual woman is depressed.
(b) To check improvement in depression with treatment or over time.
(c) As a routine screen for all postnatal women.

Advantages of giving the EPDS routinely to all women are that an individual woman does not feel singled out, and early problems can be picked up, giving the opportunity for preventive interventions.

Intervention

To administer a screening test carries the implication that treatment will be available for those found to be suffering from the condition. Before starting to use the EPDS routinely, therefore, careful thought should first be given to the adequate provision of intervention strategies. Regular non-directive counselling by health visitors has been shown to lead to the recovery of many depressed postnatal women and to have been helpful in supporting those who did not recover (Holden *et al*, 1989; see also Chapter 5). Other treatments include antidepressants. If these are needed, it is important that they be given in an adequate dosage to be effective, and that the woman also receives regular support and encouragement to persevere with treatment.

If a woman still does not seem to be recovering, she should be referred for specialist advice and/or treatment.

When should the EPDS be given?

Our original advice (Cox *et al*, 1987) was that the EPDS could be given at the postnatal check-up at about six weeks. However, in practice it became apparent that this would not pick up all depressions, as the onset of depression for any individual woman could be any time during the postnatal months. However, as half the cases of postnatal depression start within the first three months and three-quarters by six months postnatal (Cooper *et al*, 1988) three contact times would maximise detection rates. In theory it should be possible to fit this extra service into existing contacts with postnatal women. Moss *et al* (1987), who studied London mothers' perceptions of health visitors in the first six months after birth, found that the mean number of home visits to each mother in the first postnatal year was 4.4, with an additional mean of 12.9 clinic visits per woman. Given a mean total of 17.3 contact times in the postnatal year, it does not seem unreasonable to include 3 EPDS screening times. In our three-centre intervention training trial the EPDS was given between 5–8, 10–14 and 20–26 weeks postnatally, with an explanatory visit during pregnancy, and an introductory letter at the first postnatal visit.

High scores at any of these occasions were followed by assessment, referral to the GP (with the mother's consent), and the offer of a set number of extra 'listening visits', after which another EPDS was given. A further high score at this time was followed by further listening visits or referral, depending on the woman's condition. This system resulted in a significant reduction in the percentage of women who scored 12 or more at six months postnatal (Gerrard *et al*, 1993).

Problems which may be experienced in routine screening

Administration

Difficulties described by health visitors in administering the EPDS were as follows:

(a) It was hard to remember when the EPDS was due, even when planned to coincide with existing contact times.
(b) At busy clinics the health visitor may forget to ask women to fill in an EPDS form.
(c) The complexities of administration and the added paper-work added significantly to the increasing time required for record-keeping.

Possible solutions to administrative problems

Much of the paper-work could be done by clerical staff. The timing of the EPDS could be added in to existing systems used in some health authorities to alert health professionals or mothers themselves to immunisations and screening test dates.

Do women answer honestly?

Health visitors are sometimes concerned that women who do not wish to admit they are depressed may conceal this and deliberately obtain a low score. A total score of zero is a particular worry, especially if the health visitor suspects the woman is experiencing problems. It is, of course, impossible to know how many women do not fill in the form honestly; on the other hand, the decision as to whether or not to reveal their feelings to a health professional is one which any individual must be free to make for themselves. The advice given when training health visitors in using the EPDS is to respect any woman's right not to complete an EPDS. If they suspect that someone is deliberately scoring low, this is also their right. The EPDS should be seen as an *offer* of help which can be accepted or not, as the woman chooses. The fact that the offer has been made may in itself indicate to women that it is appropriate to discuss their feelings with a health professional, which they may take advantage of on a subsequent occasion.

Medicalisation of low mood

Elliott (Chapter 14) and Thome (1991) have discussed the question of whether women may become more depressed by being told that they are suffering from depression. Thome found that Icelandic mothers who scored high on the EPDS did not see their distress as 'mental disturbance', and neither did the nurses who administered the scale and supported them. The nurses in fact admired some mothers for their strength in living through very difficult life situations and not showing more distress than they actually did.

It is difficult to know what the word 'depression' means to individuals or to establish whether this word does in fact carry a worrying stigma. The fact that compliance with completion of the EPDS has been consistently high in published studies seems to imply that women do not find this a problem.

Small (1994), in Victoria, Australia, followed up 45 women who scored high on the EPDS at 8–9 months postnatal and 45 controls. When women in the case-group were asked at follow-up whether they had been depressed at the time of their high EPDS score, only one disagreed with this assessment. However, one-third of all women who had felt depressed since the birth did not agree with naming this experience postnatal depression; they explained their feelings in terms of added workload or tiredness.

'Depression about depression' did not seem to be an issue with the women who were interviewed after our own intervention study (Holden *et al*, 1989). The knowledge that they were depressed seemed to have directly helped some women to confide in other people. This excerpt from an interview with one of the respondents, Cathy, clearly illustrates the beneficial effect of having an explanation for the way she was feeling, and her remarks were typical of what many of the women described. Cathy said:

> "Being told that I was depressed helped in so many ways. It meant I could tell other people when they asked how I was. I was amazed how many people said they had had it themselves, or knew someone who had had it. Before, I couldn't tell anyone how I was feeling. I just pretended I was fine. I thought no one would understand. But everyone seemed to have a story about someone they had known who was depressed. If everyone was more open about it, people could help each other more."

Anxiety about waiting to take action on a high score

When the EPDS is given at a busy clinic, the health professional may not be able to check the score of each woman immediately. Some health visitors prefer to give the EPDS at a home visit where there is the opportunity for immediate discussion of any problems. For others, if the EPDS was not given at a clinic it would not be given at all. The scores should be checked and high-scoring women should be interviewed as soon as possible. Depressed women may be unable to get to the clinic, and the importance of giving an EPDS at home to non-attenders at clinics should be emphasised.

Alerting health professionals to suicidal thoughts

One area which causes health visitors considerable anxiety is what action should be taken when a woman responds positively to item 10, which relates to thoughts of 'self-harm' or suicide. In giving the opportunity for preventive action, this is an advantage rather than a problem of using the EPDS.
Item 10 on the EPDS reads:

10. The thought of harming myself has occurred to me:
    Yes, quite often   3
    Sometimes   2
    Hardly ever   1
    Never   0

Any positive score on this item should be taken seriously. Using the EPDS routinely may reveal suicidal feelings before a woman feels desperate enough to act on them. It takes courage to acknowledge feeling suicidal, but women do admit to this on the EPDS. Even if a woman scores only 1, the fact that she has put this down in writing indicates that she is having problems which need to be discussed as soon as possible. A score of 2 or more should be interpreted as a cry for help. Scores on the self-harm item in our sample of depressed women (Holden *et al*, 1989) were associated with severity of depression, and the only two women to score 3 at 6 weeks actually attempted suicide.

Deciding policy

Before adopting the EPDS for routine screening in primary care, the implications of a high score on item 10 should be discussed at a meeting between members of the primary care team, nurse management, and members of the psychiatric and psychology services to decide on a policy of action. For example, in an emergency, could a health visitor phone a psychiatrist directly?

Implications for practice

Health visitors giving the EPDS routinely at the clinic have told us that they do not always have time to look at the scores until the next day, or perhaps even longer. They are understandably worried about a delay in seeing women who have scored positively on the self-harm item. Without the EPDS, however, the health professional may never have learned how the women were feeling; one woman in Stoke-on-Trent who told her health visitor that she had ''felt a bit low'' during her pregnancy later admitted that she had actually tried to hang herself on two occasions. Seeing the question on the EPDS may give a woman who is feeling desperate the courage to say so. This knowledge does, however, place the health professional in a unique position of responsibility. What action should be taken?

What to do if someone scores on item 10

If the EPDS forms are given at a busy clinic it is important to screen them for high scoring women and especially for positive responses to the self-harm item. Women with scores on item 10 (especially when combined with a high overall score) should be seen as soon as possible, and their doctor should be informed. Ideally, this should not be done without the woman's consent. If, however, the health professional knows that she/he will not be able to see the woman within 48 hours (for example, if the clinic was late on a Friday afternoon), the doctor should be told and asked to visit.

Discussion of a positive score on item 10

Some health professionals understandably feel they are 'out of their depth' in discussing suicidal feelings, or in making an assessment of risk. Most women who have admitted to such feelings are, however, sufficiently disturbed to find discussion a relief. Talking to someone who validates her feelings in a non-judgemental way may in itself be therapeutic and preventive. It is inappropriate to try to cheer the woman by suggesting that things aren't as bad as she thinks. It is, however, important to establish what the woman meant by answering as she did. She may have misinterpreted the question. Having established that she does have suicidal thoughts, it is necessary to find out how serious these are.

Areas to discuss in talking to a woman who scores on item 10

1. How often and how severe is the feeling?
2. Has she made any previous attempts?
3. Has she thought how she would go about it?
4. Has she got the means? (And are these likely to be effective?)
5. What has she got to live for?
6. What support does she have at home?
7. If she has a partner, has she told him how she is feeling?
8. Can she count on him to understand and give her emotional support?
9. If she hasn't told him, would she like you or her doctor to help her to explain how she is feeling?
10. If she doesn't have a partner or feels that she really can't tell him, is there anyone else who would be understanding (and not judgemental) and whose support she could realistically call on?
11. Has she told this person or anyone else about her feelings?
12. Could she phone this person and would they come if she feels bad?
13. Do her parents know? (Is she close to them?)

Let the woman know that it is important to seek help, and that help is available. If you are not her doctor, try to persuade her to agree that you tell her doctor how she is feeling and ask her or him to call. Although it is necessary to assess risk and the availability of support, this should not be an interrogation! Encourage the woman to talk in her own way.

The need for clearly identified referral systems

Before starting to use the EPDS as a routine screen for all women, it is essential to tell other services what is involved, to gain their cooperation, and to ensure that community psychiatrists, psychologists and psychiatric nurses will be willing and able to accept referrals and that they are aware of the special requirements of postnatal women. As mentioned earlier, using the EPDS can effect a general increase in awareness of postnatal depression, among both professionals and the women themselves. Ideally this can lead to the promotion of closer interdisciplinary links and clearer lines of referral. Increased professional alertness may in itself be preventive.

Advantages of using the EPDS routinely

Creating a climate of openness

Introducing the EPDS into a primary care setting may have more widespread effects than simply increased efficiency, important though that is. As mentioned in the introduction, postnatal women often find it difficult to tell health professionals that they are depressed. They may even feel that it is dangerous to do so – fearing that the professional has the power to take the baby away, or at least regard them as an inadequate mother. Using the EPDS is a positive and tangible statement to postnatal women not only that it's alright to have negative feelings but that it's alright to talk about them. It is a clear indication that health professionals are interested in them as a person, not just as the mother of an infant.

It can also be a consciousness-raising exercise for the professional. In our counselling intervention (Holden *et al*, 1989) health visitors administered the scale but did not see the scores. Nevertheless, both they and family doctors reported increased awareness of the possibility of depression generally, and heightened sensitivity to signs that all was not well with individual women. The EPDS not only gives women 'permision to speak'; it also gives the professional 'permission to listen'. Taylor (1989) found that the health visitors in her study used women's EPDS responses as a starting point for a discussion of their feelings whether they scored high or not. Stoke-on-Trent health visitors also reported that giving the EPDS routinely was an unobtrusive way to approach the subject of how women are feeling, and that giving the scale at definite contact times gave them a structured approach to the problem of postnatal depression, a state which many had found overwhelming previously (Gerrard *et al*, 1993). Ring & McLean (1994) reported that routine screening encouraged postnatal women to seek help with emotional problems at other than the actual contact times the EPDS was being administered.

Summary of advantages

    (a) Raises awareness among:
        (i) health professionals
        (ii) women themselves
        (iii) their families
    (b) (i) Gives women 'permission to speak'
        (ii) Gives health professionals 'permission to listen'
        (iii) Encourages women to seek help from others
    (c) Legitimises the woman's feelings, enabling her to seek help from others as well as health professionals
    (d) Changes women's perception of what health professionals can offer in the way of emotional support

(e) Gives health professionals a structured approach to:
    (i) identification of low mood or depression
    (ii) intervention
(f) Gives weight to a 'hunch' that a woman is depressed
    (i) clarifies the situation for woman and professional
    (ii) allows discussion of intervention
    (iii) validates referral
(g) Gives the opportunity for early preventive intervention
(h) May help to prevent suicide
(i) Can lead to improved sensitivity to the needs of postnatal women
(j) Can lead to improved liaison with other professionals
(k) Evidence of the number of high-scoring women may alert health authorities and management to the need for extra provision of services, or redeployment of existing services.

Intervention

To administer a screening test carries the implication that treatment will be available for those found to be suffering from the identified condition. Before starting to use the EPDS routinely, therefore, careful thought should first be given to the adequate provision of intervention strategies, including support, counselling, antidepressants and therapy or support groups. (Intervention is discussed in Chapter 5.)

Support for the carers

Dealing with other people's problems can be very taxing, especially if this 'taps in' to the helper's own insecurities or sadness. Professionals who take on this work may need to be supported themselves. One way to do this is to set up a support group; if possible this should be led by a mental health nurse. In practice, many health visitors working in primary care developed their own informal support system. Health visitors or other professionals who do not work as part of a team may need a more formalised support structure.

Conclusions

The EPDS is an acceptable and simple means of identifying postnatal women who are experiencing emotional distress. Its routine use in health care settings may prevent much suffering, and may also encourage a climate in which even negative feelings are seen as a legitimate subject for discussion. It would indeed be worrying, however, if the EPDS were to be used as a replacement for clinical judgement. One of its important functions is to facilitate the opening of a dialogue between a woman and someone who can help her. All women who have scored above threshold on the EPDS should be encouraged as soon as possible to elaborate on why they completed items in a particular way, given a full opportunity for discussion of their problems and/or feelings, be offered a suitable intervention and carefully monitored in the following weeks.

To encourage health professionals to detect postnatally depressed women in a climate of reducing health care provision may seem over-optimistic. Changing systems is by no means easy, especially when health service cutbacks mean that personnel are already stretched, sometimes to the limit of their capacity. To engage them in the extra work and change in routine which is an inevitable consequence of introducing EPDS screening could be seen as adding to existing overload. Health professionals are, however, already considerably involved with women they suspect of being depressed. Developing a structured and effective approach to promoting the psychological well-being of postnatal women can help to maximise the time they have available to invest and provide a clear definition of their role with this client group. Not only can this actually save on resources but it can give health professionals increased confidence in their ability to offer constructive help. Routine use of the EPDS may also be a way to produce evidence of need to promote the allocation of appropriate resources.

Health professionals wishing to introduce this service need the informed support of management, who should take into account exactly what is involved in terms of extra work and time, especially in the initial stages of setting up the service. The primary care team need to work together to ensure that the service works efficiently. Other services, including midwives, obstetricians, community psychiatric nurses, counsellors, psychologists, psychiatrists and voluntary agencies such as the National Childbirth Trust, should also be alerted and informed. Extra clerical and/or auxiliary staff may be needed to help with implementation.

The possible long-term consequences (chronic depression, separation, divorce, effects on children) cannot be measured financially or in terms of human misery. There is evidence that the introduction of a structured programme including the use of the EPDS in clinical practice and early intervention can reduce the number of women with high scores at around six months postnatal (Gerrard *et al*, 1993). Surely this is worth aiming for.

Appendix I. A system for using the EPDS as a routine screen for the detection and prevention of postnatal depression

Contact times

These should be chosen to fit in with times mothers are routinely seen, such as at postnatal check-up, immunisation clinics, or developmental screening.

(a) *Explanatory visit during pregnancy*
   If possible, arrange to see both prospective parents. Discuss possible emotional responses including low mood and depression, and explain the usefulness of the EPDS. Discuss the benefits of rallying practical and emotional support during pregnancy and after baby comes, from friends and family, and allocation of specific tasks to partner. Explain roles of health professionals, leave telephone number and contact times.

(b) *First postnatal visit*
   See both parents if appropriate. Encourage the mother to talk about her response to the birth of her baby. Tell her about the EPDS. Give your telephone number and time(s) she can contact you.

(c) *Give an EPDS to all women* between 5–8, 10–14 and 20–26 weeks postnatal.

   (a) At 5–8 weeks high scorers may be still adjusting to the baby, and only need information and reassurance. Intervention in the form of listening and support may prevent long-lasting depression.

   (b) Low scoring women may become depressed later, so all women should be asked to complete a second EPDS at 10–14 weeks.

   (c) A third EPDS given to all mothers at 20–26 weeks should pick up any problems requiring referral.

Early recognition and intervention should lead to fewer depressed mothers at 3 and 6 months, which should be reflected in lower EPDS scores at these times.

The EPDS forms

It is helpful to obtain sets of three EPDS forms in different colours marked '5–8 weeks', '10–14 weeks' and '20–26 weeks'. As each birth is notified, the top of each EPDS form can be completed with the date due, and the complete set kept in the record notes. Administrative tasks could be done by a clerical or auxiliary worker, who could also be trained to give out the forms.

Where to give the EPDS

(a) At the clinic. Privacy can be provided by screening a table and chair in a corner of the room, with a closed 'post-box' for EPDS forms.

(b) Non-attenders may be depressed. The EPDS may be given at home or posted with an explanatory letter (and a stamped addressed envelope).

Completing the EPDS

(a) The EPDS only takes one or two minutes to complete.
(b) It should be filled in by the woman herself without discussion with other people.
(c) Make sure that both sides of the EPDS are completed.
(d) Discreet help may be offered if the woman has reading difficulties.

Scoring

The EPDS items are scored from 0–3; the normal response scores 0, and the 'severe' response scores 3. (See EPDS scoring sheet.) Total the individual item scores.

Action

Anyone who scores on item 10 (especially with a high overall score) should be seen immediately and assessed by a doctor as soon as possible.
Women who score 12 or more on the EPDS should be given the opportunity for discussion and assessment with a health professional as soon as possible.

(a) The woman may have been unhappy for a particular reason at the time of completion. Let her know how to contact you if she needs more help.
(b) Women who have more than transient low mood should be monitored, seen by a doctor, and asked to complete another EPDS after two weeks. Women with two high scores need further assessment and intervention.
(c) The woman may be offered a set number of extra weekly supportive 'listening' visits and/or may be prescribed antidepressants if appropriate. Review using the EPDS after an appropriate time interval.
(d) Women who do not respond to simple treatment will need to be reassessed and may need further referral to psychiatric or psychology services.

Non-English speakers

(a) Although the EPDS has been translated into other languages (see pp. 248–270), there may be cultural differences in interpretation, and the score may not accurately reflect the mother's mood.
(b) *Using a translated EPDS or an English EPDS explained by an interpreter* The EPDS can be used to open the subject for discussion, but unless the EPDS has been validated for use in that language, the score should not be assumed to have the same meaning.

Appendix II. Edinburgh Postnatal Depression Scale

Today's date......................... Baby's age ....

Baby's date of birth................ Birth weight ....

Triplets/twins/single................ Male/female ....

Mother's age.........................

Number of other children: 0 1 2 3 4 5 5 +

HOW ARE YOU FEELING?

As you have recently had a baby, we would like to know how you are feeling now. Please underline the answer which comes closest to how you have felt in the past 7 days, not just how you feel today.

Here is an example, already completed:

I have felt happy:

   Yes, most of the time
   Yes, some of the time
   No, not very often
   No, not at all

This would mean: "I have felt happy some of the time" during the past week. Please complete the other questions in the same way.

IN THE PAST SEVEN DAYS

1. I have been able to laugh and see the funny side of things:
      As much as I always could
      Not quite so much now
      Definitely not so much now
      Not at all

2. I have looked forward with enjoyment to things:
      As much as I ever did
      Rather less than I used to
      Definitely less than I used to
      Hardly at all

3. I have blamed myself unnecessarily when things went wrong:
      Yes, most of the time
      Yes, some of the time
      Not very often
      No, never

Please continue overleaf

4. I have felt worried and anxious for no very good reason:
   No, not at all
   Hardly ever
   Yes, sometimes
   Yes, very often

5. I have felt scared or panicky for no very good reason:
   Yes, quite a lot
   Yes, sometimes
   No, not much
   No, not at all

6. Things have been getting on top of me:
   Yes, most of the time I haven't been able to cope at all
   Yes, sometimes I haven't been coping as well as usual
   No, most of the time I have coped quite well
   No, I have been coping as well as ever

7. I have been so unhappy that I have had difficulty sleeping:
   Yes, most of the time
   Yes, sometimes
   Not very often
   No, not at all

8. I have felt sad or miserable:
   Yes, most of the time
   Yes, quite often
   Not very often
   No, not at all

9. I have been so unhappy that I have been crying:
   Yes, most of the time
   Yes, quite often
   Only occasionally
   No, never

10. The thought of harming myself has occurred to me:
    Yes, quite often
    Sometimes
    Hardly ever
    Never

(Cox, J. L., Holden, J. M. & Sagovsky, R. (1987) Detection of postnatal depression: development of the 10-item Edinburgh Postnatal Depression Scale. *British Journal of Psychiatry*, **150**, 782–786.)

Edinburgh Postnatal Depression Scale: Scoring Sheet

1. I have been able to laugh and see the funny side of things:
   As much as I always could   0
   Not quite so much now   1
   Definitely not so much now   2
   Not at all   3

2. I have looked forward with enjoyment to things:
   As much as I ever did   0
   Rather less than I used to   1
   Definitely less than I used to   2
   Hardly at all   3

3. I have blamed myself unnecessarily when things went wrong:
   Yes, most of the time   3
   Yes, some of the time   2
   Not very often   1
   No, never   0

4. I have felt worried and anxious for no very good reason:
   No, not at all   0
   Hardly ever   1
   Yes, sometimes   2
   Yes, very often   3

5. I have felt scared or panicky for no very good reason:
   Yes, quite a lot   3
   Yes, sometimes   2
   No, not much   1
   No, not at all   0

6. Things have been getting on top of me:
   Yes, most of the time I haven't been able to cope at all   3
   Yes, sometimes I haven't been coping as well as usual   2
   No, most of the time I have coped quite well   1
   No, I have been coping as well as ever   0

7. I have been so unhappy that I have had difficulty sleeping:
   Yes, most of the time   3
   Yes, sometimes   2
   Not very often   1
   No, not at all   0

8. I have felt sad or miserable:

Yes, most of the time	3
Yes, quite often	2
Not very often	1
No, not at all	0

9. I have been so unhappy that I have been crying:

Yes, most of the time	3
Yes, quite often	2
Only occasionally	1
No, never	0

10. The thought of harming myself has occurred to me:

Yes, quite often	3
Sometimes	2
Hardly ever	1
Never	0

EPDS Record Sheet

Health professional...............................   District..............

| Name | Baby's D.O.B. | 5–8 wk EPDS | | 10–14 wk EPDS | | 20–26 wk EPDS | | Counselling support | | Referred? |
		Date	Score	Date	Score	Date	Score	Start	End	Date

References

ANGELI, N. & GRAHAME, K. (1990) Screening for postnatal depression. *Midwife, Health Visitor and Community Nurse*, **26**, 428–430.

COMPORT, M. (1987) *Towards Happy Motherhood: Understanding Postnatal Depression*. London: Corgi.

COOPER, P. J., CAMPBELL, E. A., DAY, A., *et al* (1988) Non-psychotic disorder after childbirth: a prospective sudy to prevalence, incidence, course and nature. *British Journal of Psychiatry*, **152**, 799–806.

COX, J. L. (1986) *Postnatal Depression: A Guide for Health Professionals*. Edinburgh: Churchill Livingstone.

——, HOLDEN, J. M. & SAGOVSKY, R. (1987) Detection of postnatal depression: Development of the Edinburgh Postnatal Depression Scale. *British Journal of Psychiatry*, **150**, 782–786.

CULLINAN, R. (1991) Health visitor intervention in postnatal depression. *Health Visitor*, **64**, 412–414.

FIELD, S. (1982) The consumer's view of the health visiting service. *Maternal and Child Health*, **23**, 44–47.

FROMMER, E. A. & O'SHEA, G. (1973) Antenatal identification of women liable to have problems in managing their infants. *British Journal of Psychiatry*, **123**, 149–156.

GERRARD, J., HOLDEN, J. M., ELLIOTT, S. A., *et al* (1993) A trainer's perspective of an innovative training programme to teach health visitors about the detection, treatment and prevention of postnatal depression. *Journal of Advanced Nursing*, **18**, 1825–1832.

GOLDBERG, D. P., EASTWOOD, M. R., KEDWARD, H. B., *et al* (1979) A standardised psychiatric interview for use in community surveys. *British Journal of Preventive and Social Medicine*, **24**, 18–23.

GRAHAM, H. & M'KEE, L. (1980) *The First Months of Motherhood*. London: The Health Education Council.

GREEN, J. M., SNOWDON, C. & STATHAM, H. (1991) EPDS by post. *British Journal of Psychiatry*, **158**, 865.

HARRIS, B., HUCKLE, P., THOMAS, R., *et al* (1989) The use of rating scales to identify postnatal depression. *British Journal of Psychiatry*, **154**, 813–817.

HOLDEN, J. M., SAGOVSKY, R. & COX, J. L. (1989) Counselling in a general practice setting: a controlled study of health visitor intervention in the treatment of postnatal depression. *British Medical Journal*, **298**, 223–226.

MOSS, P., BOLLAND, G., FOXMAN, R., *et al* (1987) The division of household work during the transition to parenthood. *Journal of Reproductive and Infant Psychology*, **5**, 71–87.

MURRAY, D. & COX, J. (1990) Screening for postnatal depression during pregnancy with the Edinburgh Postnatal Depression Scale (EPDS). *Journal of Reproductive and Infant Psychology*, **8**, 99–109.

—— & CAROTHERS, A. D. (1990) The validation of the Edinburgh Postnatal Depression Scale on a community sample. *British Journal of Psychiatry*, **157**, 289–290.

RING, N. & MCLEAN, T. M. (1994) Routine postnatal depression screening and the effects on health visitor practice. *Journal of Advanced Nursing* (in press).

SMALL, R. (1994) Missing voices: what women say and do about depression after childbirth. *Australian and New Zealand Journal of Psychiatry* (in press).

SPITZER, R., ENDICOTT, J. & ROBINS, E. (1975) *Research Diagnostic Criteria. Instrument No. 58*. New York: New York Psychiatric Institute.

TAYLOR, E. (1989) Postnatal depression: what can a health visitor do? *Journal of Advanced Nursing*, **14**, 877–886.

THOME, M. (1991) Emotional distress during the postpartum period, from the second to the sixth month, assessed by community nurses. *Nordic Midwives and Research Oslo*, **9**, 25–27.

WING, J. K., COOPER, J. G. & SARTORIUS, N. (1974) *Measurement and Classification of Psychiatric Symptoms*. Cambridge: Cambridge University Press.

10 Postpartum depression: identification and measurement in a cross-cultural context

MICHAEL W. O'HARA

The Edinburgh Postnatal Depression Scale (EPDS) was developed specifically to screen women for postpartum depression (Cox *et al*, 1987). Because it is one of the few (if not the only) instrument developed to assess depression in recently delivered women and because research evidence has suggested that it is reliable and valid as a screening tool (Cox *et al*, 1987; Harris *et al*, 1989; Murray & Carothers, 1990), it has been used in a number of international settings (e.g. in the US, the Netherlands, Iceland, Australia, Sweden), in English and translated versions. The desire of clinicians and researchers, outside of Great Britain, to take advantage of the special features of the EPDS in their own countries is understandable. However, many questions can be raised regarding the appropriateness of using the EPDS in countries other than Great Britain before it is validated for use in those settings (Draguns, 1982). These concerns reflect the conclusions of a rather large literature in the area of cross-cultural psychopathology (Al-Issa, 1982; Littlewood, 1990).

Before explicitly considering the applicability of the EPDS for use outside Great Britain, several issues that bear on assessing psychopathology in a cross-cultural context will be discussed. The first section of this chapter will briefly consider the issue of the influence of culture on psychopathology. The second section will address the issue of the cross-cultural expression and measurement of postpartum depression in particular. The fourth section will address specifically the use of the EPDS in cross-cultural settings. Finally, I will make recommendations for future research on cross-cultural uses of the EPDS.

Culture and psychopathology

There have been many definitions of culture and over 150 definitions have been identified by Kluckhohn & Kroeber (1952). In the most general sense, features of culture include: (a) aspects of our physical environment such as roads, bridges and buildings; and (b) aspects of our internal or cognitive environment such as beliefs, norms, and myths which are shared by a group (Al-Issa, 1982). Culture may be regarded as a schema which filters and organises our experience in particular ways that tend to link us to other members of our own culture and separate us from members of other cultures (Marsella, 1987). The potential implications of cultural differences for understanding the aetiology, symptomatology, and measurement of psychopathology will depend upon the extent to which these aspects of psychopathology are affected by culture (Littlewood, 1990).

Cross-cultural approaches to the study of psychopathology have a variety of goals. Examples include developing a unified understanding of psychopathology, comparing rates of disorders across cultures, determining the extent to which symptom features differ across cultures for particular disorders, and identifying cultural characteristics that may lead to higher or lower rates of certain disorders (Draguns, 1982; Littlewood, 1990; Marsella, 1987). The purpose most relevant to this chapter is that of applying a measure developed in one culture (the EPDS) for use in another culture. Although this issue could be construed simply as a matter of rendering an accurate translation of the EPDS, there are other factors that may affect the reliability and, importantly, the validity of the EPDS in other cultural settings (Marsella, 1987).

There are two basic approaches to the study of other cultures, the etic and the emic. The etic approach involves the study of one culture from the perspective of another culture. In psychopathology research the etic approach is most common (Draguns, 1982; Leff, 1990; Marsella, 1987). Much of this work has been dominated by US and British researchers applying their concepts and measures to study psychopathology in other countries. The emic approach involves the study of psychopathology from within the culture and from the perspective of that culture, an approach most commonly taken by medical anthropologists (Littlewood, 1990). However, investigators who are indigenous to the culture being studied may still use an etic approach, particularly if they were trained in another cultural setting (e.g. in the US or Great Britain) (Leff, 1990).

Depression – a world context

Depression would seem to be ubiquitous in the United States and Great Britain. However, early research suggested that it might not be so common in other countries of the world, particularly those of Africa (Engelsmann, 1982; Laubscher, 1937; Singer, 1984). As I suggest above, it is Western investigators, particularly the Americans and the British, who have conducted the studies aimed at determining the prevalence of depression and its typical symptomatology around the world. In this section I will briefly comment on the prevalence and expression of depression in selected cultures.

Depression in non-Western cultures

Although early research in Africa suggested that depression was rare (Laubscher, 1937), more recent research has suggested that depression is relatively common in African countries such as Benin, Lesotho, Nigeria, Senegal, Ghana, Ethiopia, Sudan, South Africa, and Uganda (Bertschy *et al*, 1992; Hollifield *et al*, 1990; Odejide *et al*, 1989; Orley & Wing, 1979; Singer, 1984). Characteristic features of depression have differed across the cultural groups that have been studied. For example, in Nigeria there is a predominantly somatic presentation, whereas in Ghana there is a high frequency of self-accusations of witchcraft (Singer, 1984). Leighton *et al* (1963) studied the Yoruba in Nigeria and found that they had no word for depression and that the concept of depression as a syndrome was unknown; nevertheless, the only symptoms common in the West that were missing were guilt and self-recrimination. In a recent review, Odejide *et al* (1989) suggest that feelings of sadness, hypochondriasis, and somatisation are the most characteristic features of depression in Africa. However, they note that the somatisation is different from that reported in Western literature. For example, somatisation often presents as paraesthesias (e.g. crawling, heat, peppery sensations). Odejide *et al* go on to suggest that many African patients with somatic symptoms do not respond to physical methods of treatment, including adequate doses of antidepressants. These observations suggest that the somatised depressions found in Africa may be quite different from Western conceptions of depression (even those with a strong somatic component).

A number of epidemiological studies have been conducted in Asia, particularly in India (Leff, 1981; Sethi, 1986). Rates of non-psychotic depression in the community, based on surveys between 1964 and 1983, range between 0.15% to 6% (Sethi, 1986). These epidemiological studies have also revealed that depression is more common in the northern and eastern parts of the country and more common in urban than rural settings (Sethi, 1986). Sethi (1986) also comments that ideas of personal guilt, self-reproach, and suicide frequently observed in Western depressives are less frequently seen in India. Symptoms such as somatisation, frequent agitation, commonly expressed suicidal ideas and attempts, and infrequent completions of suicide attempts are the common features in Indian depressives (Sethi, 1986). Gupta *et al* (1991), in a report of a systematic study of symptoms in a sample of depressed out-patients using the cross-culturally standardised WHO–SADD interview (Jablensky *et al*, 1986) made many of the same observations about their depressed patients in summarising the epidemiological literature for India.

The older literature for Japan, Korea, and China, much like Africa and India, suggests that depression was relatively uncommon, under 1% (Kato, 1969; Lin, 1953; Lin *et al*, 1969; Nakane *et al*, 1988). More recent work suggests prevalence rates that are higher but are still below those commonly observed in the West (Nakane *et al*, 1988). In a recent study, Nakane and his colleagues (Nakane *et al*, 1988, 1991) attempted to determine diagnostic differences among Japanese, Korean, and Chinese psychiatrists and symptom differences among Japanese, Korean, and Chinese depressives. For example, they found that Korean psychiatrists were much more likely to diagnose neurotic depression relative to major depression (based on ICD–9) compared with the Japanese and Chinese psychiatrists (even when common patients were diagnosed) (Nakane *et al*, 1991). Surprisingly, Korean patients had the highest levels of depressive symptomatology indexed by the Hamilton Rating Scale for Depression (HRSD). Although there were many differences with respect to depressive symptoms across the patients from the three countries, it was difficult to interpret these differences with respect to patient, psychiatrist, or cultural factors that might have been responsible. The authors offer a number of explanations for their cross-cultural differences that include: (a) variability in the type of training received by psychiatrists in each of the countries; (b) the problem of symptom demarcation, particularly the distinction between neurotic and major depression; (c) cultural differences in openness; and (d) the varying natures of the centres where the study was completed. Interestingly, a study of Hawaiian university students of Japanese, Chinese, and Caucasian ancestry found that Asian students, particularly females, had a significantly higher prevalence of depression than Caucasians, in contrast to the relatively low rates observed in Asia (Kinzie *et al*, 1973). These findings again highlight the importance not only of one's cultural group but of one's cultural setting.

Methodological issues in cross-cultural measurement

Several methodological issues bear on the appropriate use of depression measures (clinical–diagnostic and self-report) in a cross-cultural context (Draguns, 1982; Jablensky *et al*, 1986; Marsella, 1987). For example, with respect to diagnosis, behaviours that are considered abnormal, symptoms that form the core of a disorder, and cultural meaning of symptoms may vary across cultures and reduce the validity of cross-cultural comparisons (Draguns, 1982; Littlewood, 1990). With respect to the use of rating scales and self-report measures, methodological issues include translation of instruments, conceptual equivalence of instrument items, and scale equivalence (Marsella, 1987).

Diagnosis

Abnormality or mental illness are central features of most concepts of a psychiatric diagnosis (Draguns, 1982). To an unknown degree, culture shapes what is considered be deviant or abnormal behaviour. Even within cultures, standards for deviance have changed over time. For example, in the United States the concept of mental illness has broadened considerably over the years (Draguns, 1982). It has been recognised that less severe forms of many types of psychopathology exist and although the afflicted individual may not seek treatment for the problem, personal suffering and social disability can often be observed. The extent to which these changes in perspective have occurred in other cultures over time is unclear. In non-Western cultures symptoms such as somatisation play a much more prominent role in the identification of depression (Odejide *et al*, 1989). For example, Bertschy *et al* (1992) proposed adding two symptoms to the DSM–III criteria for major depression to make them more applicable for use in black Africa: (a) aches and 'toilsome' physical sensations; and (b) ideas of persecution. Finally, given that so many symptoms of depression are subjective and cannot be objectively measured or observed, cultural influences which impinge on both the mental health specialist and the patient will be hard to detect and overcome (Draguns, 1982).

Rating scales and self-report measures

Researchers in cross-cultural psychopathology have argued that measuring symptoms in cross-cultural contexts rather than attempting diagnoses has some distinct advantages (Draguns, 1982). For example, conducting investigations at the level of symptoms rather than diagnosis decreases problems associated with variability in diagnostic terms. Also, problems associated with determining a common threshold for determination of clinical significance of symptoms in making a diagnosis are reduced. In turn, problems associated with defining the overall configuration of symptoms and the level of deviance necessary for a diagnosis are eliminated. In terms of level of abstraction, individual symptoms are closer to the experience of the individual patient than is a diagnosis of depression, which is to some degree an abstraction reflecting an understanding of the meaning of various complexes of symptoms. Focus on symptoms also serves to reduce the possibility that cultural factors affecting the expression of core symptoms of depression would lead to estimates of the prevalence of depression that may be inappropriately high or low. Despite some advantages of the use of rating scales and self-report measures of symptomatology, there are methodological problems inherent in their use as well.

Translation of an instrument is usually the first problem to be solved in cross-cultural studies of depressive symptomatology (Marsella, 1987).

For research purposes an accurate translation of an instrument into a new language requires two steps. The first step requires that a bilingual individual translates the measure into the appropriate language. The second step requires a second individual to translate the translated version back to its original language. The process is called 'back translation' (Marsella, 1987). The purpose of back translation is to ensure that the denotative and connotative meanings of the measure are not changed in translation. Unfortunately, even when the denotative meaning of a measure is preserved in translation, its connotative meaning may not be preserved. Some English words or concepts have no equivalent meaning in another language. For example, depression and anxiety do not have good equivalents in Yoruba, a Nigerian language (Leff, 1977). The words eventually chosen in a WHO study to represent depression were back translated into English as "the heart is weak" (Leff, 1977). These problems of translation are particularly acute when abstract concepts like emotions (e.g. depression and anxiety) are studied (Leff, 1977; Marsella, 1987).

The problem of connotative differences in meaning have to do with conceptual equivalence of words or constructs. Marsella (1987) gives the example of the differing meanings of dependency in Anglo-American and Japanese cultures. Whereas in traditional Anglo-American culture, dependency is associated with psychopathology, in Japanese culture, the closest equivalent term, *amae*, has no such meaning. It is highly valued because Japanese culture values group cohesion much more so than the Anglo-American ideal of individualism. These cultural differences would suggest that even an accurate translation of dependency into Japanese would convey an unintended meaning and would lack conceptual equivalence.

There are several approaches that are used to establish conceptual equivalence between measures (Marsella, 1987; Triandis, 1972). These procedures include defining the domain (e.g. through interviewing to determine what characterises depression), determining the domain's organisation (e.g. ranking or scaling characteristics of depression), analysing meaning (e.g. using semantic differential, attribute interviews), and analysing behaviour (e.g. behavioural observation and analysis) (Marsella, 1987). All of these procedures require study within the culture itself (i.e. the emic approach).

After conceptual equivalence has been established, the investigator must confront the problem of scale equivalence (Marsella, 1987). Common scale formats in the West such as Likert scales, true–false ratings, multiple choice items, and visual analogue scales that are used to quantify depressive symptomatology may be unfamiliar to the culture to which the measure is to be applied. In these cases even though the instrument may be perfectly understandable to an individual of the target culture, the options that he/she has for responding may be quite foreign, thus reducing the validity of the measure.

Measures of depression

Many depression measures developed in the US and Great Britain have been adapted for use in cross-cultural contexts (Sartorius & Ban, 1986). Moreover, investigators indigenous to other countries have developed depression measures specifically for use in their own culture. However, the vast majority of this work has been done in Western countries (e.g. Germany, France, Italy, Scandinavia).

Self-report measures

Two of the most commonly used self-report measures of depression are the Beck Depression Inventory (BDI; Beck *et al*, 1961) and the Zung Self-Rating Depression Scale (SDS; Zung, 1965). These two measures, both developed in the US, have been translated into several languages and have been used in cross-cultural research (Steer *et al*, 1986; Zung, 1986). The BDI is a 21-item self-report scale that assesses cognitive, affective, and physiological symptoms of depression. Each item is rated by the patient on a 4-point scale which ranges from absence of symptom (score of 0) to a severe level of symptom (score of 3). Numerous studies have documented the reliability of the BDI and its validity as an indicator of depression severity (Beck *et al*, 1988). In cross-cultural contexts its Spanish language version has been used extensively (Comas-Diaz, 1981; Lopez *et al*, 1976; Steer *et al*, 1986). The BDI has been translated into the languages of several other countries including Germany (Lukesh, 1974), India (Ajmany & Nandi, 1973), Denmark (Bech *et al*, 1975), and Japan (Shinfuku, 1973). Symptom levels do vary across cultural groups and cultural norms for the BDI are necessary (Steer *et al*, 1986).

The SDS is a 20-item self-report measure that assesses symptoms of depression similar to the BDI (Zung, 1986). Rather than asking the patient to rate the severity of each symptom, the SDS asks the patient to rate on a 4-point scale how much of the time during the past week the symptom was present (ranging from "None or a little of the time" to "Most or all of the time"). Like the BDI, the SDS has demonstrated reliability and validity as a measure of depression severity (Zung, 1986). Normative data for normal and depressed subjects for the SDS have been established for several countries including Australia, Czechoslovakia, England, Germany, Spain, Sweden, India, Japan, Korea, The Netherlands, and the US (Zung, 1986). Altogether the SDS has been translated into 30 languages (Zung, 1986).

Rating scales and interview schedules

Clinician-administered scales have the advantage of bringing expert judgement to bear regarding the presence and severity of depression symptomatology.

Clinician-administered scales are particularly important with patients who may be unfamiliar or not comfortable with self-report measures. The most widely used clinician-administered measure of depression severity is the Hamilton Rating Scale for Depression (HRSD; Hamilton, 1967). The HRSD contains 21 items, of which the first 17 items are counted for total severity score. The last four items describe symptoms that either occur very infrequently or describe the quality of the depression (Hamilton, 1986). The HRSD is heavily oriented toward somatic symptoms of depression, which may in part explain its popularity around the world. The reliability of the HRSD has been assessed in a large number of studies (Hamilton, 1986) and although found to be acceptable, the HRSD has been improved by the development of a structured interview in which to embed the measure (Williams, 1988). The validity of the HRSD for assessment of depression severity has also been established in a large number of studies (Hamilton, 1986). The HRSD has been widely used and validated for use in other cultural contexts and countries including Germany (Fähndrich *et al*, 1986), France (Bobon, 1986), Spain (J. J. López-Ibor & J. M. López-Ibor, 1986), Czechoslovakia (Skoda & Vinar, 1986), Scandinavia (Lingjaerde, 1986), Japan (Takahashi, 1986), Italy (Cassano *et al*, 1986), and Nigeria (Odejide, 1986).

The WHO developed a clinician-administered measure of depression symptoms to be used in cross-cultural contexts, the Schedule for Standardised Assessment of Depressive Disorders (WHO–SADD; Jablensky *et al*, 1986). The WHO–SADD includes 40 symptoms that are rated on 3-point scales (ranging from 'Absent' to 'Present, continuously or in severe form'). The measure was developed specifically to study depressive disorders in different cultures. The original sites for measure development and use included Basle (Switzerland), Montreal (Canada), Nagasaki and Tokyo (Japan), and Tehran (Iran). The measure has since been used for research purposes in several other countries including Austria, Bulgaria, Denmark, Finland, France, Germany, Ghana, India, Poland, and Great Britain (Jablensky *et al*, 1986). The WHO–SADD has many attractive features for use in cross-cultural context including systematic translation and back translation to ensure textual and semantic equivalence across versions of the measure and comparable reliability data from the different settings in which it has been used (Sartorius *et al*, 1983).

More recently, the WHO has developed the Composite International Diagnostic Interview (CIDI; Robins *et al*, 1988; Wittchen *et al*, 1991) which can be administered by lay interviewers and was designed to provide DSM–III–R and ICD–10 diagnoses of a wide range of mental disorders across cultural settings. The CIDI has been field tested in Europe, Asia, North America, South America, and Australia (Wittchen *et al*, 1991). Evidence from initial studies suggests that the CIDI is a reliable and valid diagnostic measure (Robins *et al*, 1988; Wittchen *et al*, 1991).

Nevertheless, some centres questioned the validity of some of the symptom questions and there was general concern that the interview was too long for populations that were studied (Wittchen *et al*, 1991). Despite these concerns, the WHO measures (the SADD and CIDI) stand as the best validated measures of depressive symptomatology and diagnosis for use in cross-cultural settings.

Postpartum depression in a cross-cultural context

Depression after childbirth has been identified and described in many different cultural settings. A partial listing of countries would include Great Britain, Canada, the US, Australia, Germany, France, Italy, The Netherlands, Sweden, Jamaica, Nigeria, Uganda, Japan, and India. In the United States and Great Britain postpartum depression has been defined in terms of standard psychiatric diagnostic criteria including the Research Diagnostic Criteria (Spitzer *et al*, 1978), the DSM–III and DSM–III–R (American Psychiatric Association, 1980, 1987), and the ICD–9 (World Health Organization, 1978). In general, investigators have found these widely used criteria suitable for use with childbearing women (Kumar & Robson, 1984; Cooper *et al*, 1988; Cutrona, 1983; O'Hara *et al*, 1990). Prevalence rates of postpartum depression based on these criteria have been in the 10% to 15% range (O'Hara, 1991*a*). The generalisability of these findings to other cultures will be discussed in the rest of this section.

Several reviews of the literature on the cross-cultural expression of postpartum depression by anthropologists and psychiatrists have been published (Bågedahl-Strindlund, 1992; Cox, 1988; Harkness, 1987; Jansson, 1987; Stern & Kruckman, 1983). Anthropologists (Harkness, 1987; Stern & Kruckman, 1983) argue that postpartum depression may be a culture-bound phenomenon peculiar to the West, much like *Amakiro* (a form of puerperal mental illness) is peculiar to the Baganda of Uganda (Cox, 1988). One of the first formulations of this perspective on postpartum depression was offered by Stern & Kruckman (1983), who argued that the anthropological ethnographic literature on childbirth shows little evidence of the phenomenon of postpartum depression. They identified six elements in the social structuring of the postpartum period common to non-Western cultures, some of which may be missing in modern Western cultures. These include (1) cultural patterning of a distinct postpartum period; (2) protective measures designed to reflect the vulnerability of the new mother; (3) social seclusion; (4) mandated rest; (5) assistance in tasks from relatives and/or midwife; and (6) social recognition of new social status (Stern & Kruckman, 1983). They argue that elements of these common patterns are missing in the US (and perhaps Great Britain) and that postpartum depression may result particularly from a lack of: (a) social structuring of postpartum events;

(b) social recognition of the role transition for the new mother; and (c) instrumental support and aid for the new mother (Stern & Kruckman, 1983).

Harkness (1987) came to very much the same conclusion as Stern & Kruckman (1983) in her study of the Kipsigis people of Kenya. She found that even though there were modern elements in the village life of these people, the practices surrounding childbirth were very traditional. Based on her discussions with informants and her own study of the dreams of ten childbearing women, she found no evidence of postpartum depression. Interestingly, she did observe that women tended to have more negative dreams during pregnancy, a finding not inconsistent with the observation of higher levels of depressive symptoms of Western women during pregnancy relative to the puerperium (O'Hara *et al*, 1990). The more general thrust of the argument of these anthropologists is that the aetiology of postpartum depression must be more in the social than in the psychological or hormonal realm because of the importance of cultural differences in the prevalence and the expression of postpartum depression.

In reviewing very much the same literature as the anthropologists, psychiatrists have come to somewhat different conclusions. Cox (1988, p. 82) noted: "However it has been shown that this disorder is not restricted to a specific cultural context, and cannot therefore be construed as a cultural artefact, universal sociocultural norms (i.e. similarities) cannot be neglected nor biological factors ignored." Bågedahl-Strindlund (1992, p. 7) similarly observed: "The general impression from the review of the literature is that there are no great differences in the frequency of severe postpartum mental disorders throughout the world. Symptomatologically, the trend seems to be that differences are diminishing." Finally, Jansson (1987, p. 23) concurred: "My general impression of the literature review is that there are no great differences as regards the frequency of mental disorders postpartum throughout the world. Symptomatological differences follow the pattern seen in mental disorders in general." In fairness to the anthropological perspective, each of these authors acknowledges the importance of studying cultural factors in the aetiology of postpartum depression; however, none of them accept the view that postpartum depression is essentially a culture-bound disorder peculiar to the West.

Several anthropological studies are commonly cited as providing evidence for the relative lack of postpartum depression in many non-Western cultures. For example, Pillsbury (1978) in research on the postpartum period (called 'doing the month') in China found no evidence of postpartum depression. He observed that during the first month postpartum Chinese mothers are lavished with attention, much more so than is the infant. He argued that this attention (i.e. social support from family and friends) acted to prevent the development of depression. It also stands in contrast to Western postpartum customs that focus attention on the baby more than the mother.

Kelly (1967) studied the obstetric practices of the Ibibio people of Nigeria and found little evidence of postpartum depression, which he attributed to their postpartum customs. For example, the new mother and baby are placed in a special hut, a 'fattening room', where they are secluded and attended to by the woman's mother for several months. Other anthropological studies also make very similar observations about childbearing practices in non-Western cultures (Jansson, 1987; Stern & Kruckman, 1983).

Many of the practices observed in traditional non-Western cultures regarding postpartum care and support of the mother are present in Japanese culture (Shimizu & Kaplan, 1987). For example, Japanese women often go to the home of their parents for about a month after delivery, where the family provides care for the mother and baby. Also, Japanese women are not as likely to be employed as American women and as a consequence they are under less pressure to arrange for alternative child-care for their child (Shimuzu & Kaplan, 1987). One early Japanese study revealed that postpartum women did not differ much from non-childbearing controls with respect to sadness on an adjective checklist (Murai *et al*, 1978). The investigators concluded that postpartum depression did not exist in Japan. To follow up this finding, Shimuzu & Kaplan (1987) compared 29 Japanese women (from Osaka) and 21 American women (from New York City) using Pitt's (1968) postpartum depression scale. The measures were translated into Japanese and back translated to ensure comparability. The authors predicted that Japanese women would have lower levels of postpartum depressive symptoms and would experience less social isolation after delivery. Contrary to their expectations, there were no differences between the American and Japanese women at four to six weeks postpartum with respect to either of these factors. The study's small sample size may have contributed to the lack of significant differences between the two populations. Nevertheless, further cross-cultural work of this sort is certainly indicated.

It should not be surprising that there is little evidence of postpartum depression in non-Western cultures. Despite the fact that postpartum psychosis has been recognised throughout the history of medicine (Turnbull, 1969), the identification of postpartum depression has had a much more recent origin. Although others had recognised postpartum depression earlier, Pitt's (1968) work can be credited with spurring a great deal of research on postpartum depression in Great Britain and the United States. A very large number of systematic studies assessing depressive symptomatology and determining the occurrence of the syndrome of depression in the puerperium presented converging evidence that depression (defined in various ways) was present in the puerperium and that its prevalence was probably in the range of 10% to 20% (O'Hara, 1991*a*; O'Hara & Zekoski, 1988). Very little systematic study of postpartum depression has occurred in non-Western cultures. Cox's (1979, 1983) pioneering work in Uganda is an outstanding exception. He found that among women of the Ganda tribe in Uganda ($n = 183$) 10% experienced a postpartum depression based on the ICD–8 criteria for depression. Using similar methods he found that 13% of Scottish women experienced a postpartum depression and argued that postpartum depression rates were similar in these two very dissimilar cultures (Cox, 1982, 1983). The major symptomatic difference between the African and Scottish women was that the African women reported much less guilt and self-blame than the Scottish women, a phenomenon observed in non-childbearing Africans as well (Odejide, 1986).

A more recent prospective study of postpartum depression included a large sample of Yoruba women from Nigeria (Jinadu & Daramola, 1990). The investigators developed their own measure of psychological complaints and included symptoms such as insomnia, anorexia, 'feeling hot-in-the-head', palpitations, awareness of increased tension and anxiety, apprehension, guilt, and nausea/vomiting. They did not attempt to diagnose depression in their subjects ($n = 348$). The investigators found that symptoms were significantly more common during pregnancy than after delivery. Nausea/vomiting and 'heat in-the-head' were the most common symptoms during pregnancy and insomnia and 'heat in-the-head' were the most common symptoms after delivery. The authors asserted that the proportion of women experiencing psychological complaints was less than that reported in the West; however, the lack of comparability between their measures and measures used in Western studies make judgements about differences in prevalence rates tenuous at best.

The final study to be discussed in this section was done in England, comparing recently delivered non-English speaking Bengali immigrants to England, a heterogeneous group of English speaking immigrants, and indigenous English women (Watson & Evans, 1986). The General Health Questionnaire (GHQ; Goldberg, 1972), interviewer judgement, and personal judgement were used to determine depression in this sample. The authors noted that some of the GHQ questions were not meaningful to the Bengali women. Despite the authors' argument that roughly the same amount of depression was observed in each of the three groups of women, there was a high level of disagreement among the three measures of depression. For example, the kappa values (reflecting agreement between the various measures) for agreement between the interviewers and the women with respect to the presence of depression ranged between 0.23 and 0.38 at the first assessment and between 0.36 and 0.54 at the second assessment. These relatively low rates of agreement make it difficult to determine the extent to which cultural differences may have affected the expression or prevalence of depression in these recently delivered women.

EPDS in cross-cultural settings

The literature on postpartum depression in non-Western cultures points to the importance of systematic and comparable surveys of postpartum depressive symptomatology and the determination of rates of diagnosed postpartum depression cross-culturally. The World Health Organization has carried out major cross-cultural studies of depression (Sartorius *et al*, 1983). Although large-scale systematic cross-cultural studies of postpartum depression probably are not feasible, the use of comparable methods of depression assessment by international investigators would certainly advance our understanding of the prevalence and expression of postpartum depression around the world. Earlier in this chapter I briefly discussed some of the depression measures that have been commonly used in cross-cultural work on depression. Certainly, when it comes to establishing depression diagnoses in cross-cultural studies, the WHO–SADD has much to recommend it (Jablensky *et al*, 1986). It was specifically developed to be used in cross-cultural research and it has good psychometric characteristics (Jablensky *et al*, 1986). In addition to its original use in Switzerland, Canada, Japan and Iran, it has also been used in Austria, Bulgaria, Denmark, Finland, France, Germany, Ghana, India, Poland, and the United Kingdom. It is currently available in at least 10 languages (Jablensky *et al*, 1986).

Although the Beck Depression Inventory (Beck *et al*, 1961) and the Zung Self-Rating Depression Scale (Zung, 1965) are widely used in cross-cultural research, they may not be the preferred measures for systematic studies of postpartum depressive symptomatology or for use as screening measures in postpartum depression research (Harris *et al*, 1989). For example, 7 of 21 items on the BDI refer to somatic symptoms of depression. Given the normal physiological changes that accompany pregnancy and childbirth (e.g. changes in appetite, sleep, energy), the BDI may not be ideally suited for use during the puerperium (O'Hara *et al*, 1990). Moreover, the sensitivity and specificity of the BDI for identifying postpartum depressed women meeting the Research Diagnostic Criteria are relatively low (Harris *et al*, 1989; O'Hara *et al*, 1984). The Zung SDS has been used much less frequently than the BDI in postpartum depression research; however, it too has a number of somatic items and may suffer from some of the same problems as the BDI.

The Edinburgh Postnatal Depression Scale (Cox *et al*, 1987) was developed specifically for use with childbearing women. Other chapters in this volume describe its development and use in a number of settings and for a number of purposes. Because of its demonstrated reliability and validity as a screening measure for postpartum depression with British women (Cox *et al*, 1987; Harris *et al*, 1989; Murray & Carothers, 1990), a consideration of its use in cross-cultural settings is indicated. Two major purposes could be served by the use of the EPDS in cross-cultural settings and they generally reflect the etic and emic approaches to the cross-cultural study of psychopathology. First, the EPDS could be an important epidemiological tool for comparing rates of postpartum depression cross-culturally. There is still a great deal of debate, as I suggested earlier, regarding the extent to which rates of depression vary across cultures. As has been suggested by anthropologists (Stern & Kruckman, 1983), differences in rates of depression across cultures that have very different social organisations may provide clues to the aetiology of the disorder. Second, the EPDS could be useful to indigenous clinicians and researchers who are interested in: (a) determining the prevalence of postpartum depression in their own communities; (b) identifying women at risk or women who are depressed; and (c) providing care for depressed women.

The importance of cross-cultural conceptual and scale comparability for these two purposes is quite different. To the extent that an investigator must measure postpartum depression in the same way across cultures (i.e. for cross-cultural epidemiological research), conceptual and scale comparability are important (Marsella, 1987). However, for the clinician or investigator who is interested in using a measure within a particular culture (e.g. for screening or measurement purposes), and does not wish to generalise results of these investigations to other cultures, issues of conceptual and scale equivalence – and translation fidelity, for that matter – are less important.

The EPDS has been used in a number of countries outside Great Britain, including the United States, Australia, Iceland, Sweden, and The Netherlands. It has also been translated into Spanish, Italian, Portuguese, French, Hebrew, and Greek (see Appendix, pp. 248–270, which gives most of the available translations of the EPDS). There is little evidence that the EPDS has yet been used in Africa, Asia, South America, or central and eastern Europe. Nevertheless, it is appropriate to examine the small literature available that bears on the cross-cultural use of the EPDS.

Scandinavian and Nordic countries

Although Swedish investigators have been active in the study of postpartum mental illness (Nilsson, 1970; Uddenberg, 1974; McNeil, 1986), Swedish approaches to measuring and diagnosing postpartum depression have not been comparable to those approaches used in the US and Great Britain. As a consequence, it has been difficult to compare rates of postpartum depression in Sweden to those in other countries. Recently, Lundh & Gyllang (1993) adapted the EPDS for use in Sweden. The EPDS was to be used to identify recently delivered women in primary care settings who might be depressed. The investigators were also interested in comparing rates of postpartum depression in Sweden to rates in other countries. The EPDS was translated into Swedish by the investigators under the supervision of a professional translator. The translator was also involved in translating the EPDS back to English. The authors did not comment on the conceptual or scale equivalence of the Swedish and English versions of the EPDS; however, there is no indication in their report that women had any difficulty comprehending or completing the measure (Lundh & Gyllang, 1993). The EPDS was validated for a Swedish population by administering it to a sample of 53 mothers who were also rated on the Comprehensive Psychopathological Rating Scale, a psychopathology rating scale commonly used in Sweden and commonly used in cross-cultural research (Perris, 1986). Although the investigators did not report the correlation between the two measures, an inspection of the plot of the subjects' scores on the two measures indicated that they were positively correlated at a reasonable level.

The participants in the study were 258 women, roughly half of whom were primiparous. Women came from two communities, one a small city and the other a rural setting. Subjects completed the EPDS on four occasions, two weeks, six weeks, three months, and eight to nine months postpartum. The investigators found that 26% of the women at two weeks postpartum, 8% at six weeks postpartum, 13% at three months postpartum, and 8% at eight to nine months postpartum had EPDS scores above the cut-off score of nine. It should be noted that the authors did not report any data regarding the sensitivity or specificity of the EPDS for identifying postpartum depressed women (based on diagnostic criteria). Overall, the investigators concluded that the EPDS was an easily administered and useful self-report measure for screening recently delivered women in primary care settings.

Thome (1991) studied 200 women from three health centres in the Greater Reykjavik, Iceland, area. The EPDS was translated into Icelandic by the author and back translated to English by a native English speaker (American) unfamiliar with the measure. Corrections to the Icelandic version were made by the author. Thome indicated that several of the items (numbers 3, 4, 7 & 9 – see pp. 139, 140) were problematic when translated into Icelandic. The author observed that two of the items (7 & 9) began with "I have been so unhappy". Evidently, the similarity in the two items made for difficulty in translation. Thome suggested that these two items eliminate the "I have been so unhappy" and just ask about difficulty in sleeping (no. 7) and crying (no. 9). The author also observed that for item 3 some mothers blame themselves for reasons not related to things that went wrong. Finally, the author indicated that on items 4 and 5 many of the mothers named good reasons for being anxious or worried or panicky. However, Thome did not suggest revisions for these latter two items.

Women participating in the study had an average age of 28.8; 31% were primiparous, 55.7% were married and 38.8% were cohabiting. Women completed the EPDS between 7 and 8 weeks postpartum and women who scored greater than 9 were re-tested at three and six months postpartum. Thome reported that the Icelandic version of the EPDS was reliable ($\alpha = 0.80$). Thome also reported that 24% of the women scored 9 or above at two months postpartum (9% scored ≥ 12) (mean EPDS = 6.0; s.d. = 3.9).

Over half of these women scored either a 9 or a 10. These women (EPDS ≥9) were greatly improved by the 3 months postpartum. Thome argued that a cut-off of 12 works well to distinguish mothers with more severe and long-term distress from mothers who suffer from short-term and milder distress. One indication of the EPDS's validity according to Thome was that in the majority of the cases women scoring at 9 or greater attributed their distress to life stressors or anxiety (i.e. they could identify some cause for their distress). Interestingly, in only five cases was depression identified by the women as the cause of their postpartum distress. However, it should be noted that a clinical assessment was not done with these women so that the proportion of women with high scores on the EPDS who would have met clinical criteria for depression is unknown.

Europe

The psychometric characteristics and the concurrent validity of the EPDS were also evaluated in The Netherlands, the only non-British European setting (Pop *et al*, 1992). The authors translated the EPDS into Dutch and it was translated back into English by a native English speaker. According to the authors there were no important differences between the original and translated versions. The EPDS and several other measures already validated for use with Dutch women (i.e. the Zung SDS, the BDI, the Symptom Checklist 90 depression subscale, and the Dutch version of the DACL) were administered to 303 women who lived in a town in the southern part of The Netherlands. The mean EPDS score for these women was 5.89 (s.d. = 4.03). The internal consistency of the measure was adequate ($\alpha = 0.80$). Also, the EPDS was significantly correlated with the other depression measures ($r = 0.57$ to 0.69, $P < 0.001$). The authors reported that their subjects had no trouble in completing the EPDS in contrast to the 12% of subjects who complained about the difficulty of the BDI. In summary, the authors argue that the EPDS is an excellent self-report scale for assessing depressive symptoms in the postpartum period.

Australia

Boyce and his colleagues have conducted several studies relevant to the use of the EPDS in Australia (Boyce, 1991; Boyce *et al*, 1991). They surveyed community users of the EPDS and found that in clinical settings it is used as a screening and assessment instrument and as a measure of change (Boyce *et al*, 1991). In research settings it is also being used as a measure of change and as an epidemiological tool. The authors indicated that the most usual cut-off score used by their respondents was 12/13, the cut-off recommended by Cox *et al* (1987). Finally, the authors note that the EPDS is well accepted by clinicians, researchers, and mothers. Boyce *et al* (1991) also conducted a study of 98 women from the Sydney area within six months of delivery who completed the EPDS and were administered the Diagnostic Interview Schedule (Robins *et al*, 1981) to assess DSM–III–R major depression. They found that the EPDS was internally consistent ($\alpha = 0.92$) and that the mean EPDS was 6.2 (s.d. = 5.1). Based on logistic regression using the DSM–III–R criterion of major depression, the authors found that the 12/13 cut-off on the EPDS was associated the highest probability of being a DSM–III–R case. In predicting DSM–III–R major depression, this cut-off had a sensitivity of 100%, a specificity of 96%, and a positive predictive value of 67%. The level of agreement between the EPDS and DSM–III–R diagnosis was 96% (kappa = 0.78).

Boyce (1991) compared the EPDS and the BDI as measures of postpartum depressive symptomatology among 161 women who were evaluated at one, three, and six months postpartum. Using a 12/13 cut-off on the EPDS and a 13/14 cut-off on the BDI, Boyce found that 11.8%, 9.9%, and 7.7% of women based on the EPDS and 10.8%, 8.4%, and 9.6% of women based on the BDI had scores above the measures' respective cut-offs at one, three, and six months postpartum. The percentage agreement between the two instruments with respect to caseness (of postpartum depression) defined by scale cut-offs ranged from 91% to 96%. Boyce observed that the highest level of agreement between the two measures was obtained at the six-month assessment and suggested that physiological symptoms which might affect BDI scores (the BDI has 7 items reflecting somatic symptoms) are much less common than earlier in the puerperium.

North America

The final study to be reviewed in this section was completed by my group at the University of Iowa in the United States (O'Hara, 1991b). We screened 193 women at approximately one month postpartum. Measures included the EPDS and the Inventory to Diagnose Depression (IDD; Zimmerman *et al*, 1986) which was designed and validated (Zimmerman & Coryell, 1988) to identify individuals meeting DSM–III criteria for major depression. Also, a subsample of women ($n = 36$) who met and did not meet depression criteria on the IDD were interviewed to determine whether or not they met the Research Diagnostic Criteria (Spitzer *et al*, 1978) for major or minor depression. Roughly 37% of subjects were having their first child; the mean age of subjects was about 29 and all were married. The mean EPDS score was 6.93 (s.d. = 4.55) and 11.9% of subjects scored above the 12/13 cut-off. The IDD identified 15.5% of subjects as depressed. The association between the EPDS and the IDD with respect to depression caseness was significant. The IDD and the EPDS agreed on 89% of cases. A total of 36 of the 193 women participated in a diagnostic interview to determine major and minor depression. The EPDS and the diagnostic interview agreed on 86% of cases. The sensitivity of the EPDS was 72%, its specificity was 100%, and its positive predictive value was 100%. These findings provide support for the reliability and validity of the EPDS for use in the United States.

Summary and recommendations

The EPDS has gained increasing acceptance in Great Britain as a screening measure for postpartum depression. As other authors in this volume have described (see Cox, Chapter 8), the EPDS is reliable and valid as a screening instrument. Moreover, its reasonably high sensitivity, specificity, and positive predictive value in identifying depressed women make it useful to the clinician and researcher alike. Much less work with the EPDS has been done in centres outside Great Britain. The work that I have reviewed is largely unpublished and although the results of these studies are promising regarding the usefulness of the EPDS in non-English cultures, the cross-cultural work is still at a very preliminary stage. A second feature of the cross-cultural work with the EPDS is that it has been done almost entirely in Western countries and cultures. The issues that I reviewed regarding the cross-cultural expression and measurement of depression and postpartum depression, in particular, should give researchers and clinicians pause before they introduce the EPDS into non-Western cultures. It is clear that an adequate translation of the EPDS will not be enough. Some of the problems noted by Thome in her translation of the EPDS into Icelandic give testimony to the potential problems that may occur in African, Asian, and possibly in Latin cultures.

An enormous amount of cross-cultural research on depression and other disorders has been and currently is being conducted. Certainly, over the past two decades the work of the World Health Organization to organise large-scale cross-cultural epidemiological studies of mental illness that are culturally informed and that take into account the sensitivities of indigenous investigators is to be applauded. However, an implicit assumption of much of this work seems to be that diagnostic systems originated in the West (i.e. DSM–III–R and ICD–10) are sufficient to characterise mental illness in non-Western cultures. Recent epidemiological research would seem to confirm this view. For example, Sartorius *et al* (1983) were able to identify a core of symptoms which characterised depressives in Japan, Iran, Switzerland, and Canada. Nevertheless, the perspective of the 'new cross-cultural psychiatry' (Leff, 1990; Littlewood, 1990) would suggest that insufficient attention is given to the cultural context in which mental disorders arise and are identified. This perspective argues that careful observation of mental disorder from within a culture is necessary to establish its presence,

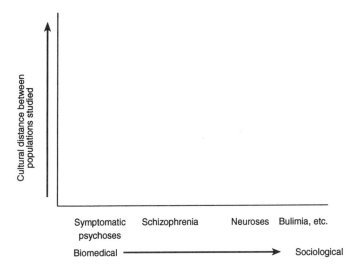

Fig. 10.1. Criteria for judging cross-cultural studies (adapted from Leff, 1990, reproduced with permission)

definition, and community response (Littlewood, 1990). Very little of this type of work has occurred in the cross-cultural study of depression.

The essential argument of the 'new cross-cultural psychiatry' is that cultural factors are particularly important in mental illness, including depression. However, it has also been argued that to the extent to which a disorder is biologically driven (smallpox being a clear example) the effect of culture is diminished (Leff, 1990; Littlewood, 1990). Disorders such as schizophrenia and perhaps bipolar depression and psychotic unipolar depression, may be less coloured by cultural factors than non-psychotic depression and most importantly, postpartum depression. Both Leff and Littlewood argue that it is important to consider the extent to which a disorder is likely to have a biological aetiology versus a social aetiology. Leff also suggests that it is important to consider the cultural distance between populations being studied. Figure 10.1, adapted from Leff (1990), illustrates this issue well. What Leff argues is that cross-cultural studies that fall into the upper-right-hand quadrant of the graph and that do not take into account indigenous belief systems would probably be fatally flawed. The greater the likely social aetiology and the greater the cultural distance between the two groups being studied, the more important it is to study the indigenous culture and the people most likely to experience the disorder being considered (Leff, 1990). I have mentioned some relevant strategies recommended by Marsella (1987) for establishing conceptual equivalence between measures earlier in this chapter.

Postpartum psychoses, as an example, would probably fall on the biomedical end of the continuum shown in the figure, somewhat reducing the need for a cross-cultural perspective. However, postpartum depression and the blues would probably fall more toward the social end of the continuum and, if African or Asian populations were being studied, this work would fall into the upper-right-hand quadrant of Figure 10.1. This analysis suggests that postpartum depression research done in other cultures, particularly non-Western ones, must be culturally informed. Obviously, studies of the EPDS in other cultures will also need to take cognizance of the cultural understanding of childbirth and its consequences for both mother and child.

References

AJMANY, S. & NANDI, D. N. (1973) Adaptation of A. T. Beck's *et al*'s An inventory for measuring depression. *Indian Journal of Psychiatry*, **15**, 386–390.

AL-ISSA, I. (1982) Does culture make a difference in psychopathology? In *Culture and Psychopathology* (ed. I. Al-Issa), pp. 3–32. Baltimore: University Park Press.

AMERICAN PSYCHIATRIC ASSOCIATION (1980) *Diagnostic and Statistical Manual of Mental Disorders* (3rd edn) (DSM–III). Washington, DC: American Psychiatric Association.

—— (1987) *Diagnostic and Statistical Manual of Mental Disorders* (3rd edn, revised) (DSM–III–R). Washington, DC: American Psychiatric Association.

BÅGEDAHL-STRINDLUND, M. (1992) Postpartum mental illness: Cross-cultural and social anthropological aspects – a review. In *Reproductive Life* (eds K. Wijma & B. von Schoultz). Carnforth, Lancs: The Parthenon Publishing Group.

BECH, P., DEIN, E., JACOBSEN, O., *et al* (1975) Correlation between clinical assessment, Beck's self-rating scale and Hamilton's objective rating scale. *Acta Psychiatrica Scandinavica*, **51**, 161–170.

BECK, A. T., WARD, C. H., MENDELSON, M., *et al* (1961) An inventory for measuring depression. *Archives of General Psychiatry*, **4**, 561–569.

——, STEER, R. A. & GARBIN, M. G. (1988) Psychometric properties of the Beck Depression Inventory: Twenty-five years of evaluation. *Clinical Psychology Review*, **8**, 77–100.

BERTSCHY, G., VIEL, J. F. & AHYI, R. G. (1992) Depression in Benin: An assessment using the Comprehensive Psychopathological Rating Scale and the principal component analysis. *Journal of Affective Disorders*, **25**, 173–180.

BOBON, D. (1986) Systems and scales for the assessment of depression in French-speaking countries. In *Assessment of Depression* (eds N. Sartorius & T. A. Ban), pp. 9–18. Berlin: Springer-Verlag.

BOYCE, P. (1991) *Limitations and Use of the Edinburgh Postnatal Depression Scale and Beck Depression Inventory in Postnatal Depression*. Paper presented at the conference on Prevention of Depression After Childbirth: Use and Misuse of the Edinburgh Postnatal Depression Scale, University of Keele, Staffordshire, UK.

——, STUBBS, J. & TODD, A. (1991) *The Use and Validation of the Edinburgh Postnatal Depression Scale in Australia*. Paper presented at the conference on Prevention of Depression After Childbirth: Use and Misuse of the Edinburgh Postnatal Depression Scale, University of Keele, Staffordshire, UK.

CASSANO, G. B., CASTROGIOVANNI, P. & RAMPELLO, E. (1986) Rating scales for depression in Italy. In *Assessment of Depression* (eds N. Sartorius & T. A. Ban), pp. 46–54. Berlin: Springer-Verlag.

COMAS-DIAZ, L. (1981) Effects of cognitive and behavioral group treatment on the depressive symptomatology of Puerto Rico women. *Journal of Consulting and Clinical Psychology*, **49**, 627–632.

COOPER, P. J., CAMPBELL, E. A., DAY, A., *et al* (1988) Non-psychotic psychiatric disorder after childbirth: A prospective study of prevalence, incidence, course and nature. *British Journal of Psychiatry*, **152**, 799–806.

COX, J. L. (1979) Psychiatric morbidity and pregnancy: A controlled study of 263 semi-rural Ugandan women. *British Journal of Psychiatry*, **134**, 401–405.

—— (1983) Postnatal depression: A comparison of African and Scottish women. *Social Psychiatry*, **18**, 25–28.

—— (1988) Childbirth as a life event: sociocultural aspects of postnatal depression. *Acta Psychiatrica Scandinavica*, **78** (suppl. 344), 75–83.

——, CONNOR, Y. & KENDELL, R. E. (1982) Prospective study of the psychiatric disorders of childbirth. *British Journal of Psychiatry*, **140**, 111–117.

——, HOLDEN, J. M. & SAGOVSKY, R. (1987) Detection of postnatal depression: Development of the 10-item Edinburgh Postnatal Depression Scale. *British Journal of Psychiatry*, **150**, 782–786.

CUTRONA, C. E. (1983) Causal attributions and perinatal depression. *Journal of Abnormal Psychology*, **92**, 161–172.

DRAGUNS, J. G. (1982) Methodology in cross-cultural psychopathology. In *Culture and Psychopathology* (ed. I. Al-Issa), pp. 33–70. Baltimore: University Park Press.

ENGELSMANN, F. (1982) Culture and depression. In *Culture and Psychopathology* (ed. I. Al-Issa), pp. 251–276. Baltimore: University Park Press.

FÄHNDRICH, E., HELMCHEN, H. & LINDEN, M. (1986) Standardized instruments used in the assessment of depression in German-speaking countries. In *Assessment of Depression* (eds N. Sartorius & T. A. Ban), pp. 1–8. Berlin: Springer-Verlag.

GOLDBERG, D. (1972) *The Detection of Psychiatric Illness by Questionnaire*. Oxford: Oxford University Press.

GUPTA, R., SINGH, P., VERMA, S., *et al* (1991) Standardized assessment of depressive disorders: A replicated study from northern India. *Acta Psychiatrica Scandinavica*, **84**, 310–312.

HAMILTON, M. A. (1967) Development of a rating scale for primary depressive illness. *British Journal of Social and Clinical Psychology*, **6**, 278–296.

—— (1986) The Hamilton Rating Scale for Depression. In *Assessment of Depression* (eds N. Sartorius & T. A. Ban), pp. 143–152. Berlin: Springer-Verlag.

HARKNESS, S. (1987) The cultural mediation of postpartum depression. *Medical Anthropology Quarterly*, **1**, 194–209.

HARRIS, B., JOHNS, S., FUNG, H., *et al* (1989) The hormonal environment of post-natal depression. *British Journal of Psychiatry*, **154**, 660–667.

HOLLIFIELD, M., KATON, W., SPAIN, D., *et al* (1990) Anxiety and depression in a village in Lesotho, Africa: A comparison with the United States. *British Journal of Psychiatry*, **156**, 343–350.

JABLENSKY, A., SARTORIUS, N., GULBINAT, W., *et al* (1986) The WHO instruments for the assessment of depressive disorders. In *Assessment of Depression* (eds N. Sartorius & T. A. Ban), pp. 61–81. Berlin: Springer-Verlag.

JANSSON, B. (1987) Post-partum mental disorder + transcultural aspects. *Marcé Society Bulletin*, 18–26.

JINADU, M. K. & DARAMOLA, S. M. (1990) Emotional changes in pregnancy and early puerperium among the Yoruba women of Nigeria. *International Journal of Social Psychiatry*, **36**, 93–98.

KATO, M. (1969) Psychiatric epidemiological surveys in Japan: The problem of case finding. In *Mental Health Research in Asia and the Pacific* (eds W. Caudill & T. Lin). Honolulu: University of Hawaii Press.

KELLY, J. V. (1967) The influence of native customs on obstetrics in Nigeria. *Obstetrics and Gynecology*, **30**, 608–612.

KINZIE, J., RYALS, J., COTTINGTON, F., *et al* (1973) Cross-cultural study of depressive symptoms in Hawaii. *International Journal of Social Psychiatry*, **19**, 19–24.

KLUCKHOHN, C. & KROEBER, A. (1952) *Culture*. New York: Vintage Press.

KUMAR, R. & ROBSON, K. M. (1984) A prospective study of emotional disorders in childbearing women. *British Journal of Psychiatry*, **144**, 35–47.

LAUBSCHER, B. J. F. (1937) *Sex, Custom, and Psychopathology: A Study of South African Pagan Natives.* London: Routledge & Kegan Paul.

LEFF, J. (1977) The cross-cultural study of emotions. *Culture, Medicine, and Psychiatry*, **1**, 317–350.

—— (1981) *Psychiatry Around the Globe: A Transcultural View.* New York: Marcel Dekker.

—— (1990) The 'new cross-cultural psychiatry': A case of the baby and the bathwater. *British Journal of Psychiatry*, **156**, 305–307.

LEIGHTON, A. H., LAMBO, T. A., HUGHES, C. C., et al (1963) *Psychiatric Disorder Among the Yoruba.* New York: Cornell University Press.

LIN, T. Y. (1953) A study of the incidence of mental disorders in Chinese and other cultures. *Psychiatry*, **16**, 313–336.

——, RIN, H., YEH, E., et al (1969) Mental disorders in Taiwan fifteen years later: A preliminary report. In *Mental Health Research in Asia and the Pacific* (eds W. Caudill & T. Lin). Honolulu: University of Hawaii Press.

LINGJAERDE, O. (1986) Standardized instruments used in the assessment of depression in the Scandinavian countries. In *Assessment of Depression* (eds N. Sartorius & T. A. Ban), pp. 30–35. Berlin: Springer-Verlag.

LITTLEWOOD, R. (1990) From categories to contexts: A decade of the 'new cross-cultural psychiatry'. *British Journal of Psychiatry*, **156**, 308–327.

LOPEZ, V. C., CHAMORRO, T. E. & SERRANO, E. U. (1976) Critical review of the Spanish adaptation of the Beck Questionnaire. *Revista de Psicología General y Aplicada*, **31**, 469–497.

LÓPEZ-IBOR, J. J., JR. & LÓPEZ-IBOR, J. M. (1986) Standardized instruments for the evaluation of affective disturbances in Spain and Spanish-speaking countries. In *Assessment of Depression* (eds N. Sartorius & T. A. Ban), pp. 19–22. Berlin: Springer-Verlag.

LUKESH, H. (1974) Test criteria of the depression inventory of A. T. Beck. *Psychologische Praxis (Basel)*, **18**, 60–78.

LUNDH, W. & GYLLANG, C. (1993) Use of the Edinburgh Postnatal Depression Scale in some Swedish child health care centres. *Scandinavian Journal of Caring Sciences*, **1**, 149–154.

MARSELLA, A. J. (1987) The measurement of depressive experience and disorder across cultures. In *The Measurement of Depression* (eds A. J. Marsella, R. M. A. Hirschfeld & M. M. Katz). Chichester: John Wiley.

MCNEIL, T. F. (1986) A prospective study of postpartum psychoses in a high-risk group. 1. Clinical characteristics of the current postpartum episodes. *Acta Psychiatrica Scandinavica*, **74**, 205–216.

MURAI, N., MURAI, N. & TAKAHASHI, I. (1978) A study of moods in postpartum women. *Tohoku Psycholgica Folia*, **37**, 32–40.

MURRAY, L. & CAROTHERS, A. D. (1990) The validation of the Edinburgh Postnatal Depression Scale on a community sample. *British Journal of Psychiatry*, **157**, 288–290.

NAKANE, Y., OHTA, Y., UCHINO, J., et al (1988) Comparative study of affective disorders in three Asian countries. I. Differences in diagnostic classification. *Acta Psychiatrica Scandinavica*, **78**, 698–705.

——, ——, RADFORD, M., et al (1991) Comparative study of affective disorders in three Asian countries. II. Differences in prevalence rates and symptom presentation. *Acta Psychiatrica Scandinavica*, **84**, 313–319.

NILSSON, A. (1970) Para-natal emotional adjustment: A prospective study of 165 women, Part I. *Acta Psychiatrica Scandinavica* (suppl. 220), 1–61.

ODEJIDE, A. O. (1986) Standard instruments used in the assessment of depression in Africa. In *Assessment of Depression* (eds N. Sartorius & T. A. Ban), pp. 55–60. Berlin: Springer-Verlag.

——, OYEWUNMI, L. K. & OHAERI, J. U. (1989) Psychiatry in Africa: An overview. *American Journal of Psychiatry*, **146**, 708–716.

O'HARA, M. W. (1991a) Postpartum mental disorders. In *Gynecology and Obstetrics* (eds. J. J. Sciarra), Volume 6, Chapter 84. Philadelphia: Harper & Row.

—— (1991b) *The Use of the Edinburgh Postnatal Depression Scale With a U.S. Sample.* Paper presented at the conference on Prevention of Depression After Childbirth: Use and Misuse of the Edinburgh Postnatal Depression Scale, University of Keele, Staffordshire, England.

——, NEUNABER, D. J. & ZEKOSKI, E. M. (1984) A prospective study of postpartum depression: Prevalence, course, and predictive factors. *Journal of Abnormal Psychology*, **93**, 158–171.

—— & ZEKOSKI, E. M. (1988) Postpartum depression: A comprehensive review. In *Motherhood and Mental Illness 2 Causes and Consequences* (eds R. Kumar & I. F. Brockington), pp. 17–63. London: Wright.

——, ——, PHILIPPS, L. H., *et al* (1990) A controlled prospective study of postpartum mood disorders: Comparison of childbearing and nonchildbearing women. *Journal of Abnormal Psychology*, **99**, 3–15.

ORLEY, J. & WING, J. K. (1979) Psychiatric disorders in two African villages. *Archives of General Psychiatry*, **36**, 513–520.

PERRIS, C. (1986) Rating of depression with a subscale of the CPRS. In *Assessment of Depression* (eds N. Sartorius & T. A. Ban), pp. 90–107. Berlin: Springer-Verlag.

PILLSBURY, B. L. K. (1978) 'Doing the month': Confinement and convalescence in Chinese women after childbirth. *Social Science and Medicine*, **12**, 11–22.

PITT, B. (1968) 'Atypical' depression following childbirth. *British Journal of Psychiatry*, **114**, 1325–1335.

POP, V. J., KOMPROE, I. H. & VAN SON M. J. (1992) Characteristics of the Edinburgh Postnatal Depression Scale in the Netherlands. *Journal of Affective Disorders*, **26**, 105–110.

ROBINS, L. N., HELZER, J. E., CROUGHAN, J., *et al* (1981) National Institute of Mental Health diagnostic interview schedule. *Archives of General Psychiatry*, **38**, 381–389.

——, WING, J., WITTCHEN, H.-U., *et al* (1988) The Composite Diagnostic Interview: An epidemiological instrument suitable for use in conjunction with different diagnostic systems and in different cultures. *Archives of General Psychiatry*, **45**, 1069–1077.

SARTORIUS, N., DAVIDIAN, H., ERNBERG, G., *et al* (1983) *Depressive Disorders in Different Cultures.* Geneva: World Health Organization.

—— & BAN, T. A. (eds) (1986) *Assessment of Depression.* Berlin: Springer-Verlag.

SETHI, B. B. (1986) Epidemiology of depression in India. *Psychopathology*, **19** (suppl. 2), 26–36.

SHIMIZU, Y. M. & KAPLAN, B. J. (1987) Postpartum depression in the United States and Japan. *Journal of Cross-Cultural Psychology*, **18**, 15–30.

SHINFUKU, N. (1973) Diagnosis of manic-depressive illness with special emphasis on the basic problems of diagnosis of depressive illness. *Japanese Journal of Clinical Psychiatry*, **2**, 5–12.

SINGER, K. (1984) Depressive disorders from a transcultural perspective. In *Culture and Psychopathology* (eds J. E. Mezzich & C. E. Berganza), pp. 360–384. New York: Columbia University Press.

SKODA, C. & VINAR, O. (1986) The area of the Bulgarian People's Republic, Czechoslovak Socialist Republic, Polish People's Republic, Union of Soviet Socialist Republics and Socialist Federative Republic of Yugoslavia. In *Assessment of Depression* (eds N. Sartorius & T. A. Ban), pp. 23–29. Berlin: Springer-Verlag.

SPITZER, R. L., ENDICOTT, J. & ROBINS, E. (1978) Research diagnostic criteria: Rationale and reliability. *Archives of General Psychiatry*, **36**, 773–782.

STEER, R. A., BECK, A. T. & GARRISON, B. (1986) Applications of the Beck Depression Inventory. In *Assessment of Depression* (eds N. Sartorius & T. A. Ban), pp. 123–142. Berlin: Springer-Verlag.

STERN, G. & KRUCKMAN, L. (1983) Multi-disciplinary perspectives on post-partum depression: An anthropological critique. *Social Science and Medicine*, **17**, 1027–1041.

TAKAHASHI, R. (1986) Instruments used in the assessment of depression in Japan. In *Assessment of Depression* (eds N. Sartorius & T. A. Ban), pp. 36–45. Berlin: Springer-Verlag.

THOME, M. (1991) *Translation of Instruments: Cultural Features Influencing Measurement of Emotional Aspects of Maternal Care.* Paper presented at the conference on Prevention of Depression After Childbirth: Use and Misuse of the Edinburgh Postnatal Depression Scale, University of Keele, Staffordshire, UK.

TRIANDIS, H. (1972) *The Analysis of Subjective Culture.* New York: John Wiley.

TURNBULL, J. M. (1969) Mental illness in the puerperium. *Canadian Psychiatric Association Journal*, **14**, 525–526.

UDDENBERG, N. (1974) Reproductive adaptation in mother and daughter. A study of personality development and adaptation to motherhood. *Acta Psychiatrica Scandinavica* (suppl. 254).

WATSON, E. & EVANS, S. J. W. (1986) An example of cross-cultural measurement of psychological symptoms in post-partum mothers. *Social Science and Medicine*, **23**, 869–874.

WILLIAMS, J. B. W. (1988) A structured interview guide for the Hamilton Depression Rating Scale. *Archives of General Psychiatry*, **45**, 742–747.

WITTCHEN, H.-U., ROBINS, L. N., COTTLER, L. B., *et al* & Participants in the Multicentre WHO/ADAMHA Field Trials (1991) Cross-cultural feasibility, reliability and sources of variance of the Composite International Diagnostic Interview (CIDI). *British Journal of Psychiatry*, **159**, 645–653.

WORLD HEALTH ORGANIZATION (1978) *Mental disorders: Glossary and Guide to their Classification in Accordance with the Ninth Revision of the International Classification of Diseases* (ICD–9). Geneva: WHO.

ZIMMERMAN, M., CORYELL, W., CORENTHAL, C., *et al*, (1986) A self-report inventory to diagnose major depressive disorders. *Archives of General Psychiatry*, **43**, 1076–1081.

—— & —— (1988) The validity of a self-report questionnaire for diagnosing major depressive disorder. *Archives of General Psychiatry*, **45**, 738–740.

ZUNG, W. W. K. (1965) A self-rating depression scale. *Archives of General Psychiatry*, **12**, 63–70.

—— (1986) Zung Self-rating Depression Scale and Depression Status Inventory. In *Assessment of Depression* (eds N. Sartorius & T. A. Ban), pp. 221–231. Berlin: Springer-Verlag.

11 The Edinburgh Postnatal Depression Scale and its predecessors

BRIAN HARRIS and NAHLA JAMIL

Research carried out over the past 25 years has led to the characterisation of the various mental states occurring in the year following delivery, together with the associations of those mental states. Such research has employed a variety of methods to define maternal depression, and experience gained has led to a general consensus that features which characterise the puerperium and following months, particularly the mother's biological changes and alterations in lifestyle, necessitate the need for extra care in defining depressed mood both in terms of its essential features and also in terms of its severity. As a general principle such care is needed wherever there may be confusing factors due to the presence of other conditions. For example, in the alcohol-dependent patient, how much 'depressive symptomatology' can be explained by a state of 'chronic intoxication' or compromised nutritional status? (Schukit, 1983); and also in the apparently depressed postnatal woman: how much symptomatology is not really depressive but can be explained by biological changes in appetite, weight, libido and so on?

In one sense, the word 'predecessors' in the title of this chapter is a misnomer, since until the Edinburgh Postnatal Depression Scale (EPDS) was produced (Cox *et al*, 1987) there was no questionnaire for depression which had been designed specially for use in the postnatal period. Some of the seminal work in this field (Pitt, 1968) had employed a 24-item self-report scale comparing antenatal and postnatal mood in a large group of women, and later the Stein questionnaire (Stein, 1980) was developed as a subject-rated checklist, useful for identifying 'maternity blues', but in terms of more severe depressive states, there was a heavy reliance on rating scales which had been designed for contexts other than the puerperium. One major study, for example (Paykel *et al*, 1980), used an observer-rated scale (the Raskin 3-area scale for depression) which had been found useful in controlled trials to monitor changes in mood in patients taking antidepressant medication (Raskin *et al*, 1970), a situation very different to that of assessment of women for depression in the postnatal year! The need for a specific instrument was therefore urgent.

In screening patients for depression, besides self-report questionnaires, there are three types of assessment (Williams *et al*, 1980): firstly, a full clinical interview with a psychiatrist; secondly, a structured clinical interview such as the Present State Examination (Wing *et al*, 1973); and, thirdly, observer-rated scales. For screening purposes there are disadvantages to all these methods in that clinical and structured interviews are time consuming (and therefore impractical), the latter requiring special training to ensure competent assessments. Similarly, observer-rated scales need some form of training for standardisation of their usage. Thus, the 10-item EPDS, which is subject-rated, has been devised as a screening tool (Cox *et al*, 1987) – that is, it is used to identify women who need further assessment because they probably are depressed.

Research into the association of mood with hormone changes occurring in pregnancy and the following year requires reliable instruments for mood assessment which not only identify 'cases' of depression, but which are sensitive to changes occurring in mood between time points with particular accuracy. As previously stated, 'biological features' may change for reasons other than depression. To illustrate this, let us take the 17-item Hamilton Rating Scale for Depression (HRSD; Hamilton, 1960) which is heavily loaded for features such as appetite and weight-loss, sleep disturbance, fatiguability, loss of libido and menstrual disturbance. In fact, food intake may rapidly change after delivery partly due to a break in the normal pattern of eating habits due to disturbance of routine, and there is normal reversion of body weight – rapid over the first 24 hours postpartum, but continuing more slowly over several months (Monheit *et al*, 1980). Similarly, changes in menstruation are partly linked to infant breast feeding and consequent hormonal changes, and therefore become unreliable as a symptom of depression in the large subgroup of breast-feeding women. Another example of the validity of such questionnaires being called into question would be that of examining the association of thyroid function and mood. Postpartum auto-immune thyroid dysfunction linked to positive thyroid antibody status in 10% of normal women is known to occur at a high rate in the six months after delivery (Amino *et al*, 1982). Theoretically, the HRSD would detect the biological changes associated with thyroid dysfunction (such as anxiety and weight-loss associated with thyrotoxicosis), producing higher ratings but which are not due to depressed mood.

Consequently, work carried out in Cardiff using a variety of questionnaires (Harris *et al*, 1989*a,b,c*, 1992), though with the primary aim of examining hormonal correlates with mood, has also enabled the comparison of various questionnaires in their abilities to identify postpartum major depressive illness.

The principle employed has been identification of depression in a structured, clinical interview situation using defined criteria with operational checklists – DSM–III criteria for major depression (American Psychiatric

Association, 1980) and Research Diagnostic Criteria (RDC; Spitzer *et al*, 1978). Both sets of criteria require the presence of depressed mood or anhedonia ("markedly diminished interest or pleasure in all, or almost all activities most of the day every day") together with a required number of other optional symptoms, four in the case of DSM–III, major depression, and five for RDC, definite major depression. Furthermore, the symptoms must have been present for a minimum of two weeks for definite major depression, and symptoms clearly due to a physical condition are not to be included. (Hence, the weight loss following delivery would not be included.) Such criteria also exclude depression due to organic causes and due to bereavement. The 'gold standard' criteria having been thus defined, the abilities of questionnaires to identify and quantify the criteria could be determined as well as their associations (correlations) one with another. In addition, in a further study, the sensitivity of the EPDS in detecting change over a six-month period postpartum could be compared with that of the 17-item HRSD and the Hospital Anxiety and Depression scale (Zigmond & Snaith, 1983).

Two research studies

Study 1

The main objectives of this study (Harris *et al*, 1989*a,b*) were to examine associations between hormonal parameters (salivary progesterone, cortisol, oestradiol, plasma thyroid antibodies, and thyroid hormones) and mood at one point in time in the postpartum period. A total of 147 mothers were screened in an out-patient situation for major depression according to DSM–III criteria, at 6–8 weeks postpartum. Using predetermined cut-off points, the EPDS and the Beck scale (BDI; Beck *et al*, 1961) were compared in their abilities to identify the 15% of subjects who had major depression according to DSM–III criteria. Since its introduction in 1961, the BDI has been widely used both as a screening instrument for depression and for assessing its severity in those known to be suffering from depressive illness (Beck *et al*, 1988). Twenty-one symptoms are assessed and, for each symptom, subjects choose a statement most appropriate for their experience over the previous two weeks, successive statements indicating increasing severity. Items 1–14 reflect mainly cognitive and affective symptoms but almost a third of the items of the BDI (mainly 15–21) cover somatic features, e.g. sleep, fatiguability and distorted body image, symptoms far more common in pregnant and postpartum women – and in that context not necessarily indicative of depression.

The Raskin 3-area scale for depression (Raskin *et al*, 1970) and Montgomery and Åsberg Depression Rating Scale (MADRS; Montgomery & Åsberg, 1979) were also completed by the assessor at the time of interview.

Table 11.1 shows a comparison of the questionnaires in their abilities to identify major depression according to DSM–III criteria using cut-off points of 13 and over for the EPDS (Cox *et al*, 1987), 8 and over for the Raskin scale (Paykel *et al*, 1980), 12 and over for the MADRS (Snaith *et al*, 1986) and 11 and over for the BDI (Nielson & Williams, 1980). The sensitivity of the EPDS was 95% and its specificity 93%, but the performance of the BDI was markedly inferior, with a sensitivity of 68% and a specificity of 88%. A similar finding had already been reported by O'Hara *et al* (1983) and an examination of some of the questions on the BDI illustrate problems which may occur in the year following delivery.

Case study examples

The symptom dealing with distorted image.

		SCORE
N.	I don't feel I look any worse than I used to.	0
	I am worried that I am looking old and unattractive.	1
	I feel that there are permanent changes in my appearance and that they make me look unattractive.	2
	I feel that I am ugly or repulsive looking.	3

Obviously changes occur in body shape during pregnancy and the postpartum period.

Again: The symptom of weight loss.

		SCORE
S.	I haven't lost much weight if any lately.	0
	I have lost more than 5 lbs.	1
	I have lost more than 10 lbs.	2
	I have lost more than 15 lbs.	3

In addition the *way* in which statements are made may lead to confusion.

For example: The statements dealing with sleep disturbance.

		SCORE
P.	I can sleep as well as usual.	0
	I wake up more tired in the morning than I used to.	1
	I wake up 1 to 2 hours earlier than usual and find it hard to get back to sleep.	2
	I wake up early every morning and can't get more than 5 hours sleep.	3

The latter can be contrasted with point 7 on the EPDS:

"I have been so unhappy that I have had difficulty sleeping."

The MADRS, which is observer-rated, is at least in theory predictably useful in the postnatal year, since it contains relatively little in terms of biological features (one question on sleep and one on appetite), i.e. it is mainly orientated towards psychic symptoms of depression including

TABLE 11.1
Ability of different rating scales to identify DSM–III major depression

Questionnaire	Number completing test	Major depression	Sensitivity	Specificity
EPDS	126	21/22	95%	97/104 : 93%
BDI	129	13/19	68%	97/110 : 88%
Raskin	146	22/22	100%	109/125 : 87%
MADRS	147	20/22	91%	118/124 : 96%

Sensitivity: the percentage of individuals with depression identified as such from the total population of depressed women.
Specificity: the percentage of individuals without depression identified as such from the total population of non-depressed women.

apparent and reported sadness, ill attention, impairment of concentration, inability to experience emotions, anhedonia, pessimism and suicidal ideation. Each of the 10 items is graded 0–6, the scale being very sensitive to change accompanying treatment response. Hence it has become widely used in antidepressant trials over the past 10 years. Bearing in mind the reservation that in the study described the MADRS was completed by the same observer as for the DSM–III criteria for major depression, the Edinburgh scale is equal to the MADRS in its usefulness.

The correlations between the various questionnaires are also shown in Table 11.2, and reflect their associations one with another, not only in the region of the cut-off points (as for sensitivity and specificity) but throughout the range of scores. Not surprisingly, the two observer-rated scales (the MADRS and Raskin) have the strongest association. The study therefore shows the unreliability of the BDI in the months following delivery. This is true at least for the full 21-item BDI, and goes some way to support the work of O'Hara *et al* (1990) who suggest that the BDI might be more appropriately used without the items reflecting somatic symptoms, i.e. 15–21. Whether other modifications such as the 13-item Beck scale will be more useful remains to be seen (Guy, 1976). The scale also omits items such as irritability and tearfulness.

Study 2

There is evidence that depressed mood is associated with thyroiditis and positive antibody status in the year following delivery (Harris *et al*, 1989*c*,

TABLE 11.2
Major intercorrelations between the depression rating scales (Pearson correlation matrix)

Questionnaire	EPDS	n^1	Raskin	n^1	MADRS	n^1
BDI	0.68*	110	0.62*	129	0.61*	128
EPDS	–	–	0.80*	126	0.79*	125
Raskin	–	–	–	–	0.92*	146

1. Number of mothers assessed.
*$P < 0.001$.

1992; Pop *et al*, 1991), the commonest disorder of thyroid function being that of hypothyroidism. Since 10% of women in the general population are thyroid antibody positive (Prentice *et al*, 1990) a small but significant subgroup of women are at risk of developing such depression, antibody levels remaining low during pregnancy itself (possibly due to the normal increase in corticosteroids) but rising after delivery to reach a peak at about four months postpatum. Worldwide studies (Gerstein, 1990) have shown that between 3 and 6% of such women develop actual thyroid dysfunction with abnormal plasma thyroid hormones. The occurrence of depression in such thyroid antibody positive women is not surprising since primary depressive disorder is often accompanied by altered thyroid function (Nemeroff, 1989), and primary hypo- and hyperthyroidism can present with depressed mood. However, the exact cause and relationship to abnormal plasma thyroid hormones is not clear (Harris *et al*, 1992). In a study involving over 700 assessments, antibody positive ($n = 110$) and antibody negative ($n = 132$) women were assessed at 8, 12, 20 and 28 weeks postpartum according to RDC for major depressive disorder (Spitzer *et al*, 1978) and were rated on the 17-item HRSD rating scale using a cut-off point of 15 and over, as consistent with major depression (Hamilton, 1960). Research diagnostic criteria for major depression are similar to but more stringent than the equivalent DSM–III criteria. In addition, a category of 'probable' (as opposed to 'definite') is allowed for individuals who have only four of the optional symptoms. Similarly, if the time the symptoms have been present is greater than one week but less than two, a diagnosis of 'probable' major depression is made. A major purpose of RDC is thus "to enable investigators to select relatively homogeneous groups of subjects who meet specified diagnostic criteria" (Spitzer *et al*, 1978). The women's antibody status was determined at the antenatal booking clinic, and on the first day after delivery. The women came from social classes 3 to 5, and there were no significant differences between the two groups in terms of parity, age, the number of life events occurring in the previous year, and smoking habits (Harris *et al*, 1992). The women completed the self-rated Hospital Anxiety and Depression Scale (HAD; Zigmond & Snaith, 1983) and the EPDS. The HAD subscales contain a total of 14 statements, each for anxiety and depression, mostly confined to the psychic aspects of both. The scale was developed as an instrument for detecting states of anxiety and depression in the setting of a hospital medical out-patient clinic, and, consequently, details about symptoms which might have an organic cause, e.g. headaches, dizziness and palpitations, have been eliminated. The HAD has also been shown to be useful as a measure of the *severity* of anxiety and depression and can be used repeatedly to check patients' progress. In theory it should be useful in detecting postnatal depression, and possess a high specificity, its authors indicating that although it was constructed from data supplied from medical out-patients between the ages of 16 and 65, there is no reason

TABLE 11.3
Major depression, definite only (RDC), by antibody status

	Specificity	Sensitivity	
EPDS	579/688 (84%)	56/59 (95%)	(n = 747)
HAD A	572/697 (82%)	53/60 (88%)	(n = 757)
HAD D	626/695 (90%)	39/60 (65%)	(n = 755)
Hamilton	636/650 (98%)	51/53 (96%)	(n = 703)
(cut-off point 15)			
Antibody-positive only			
EPDS	260/320 (81%)	28/30 (93%)	(n = 350)
HAD A	262/325 (81%)	25/30 (83%)	(n = 355)
HAD D	294/324 (91%)	19/30 (63%)	(n = 354)
Hamilton	302/306 (99%)	33/34 (97%)	(n = 340)
Antibody-negative only			
EPDS	319/368 (87%)	28/29 (97%)	(n = 397)
HAD A	310/372 (88%)	28/30 (93%)	(n = 402)
HAD D	332/371 (89%)	20/30 (66%)	(n = 401)
Hamilton	334/344 (97%)	18/19 (95%)	(n = 363)

to suppose that its use would be invalid in patients attending other hospital clinics. A score of over 10 on either subscale identifies a 'potential case'. (In the development of the EPDS, the influence of the HAD is obvious in that some of the statements on the two scales are virtually identical, e.g. ''I have been able to laugh and see the funny side of things.'')

The ability of both scales to identify RDC major depression, and RDC major and probable major depression, are summarised in Tables 11.3 and 11.4, respectively. The EPDS has a high sensitivity and specificity and so also does the anxiety component of the HAD, indicating that anxiety is a major component of postnatal depression. Surprisingly, the depression scale of the HAD was lacking in sensitivity. These findings held regardless of antibody status and are therefore representative of the normal population. Two questions arise from these results. Firstly, why is the depression subscale of the HAD performing badly in terms of having a low sensitivity, and consequently missing many cases of RDC major depression? One possibility could be the cut-off point chosen. Zigmond & Snaith (1983) suggest the possibility of two cut-off points. We have used the higher cut-off point of 10/11 to avoid false positives as far as possible. Had the lower cut-off points of 8/9 been used, obviously the sensitivity of the depression subscale would have been higher, but with possibly some loss of specificity. Another possibility may lie in the actual items included in the HAD depression subscale. Five of its seven items are related to the loss of pleasure response (anhedonia) rather than items such as sadness, tearfulness and self-harm. The latter may represent essential 'core' features of postnatal depression, identified by RDC but therefore missed by the HAD. A second question concerns the anxiety subscale of the HAD. Why is its performance superior to the depression

TABLE 11.4
Major depression definite and probable, by antibody status

	Specificity	Sensitivity	
EPDS	575/664 (87%)	76/83 (92%)	($n = 747$)
HAD A	567/673 (84%)	72/84 (86%)	($n = 757$)
HAD D	612/671 (91%)	49/84 (58%)	($n = 755$)
Hamilton	624/629 (99%)	60/74 (81%)	($n = 703$)
Antibody-positive only			
EPDS	260/311 (84%)	37/39 (95%)	($n = 350$)
HAD A	260/316 (82%)	32/39 (82%)	($n = 355$)
HAD D	290/315 (92%)	24/39 (62%)	($n = 354$)
Hamilton	302/306 (99%)	33/34 (97%)	($n = 340$)
Antibody-negative only			
EPDS	315/353 (89%)	39/44 (89%)	($n = 397$)
HAD A	307/357 (86%)	40/45 (89%)	($n = 402$)
HAD D	322/356 (90%)	25/45 (56%)	($n = 401$)
Hamilton	328/332 (99%)	24/31 (77%)	($n = 363$)

subscale, at least in terms of sensitivity? This is more difficult to answer but may be due to the fact that anxiety features are an essential component of postnatal depression. Such features are included in items 4 and 5 of the EPDS, but in comparison with the number of studies carried out in terms of postnatal depression, the amount of attention given to anxiety has been relatively small.

Further work to clarify these points is obviously necessary, but in the meantime care should be taken in using the HAD in the context of postnatal depression, and the lower suggested cut-off point for the depression subscale should be used.

Furthermore, the study was able to address the question of whether or not the Edinburgh scale is sensitive to change in mood state and whether or not it measures such change in any meaningful way. This can be assessed by looking at the abilities of the 17-item HRSD (a validated observer-rated scale for measurement of mood change – Hamilton, 1960) and the EPDS in terms of their ability to identify RDC depression with the passing of time, i.e. over the 8, 12, 20 and 28 week assessments. Table 11.5 indicates that the Hamilton and Edinburgh scales remain consistent in that the sensitivity of the EPDS is higher (possibly due to its cut-off point) whereas its specificity is lower. This is in keeping with the fact that it is essentially a screening instrument by design. The Pearson rank correlation coefficient remains the same over the four assessments indicating that the Edinburgh scale retains its efficacy (at least in terms of the HRSD) over the whole range of scores.

It will also be noted from Table 11.5 that there were slight variations in numbers of subjects assessed by the HRSD and EPDS scale at the various time points, there always being more subjects with data for the latter. This is

TABLE 11.5

Comparison of the EPDS and HRSD in terms of specificity and sensitivity for definite and probable RDC major depression at the four time points of the study

	8 weeks		12 weeks		20 weeks		28 weeks	
EPDS								
Specificity	87/101	(86%)	120/132	(91%)	120/123 (90%)		111/129	(86%)
Sensitivity	8/8	(100%)	16/17	(94%)	15/18	(83%)	14/15	(93%)
HRSD								
Specificity	97/98	(99%)	126/126 (100%)		122/123 (99%)		122/122 (100%)	
Sensitivity	8/10	(80%)	13/15	(87%)	9/12	(75%)	9/13	(69%)
Rank correlations* between EPDS and HRSD (*r* values)	0.76		0.78		0.78		0.75	

*For all correlations $P < 0.001$.

because women who did not turn up at the clinic or could not be contacted were sent the EPDS by post and completed it in that way. Further information is also available by looking at the two scales in terms of their misidentification rates, i.e. for subjects who had both scales administered at the same point in time. Results are presented in Table 11.6 for the study overall. It can be seen therefore that the concordance rate is in keeping with the high correlation coefficient (i.e. 78.3%), indicating that the EPDS is at least equal to the HRSD in the region of the cut-off point for the HRSD in identifying depressed women.

We have thus shown that the EPDS can be used to monitor change in the spectrum of women examined postnatally, some of whom may also be suffering from postnatal depression linked to thyroid dysfunction. The different results obtained by the various scales considered are partly due to the position of the cut-off points. Hence, for example, the specificity of the HRSD is generally higher than that of the EPDS (Table 11.5) but the

TABLE 11.6

Concordance or discrepancies between EPDS and HRSD in terms of ratings above and below their respective cut-off points*

Assessments	1 to 2	2 to 3	3 to 4	Total
Complete concordance	123	111	80	314
No change in patient status but complete divergence of scales	10	5	3	18
Reversals of patient status in opposite directions by both scales	0	1	0	1
Reversals of patient status by EPDS not HRSD	16	17	14	47
Reversals by HRSD not EPDS	7	7	7	21
Total	156	141	104	401

*Overall concordance re: mood state at 'follow-up' appointments: 78.3%.
Over the course of the study there were 401 'follow-up' appointments where results of assessments are compared with the previous assessment.

reverse is true for sensitivity, reflecting the comparatively lower cut-off points for the EPDS. In other words, if the cut-off point of the HRSD were lowered, its sensitivity would increase. Accurate determination of the best cut-off points is necessary by further analyses of such data, constructing receiver operator characteristic curves for each time point where sensitivity is plotted against specificity using varying cut-off points for each questionnaire. Comparison of such curves using appropriate statistical tests would be a way forward in confirming the impression gained that the EPDS is at least equal and probably superior to the other questionnaires examined. The whole question of so-called 'endogenous' symptoms has not been considered, and the studies described were mostly concerned with mild/moderate depressive illness. However, what if biological features *are* due to depression? There is good evidence that more severe episodes of puerperal mental illness are mostly variants of manic–depressive psychosis, in which severe biological symptoms may abound. Severe weight loss would be a classical example, and would obviously not be picked up by the EPDS.

In conclusion, the Edinburgh Postnatal Depression Scale has shown itself, in the two studies reported, to be superior to the Beck Depression Inventory and the Hospital Anxiety and Depression scale, both of which are commonly used to assess mood. The whole question of anxiety and the contribution it makes to postnatal depression has also been raised. The use of the Edinburgh scale has proved that there is little to choose between it and the other scales which are observer-rated – such as the Montgomery and Åsberg Depression Rating Scale and Hamilton Rating Scale for Depression – since it matches these in terms of sensitivity and specificity. Further analyses are necessary to assess its efficacy in identifying minor depressive states during the postnatal time period, and in measuring change in mood in individuals exhibiting biological symptoms actually due to depression.

References

AMERICAN PSYCHIATRIC ASSOCIATION (1980) *Diagnostic and Statistical Manual of Mental Disorders* (3rd edn) (DSM–III). Washington, DC: American Psychiatric Association.

AMINO, N., MORI, H., IWATANI, Y., *et al* (1982) High prevalence of transient post partum thyrotoxicosis and hypothyroidism. *New England Journal of Medicine*, **306**, 849–852.

BECK, A. T., WARD, C. H., MENDELSON, M., *et al* (1961) An inventory for measuring depression. *Archives of General Psychiatry*, **4**, 561–571.

——, STEER, R. A. & GARBIN, M. G. (1988) Psychometric properties of the Beck Depression Inventory: Twenty five years of evaluation. *Clinical Psychology Review*, **8**, 77–100.

COX, J. L., HOLDEN, J. M. & SAGOVSKY, R. (1987) Detection of post natal depression – development in the 10-item Edinburgh Postnatal Depression Rating Scale. *British Journal of Psychiatry*, **150**, 782–786.

GERSTEIN, H. C. (1990) How common is post partum thyroiditis? *Archives of Internal Medicine*, **150**, 1397–1400.

GUY, W. (1976) *E.C.D.E.U. Assessment Manual for Psychopharmacology*, pp. 541–545. US Department of Health, Education and Welfare. Rockville, MA.

HAMILTON, M. (1960) A rating scale for depression. *Journal of Neurology, Neurosurgery and Psychiatry*, **23**, 56–62.

HARRIS, B., JOHNS, S., FUNG, H., *et al* (1989*a*) The hormonal environment of postnatal depression. *British Journal of Psychiatry*, **154**, 660–667.

——, FUNG, H., JOHNS, S., *et al* (1989*b*) Transient post partum thyroid dysfunction and post natal depression. *Journal of Affective Disorders*, **17**, 243–249.

——, HUCKLE, P., THOMAS, R., *et al* (1989*c*) The use of rating scales to identify post natal depression. *British Journal of Psychiatry*, **154**, 813–817.

——, OTHMAN, S., DAVIES, J. A., *et al* (1992) Association between post partum thyroid dysfunction and thyroid antibodies and depression. *British Medical Journal*, **305**, 152–156.

KENDELL, R. E. (1985) Emotional and physical factors in the genesis of puerperal mental disorders. *Journal of Psychosomatic Research*, **29**, 3–11.

MONHEIT, A. G., COUSINS, L. & RESNICK, R. (1980) The puerperium, anatomic and physiologic readjustments. *Clinical Obstetrics and Gynecology*, **23**, 973–984.

MONTGOMERY, S. A. & ÅSBERG, M. (1979) A new depression scale designed to be sensitive to change. *British Journal of Psychiatry*, **134**, 382–389.

NEMEROFF, C. B. (1989) Clinical significance of psychoneuroendocrinology in psychiatry: focus on the thyroid and adrenal. *Journal of Clinical Psychiatry*, **50** (suppl. 5), 13–20.

NIELSON, A. C. & WILLIAMS, T. A. (1980) Depression in ambulatory medical patients. *Archives of General Psychiatry*, **37**, 999–1004.

O'HARA, M. W., REHM, L. P. & CAMPBELL, S. B. (1983) Post partum depression: a role for social network and life stress variables. *Journal of Nervous and Mental Disease*, **171**, 336–341.

——, ZEKOSKI, E. M., PHILIPPS, L. H., *et al* (1990) Controlled prospective study of post partum mood disorders: comparison of child bearing and non-child bearing women. *Journal of Abnormal Psychology*, **99**, 3–15.

PAYKEL, E. S., EMMS, E. M., FLETCHER, J., *et al* (1980) Life events and social support in puerperal depression. *British Journal of Psychiatry*, **136**, 339–346.

PITT, B. (1968) 'Atypical' depression following childbirth. *British Journal of Psychiatry*, **114**, 1325–1335.

POP, V. J. M., DE ROOY, H. A. M., VADER, H. L., *et al* (1991) Post partum thyroid dysfunction and depression in an unselected population. *New England Journal of Medicine*, **324**, 1815–1816.

PRENTICE, L. M., PHILLIPS, D. I. W., SARSERO, D., *et al* (1990) Geographical distribution of subclinical auto immune thyroid disease in Britain. A study using highly sensitive direct assays for autoantibodies to thyroglobulin and thyroid peroxidase. *Acta Endocrinologica*, **123**, 493–498.

RASKIN, A., SCHULTERBRANDT, J., REATIG, N., *et al* (1970) Differential response to chlorpromazine, imipramine and placebo – a study of sub groups of hospitalised depressed patients. *Archives of General Psychiatry*, **23**, 164–173.

SCHUCKIT, M. (1983) Alcoholic patients with secondary depression. *American Journal of Psychiatry*, **140**, 711–714.

SNAITH, R. P., HARROP, F. M., NEWBY, D. A., *et al* (1986) Grade scores of the Montgomery–Åsberg Depression and the clinical anxiety scales. *British Journal of Psychiatry*, **148**, 599–601.

SPITZER, R. L., ENDICOTT, J. & ROBINS, S. (1978) Research diagnostic criteria. *Archives of General Psychiatry*, **35**, 773–782.

STEIN, G. S. (1980) The pattern of mental change and body weight change in the first post partum week. *Journal of Psychosomatic Research*, **24**, 165–171.

WILLIAMS, P., TARNPOLSKY, A. & HAND, D. (1980) Case definition and case identification in psychiatry epidemiology – review and assessment. *Psychological Medicine*, **10**, 101–114.

WING, T. K., COOPER, J. E. & SARTORIUS, N. (1973) *Present State Examination*. Cambridge: Cambridge University Press.

ZIGMOND, A. S. & SNAITH, R. P. (1983) The hospital anxiety and depression scale. *Acta Psychiatrica Scandinavica*, **67**, 361–370.

12 The use of the Edinburgh Postnatal Depression Scale in research to explore the relationship between antenatal and postnatal dysphoria

**JOSEPHINE M. GREEN and
DECLAN MURRAY**

Major psychiatric disturbance after childbirth drew the attention of researchers a long time ago (Esquirol, 1845), and led to the study of less dramatic disorders such as postnatal depression. As a part of the natural broadening of the field some attention has been paid to psychiatric disorders occurring during pregnancy. This chapter argues, on the evidence of published data, that antenatal depression ranks closely with postnatal depression as a health problem of importance. The special issues in the use of the EPDS in pregnancy are discussed and new data from a recent community-based research study are presented.

Why does antenatal depression matter?

'Postnatal depression' is a label which will quickly be applied to any unhappy woman who has recently had a baby. In contrast, unhappy pregnant women, even if their condition is recognised, are likely to be told that their feelings are of little significance and that all will be well once the baby arrives. Is antenatal depression less common, less severe and more transitory than its 'big sister', postnatal depression? Is it associated with different factors? Could it have implications for foetal development?

Prevalence, severity and duration

All studies using self-report symptom rating scales show a consistent pattern of higher scores in pregnancy than postnatally. Ancill *et al* (1986) used a computerised version of the Hamilton Rating Scale for Depression (Hamilton, 1960) and found an antenatal to postnatal drop in mean score from 10.2 to 7.7; Gotlib *et al* (1989), using the Beck Depression Inventory (BDI; Beck *et al*, 1961), from 7.38 down to 6.17; Atkinson & Rickel (1984) BDI from 7.51 to 6.65; Pitt questionnaire (Pitt, 1968) 14.86 down to 11.82; Rees &

TABLE 12.1
Prevalence rates of antenatal and postnatal depression in 9 studies using recognised diagnostic criteria

Author/Year	n	Antenatal Timing	Prevalence	n	Postnatal Timing	Prevalence
Wolkind *et al*, 1980	117	7 months	16%	102	4 months	10%
Cox *et al*, 1982	105	2 assessments	4%	103	3–5 months	13%
Cutrona, 1983	85	3rd trimester	3.5%	85	2 months	3.5%
Kumar *et al*, 1984	111	36th week	6.3%	114	12 weeks	15%
O'Hara, 1986	99	2nd trimester	9%	99	9 weeks	12%
Watson *et al*, 1984	128	16 weeks	4%	128	6 weeks	16%
Cooper *et al*, 1988	483	3rd trimester	6%	460	3 months	8.7%
Gotlib *et al*, 1989	295	5 weeks antenatally	8%	295	4–5 weeks	6.8%
O'Hara *et al*, 1990	182	2nd trimester	7.7%	182	9 weeks	10.4%

Lutkins (1971) BDI 8.5 down to 7.4; and O'Hara *et al* (1990) BDI 8.5 down to 4.5. Several studies using interviews to assess symptoms have found no increase from antenatal to postnatal depression (Nilsson & Almgren, 1970; Uddenberg, 1974; Sharp, 1989).

Nine studies using recognised diagnostic criteria to assess the prevalence of depression during pregnancy as well as postnatally are summarised in Table 12.1. In some of the studies several assessments were carried out both antenatally and postnatally. From these we have cited the last assessment in pregnancy and the first postnatal assessment (except where these were in the first postnatal week in order to avoid contamination by 'the blues'). It is clear from these studies that prevalence rates of depression in pregnancy are

TABLE 12.2
Severity of antenatal versus postnatal depression

	Antenatal	Postnatal
Wolkind *et al*, 1980	"Definitely handicapping"	"Definitely handicapping"
Cox *et al*, 1982	SPI total score 4.2	SPI total score 4.0
Cutrona, 1983	DSM–III major depression 3	DSM–III major depression 3
Kumar *et al*, 1984	RDC major/minor[1] 2/13	RDC major/minor[2] 5/12
O'Hara, 1986	RDC major/minor 6/3 Symptom severity 30.78	RDC major/minor 8/4 Symptom severity 25.33
Watson *et al*, 1984	ICD–9	ICD–9
Cooper *et al*, 1988	PSE (ID>5) 5	PSE (ID>5) 13
Gotlib *et al*, 1989	RDC depression, severity not given	

1. Includes two intermittent depressions.
2. Includes three intermittent depressions.

comparable with those found after delivery. These studies have reported little data on the relative severity of antenatal and postnatal depression (Table 12.2) so on this matter the jury is still out. (The puerperal psychoses, although severe, are relatively uncommon – 0.1–0.2% of live births – and will affect the overall figures very little.) Furthermore, the duration of depression reported (Kumar & Robson, 1984; Watson *et al*, 1984) suggests that antenatal and postnatal depression are of similar duration.

With regard to different factors being associated with ante- and postnatal symptoms Cox *et al* (1982) found "always been a worrier" to be significantly associated with high symptom scores before and after delivery. Although deteriorating marital relationship and decrease in sexual satisfaction were associated with postnatal symptoms, these factors were not assessed antenatally. Kumar (1982) reports differences in the factors associated with antenatal and postnatal depression. On closer examination, however, they were perhaps not so different: "anxieties about the foetus" antenatally, for example, might be thought to be equivalent to "mixed feelings and worries about baby" postnatally. Other antenatal factors were: still smoking at end of pregnancy and thought about termination, which both relate fairly specifically to pregnancy. The fact that previous psychiatric history was not associated with postnatal depression was unusual, as was their association with age over 30. Other reported factors specifically associated with postnatal depression were: a prior psychiatric disturbance in the husband; infrequent sexual intercourse; dissatisfaction with leisure activities antenatally; and poor relationship with mother antenatally.

Adverse effect on the foetus

The importance of postnatal depression has increased with the growing body of evidence that it has a deleterious effect not only on the mother but also on the child (e.g. Stein *et al*, 1991; Murray & Stein, 1991). There is some evidence that depression during pregnancy may also pose hazards for the baby. Wolkind (1981), for example, found that depressed women were poor antenatal clinic attenders and Zuckerman *et al* (1989) found associations between depressive symptoms, poor weight gain and health behaviours likely to have an adverse effect on the foetus such as smoking and the use of alcohol and cocaine. As well as these indirect effects, mediated via the depressed mother's adverse health behaviour, there may be direct effects such as the suggestion by Bragonier *et al* (1984) of placental hypoperfusion due to catecholamines released in response to maternal stress/depression. There is also the largely unexplored question of the development of a mother's feelings towards her unborn child at a time when she is depressed.

Use of the EPDS in pregnancy

If it is accepted that antenatal depression is an important topic worthy of further research and clinical effort the EPDS can fulfil two roles. It can be used as a screening instrument for diagnosable depressive episodes and, in its own right, for assessing dysphoria throughout pregnancy and the postnatal period.

Depressive illness

Any scale to be used should be validated against clinical diagnosis in the relevant population – in this case pregnant women – as measures validated in one situation (e.g. postnatally or with non-pregnant subjects) are not necessarily valid in another. Most of the commonly used scales, e.g. Hamilton (1960); BDI (Beck *et al*, 1961); HADS (Zigmond & Snaith, 1983), have not been validated for antenatal use. The GHQ–30 (Goldberg, 1972) has been validated (Sharp, 1988), but was found not to be suitable postnatally (Nott & Cutts, 1982). The EPDS, which covers the main symptoms of depression but excludes somatic symptoms such as fatigue and appetite (Cox *et al*, 1987), has been validated for use in pregnancy (Murray & Cox, 1990). In that study, 100 women between 28 and 34 weeks gestation completed the EPDS and were then interviewed using a standardised psychiatric interview (SPI; Goldberg *et al*, 1970). EPDS scores were compared with Research Diagnostic Criteria (RDC; Spitzer *et al*, 1978) diagnosis of major and minor depression derived from the interview. Of these women, 6% were diagnosed as having RDC major depressive disorder and 8% as having minor depressive disorder. A cut-off of 14/15 was found to be optimal for RDC major depression. The sensitivity was 100%, false positive rate 4% and the positive predictive value 60%. At the 12/13 cut-off (optimal in the postnatal validation of Cox *et al* (1987)), the sensitivity was 100% and there were 12 false positives (including 3 minor depressions). Considering all RDC (major plus minor) depression, and using the 12/13 cut-off as in the postnatal validation, 9 of the 14 women with RDC (major or minor) depression were correctly identified (sensitivity 64%). This apparently low figure occurs because only 3 of the 8 RDC minor depressions are detected. Lowering the cut-off to 10/11 increases the sensitivity to 71% but generates false positives such that if all women who scored 11 or more were interviewed, 29% would have RDC (major or minor) depression (positive predictive value = 29%).

An interesting footnote has been added to this study regarding item 10 of the EPDS ("The thought of harming myself has occurred to me"). This item is aimed at detecting suicidal thoughts, but, to a woman well advanced in pregnancy it could be read as "I am preoccupied by the possibility of falling and hurting myself" or even as concern that harm might befall her during labour and delivery (Green *et al*, 1991*a*). Some women added explicit comments indicating this has occurred and in a sample of 1335 women, 191 (14%) gave a non-zero reponse to this item at 35 weeks, compared with only 6% postnatally. Over one-third of these women scored 9 or less on the remaining 9 items. Overall however the EPDS is a valid instrument for clinical and research work on antenatal depression. Clinical use of the EPDS in pregnancy is dealt with in the discussion at the end of the chapter and its use in research is now described.

Research use of the EPDS in pregnancy

In addition to the clinical applications for which it was designed, the EPDS has much potential as a research tool. There are two main ways in which it can be used. One is as a screening tool for case finding: for example, for an intervention research trial or epidemiological study. The other is to regard scores not simply as a possible marker of a psychiatric diagnosis, but as a valid measure in their own right of what Kendall *et al* (1987) have termed 'dysphoria'. Used in this way it becomes an economical means of tracking dysphoria in large samples through the various stages of pregnancy and the puerperium. Although lacking the rigour of clinical diagnosis, it is possible in this way to illuminate some of the relationships between antenatal and postnatal symptoms and other associated factors, albeit based solely on self-reported symptoms.

Use of the EPDS in a longitudinal research study

In this section we will report data that illustrate an application of the EPDS in tracking antenatal–postnatal dysphoria. The data are taken from a longitudinal study of the social and psychological effects of prenatal screening for foetal abnormality (Green *et al*, 1994). The overall aim of the study was to examine women's experiences of screening for foetal abnormality in the context of other aspects of their lives. The EPDS was one of a number of assessments used. Here we will focus on the relationship between antenatal and postnatal EPDS scores and on how women with depressive symptoms antenatally differ from those who have them postnatally.

Data were collected via postal questionnaires in each trimester of pregnancy and six weeks after the birth. The EPDS was included in the third trimester and postnatal assessment and EPDS data were available for 1272 women. Item 10 was omitted from the antenatal scoring in view of the observations of Green *et al* (1991*a*) described above. Antenatal scores are therefore based on only 9 items and are thus an underestimate for the

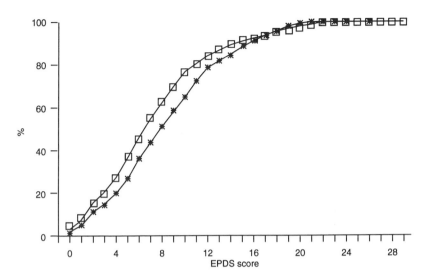

Fig. 12.1. Cumulative frequency of EPDS scores antenatally (—*—) and postnatally (—□—)

14% of women with non-zero scores on that item. However, because 86% of women scored zero on item 10, the effect on the mean score for the sample is small: 8.52 without item 10 and 8.75 with it.

There was a drop in mean EPDS score after birth, a finding consistent with the findings reported above. The frequency distribution of scores (Fig. 12.1) was very similar antenatally to that reported by Murray & Cox (1990).

Relationship between antenatal and postnatal scores

The overall correlation between ante- and postnatal scores was 0.49 ($P < 0.0001$). Ten per cent of women scored the same both antenatally and postnatally; 55% dropped and 35% rose. A total of 72% had a postnatal score that was within three points of their antenatal score.

Scores were categorised as above and below cut-off at each time point. A cut-off of 12/13 was used for postnatal scores (Cox *et al*, 1987) and 14/15 for antenatal scores (Murray & Cox, 1990). Of a sample of 1272, 1016 women (80%) scored consistently below cut-off, while 256 (20%) scored above cut-off on at least one occasion (Fig. 12.2).

Table 12.3 shows that, overall, 12% scored above cut-off antenatally and 14% postnatally. Of the 157 women who scored above cut-off antenatally, 66 (42%) also scored above cut-off postnatally, compared with only 10% of the 1125 who scored below cut-off antenatally. Clearly, then, antenatal scores do have predictive power, even though over half of antenatal

186 *The EPDS*

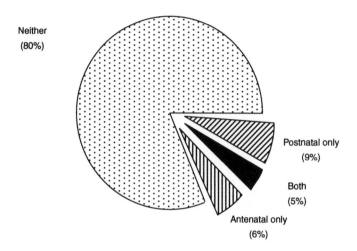

Fig. 12.2. Proportion of women scoring above cut-off on the EPDS antenatally/postnatally (n = 1272)

high-scorers do not score above cut-off postnatally. However, looked at the other way round, only 66 (38%) of the 175 women who scored above cut-off postnatally had high antenatal scores. In other words, over 60% of postnatal high scorers were not above cut-off antenatally. The fact that there seems to be a continuity for some women and not for others suggests the possibility of different aetiologies. Are there different factors contributing to the mood of these different groups of women who have high EPDS scores at different times which might shed light on the particular characteristics of antenatal and postnatal depression? In the following section we shall explore what it is that distinguishes the four groups of women represented

TABLE 12.3
Number of women scoring above and below cut-off on the EPDS antenatally (35 weeks) and postnatally (6 weeks). (Percentages are of the whole sample.)

| | Antenatal | | |
	Below cut-off	Above cut-off	Total
Postnatal	'Neither'	'Ante'	
below cut-off	1016 (80%)	81 (6%)	1097 (86%)
	'Post'	'Both'	
above cut-off	109 (9%)	66 (5%)	175 (14%)
total	1125 (88%)	157 (12%)	1272 (100%)

N.B. Percentages do not always add up due to rounding errors.
$\chi^2 = 135.8$, d.f. = 1, $P < 0.0001$.

TABLE 12.4
Mean EPDS scores of groups scoring above EPDS cut-off at different points

	Neither (n = 1016)	Ante (n = 81)	Post (n = 109)	Both (n = 66)	Significance*
At 35 weeks antenatal					
mean	7.15	16.94	9.67	17.36	0.0001
s.d.	3.67	2.25	3.44	2.28	
At 6 weeks postnatal					
mean	5.97	8.05	16.01	15.95	0.0001
s.d.	3.14	3.16	3.90	3.08	

*All groups are significantly different from each other at each time point except 'ante' and 'both' antenatally and 'post' and 'both' postnatally.

in Table 12.4: those who always scored below cut-off, those who never did, and the two groups who were above cut-off either antenatally or postnatally, but not on both occasions. We will refer to these groups as 'neither', 'both', 'ante' and 'post' respectively.

Table 12.4 gives the mean EPDS score of each group antenatally and postnatally. Note that the mean score of the 'both' group does not differ significantly from that of the 'ante' group antenatally or from the 'post' group postnatally. In other words the groups who are scoring above cut-off on only one occasion are still scoring just as high as the persistently high scorers on these occasions: the difference between the groups is not one of degree. On the other hand, when we look at the 'ante' group *post*natally and the 'post' group *ante*natally (i.e. the occasions when these two groups are *not* scoring above cut-off), we find that they do have significantly higher scores than the 'neither' group. So, on these occasions, there is a difference of degree. These groups may not be scoring above cut-off but they still have significantly higher scores than women who are never above cut-off. This should be borne in mind when interpreting the data that follow.

Demographic characteristics of groups with different scores

The 'both' group tended to be more socially disadvantaged: they were more likely to have only minimum education (76% v. 55%); to be unemployed at the start of pregnancy (56% v. 39%); not to have a partner (18% v. 5%); or to have an unemployed partner (12% v. 4%). The groups also differed slightly in age with the 'both' group having a mean age of 25.9 years compared with 27.3 for the 'neither' group, and the other two groups falling in between. Parity, number of previous pregnancies and other aspects of reproductive history were not significantly different between the groups (Table 12.5).

TABLE 12.5
Demographic characteristics of groups scoring above EPDS cut-off at different points

	Neither (n = 1016)	Ante (n = 81)	Post (n = 109)	Both (n = 66)	Significance
Minimum education	54%	59%	57%	76%	0.05
No partner	4%	9%	10%	18%	0.0001
Unemployed partner	4%	3%	4%	12%	0.0001
Age <21 years	8%	10%	11%	18%	NS
First pregnancy	35%	30%	39%	33%	NS
>2 previous pregnancies	16%	19%	15%	14%	NS
Mean age: years	27.3	26.8	26.3	25.9	0.05

Feelings at the start of pregnancy

Although the EPDS was not administered until 35 weeks, women had also completed questionnaires at approximately 12 and 22 weeks of pregnancy. These questionnaires included a number of assessments of feelings.

The first of these was "How did you feel about finding that you were pregnant?" The 'neither' group were the most likely to give a positive response (74%), and the 'both' group least likely (53%). For the 'ante' and 'post' groups the proportions were 67% and 64%. The groups also differed in their descriptions of how they were feeling physically, with the 'both' and 'ante' groups being more likely than other women to rate themselves as sick or tired 'most of the time'.

All of the questionnaires included an adjective checklist on which women were asked to indicate all the words that described their current feelings. Most of the differences in early pregnancy were between the 'neither' group and the other three. The word 'depressed', however, was chosen significantly more often by women in the 'both' group (33%) than by women in the 'ante' (19%) or 'post' (17%) groups. Only 7.5% of women in the 'neither' group chose the word 'depressed' at this stage. Total scores were calculated counting $+1$ for positive adjectives and -1 for negative ones. Scores for the four groups are shown in Figure 12.3. In early pregnancy, the 'neither' group has a significantly higher score than the other three groups, which do not differ significantly from each other.

Screening for foetal abnormalities was a central issue in this study. At 12 weeks nearly a quarter of the women in the 'ante' group thought that there was a higher than average probability that there would be something wrong with their baby, compared with only 7% of 'both' women and 14% and 18% of the other two groups.

Thus we can see that in early pregnancy, women who subsequently have high EPDS scores both at 35 weeks and postnatally are more likely to be socially disadvantaged, less happy to be pregnant, and already showing signs of low emotional well-being. Women who subsequently have high EPDS

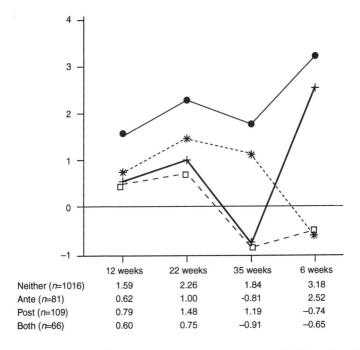

	12 weeks	22 weeks	35 weeks	6 weeks
Neither (*n*=1016)	1.59	2.26	1.84	3.18
Ante (*n*=81)	0.62	1.00	-0.81	2.52
Post (*n*=109)	0.79	1.48	1.19	-0.74
Both (*n*=66)	0.60	0.75	-0.91	-0.65

Fig. 12.3. Mean adjective checklist scores at four time points for groups above EPDS cut-off at different times (—●— neither (n = 1016), —+— ante (n = 81), --*--- post (= 109), - - -□- - - both (n = 66))

scores on only one of these occasions show equally low emotional well-being and are not distinguishable from each other at this point. The measure that does distinguish them is physical well-being: both of the groups with high EPDS scores at 35 weeks are reporting worse physical symptoms at 12 weeks. The other measure that distinguishes them is the belief that their baby is at above average risk of having a problem. So, although groups with different prognoses are not distinguishable at this early stage on the basis just of low emotional well-being (as measured by the adjective checklist), knowledge of the possible origins of that low well-being (social problems, physical problems, anxiety about the baby) provide common-sense predictors of its likely duration.

Feelings in mid-pregnancy

Women completed a second questionnaire at 22 weeks. As earlier, the 'both' group, and, to a lesser extent, the 'ante' group, reported much lower levels of physical well-being than the other two groups. The adjective checklist showed stronger differences between the groups than at 12 weeks, as Figure 12.3 shows. All groups show a trend to more positive adjectives, but the difference is smallest for the 'both' group. The 'neither' group still has significantly higher scores than the other three groups, which are not significantly different from each other.

The 22-week questionnaire also explored areas of social support, particularly relationship with husband or partner. Perceived support from partner was one of the most significant variables distinguishing the groups. Only 40% of the 'both' group felt that they always got the support that they wanted compared with 71% of the 'neither'.

Feelings in later pregnancy

At 35 weeks, adjective scores distinguished the groups still more strongly than earlier in pregnancy. All groups had more negative scores than at 22 weeks, but those of the 'ante' and 'both' groups dropped most (Fig. 12.3).

Perceptions of partner support were lower for all groups than they were at 22 weeks, but were particularly low for the 'both' group: only 25% were getting the support they would like. Women were also asked whether their relationship with their partner had changed during the pregnancy. Two-thirds of the 'neither' group reported either no change or an improved relationship, while the same proportion of the 'both' group reported some deterioration. The 'ante' and 'post' groups were, once again, between the other two, although there was more perception of positive change in the 'post' group.

Physical feelings continued to distinguish between the groups. Only 29% of women in the 'ante' and 'both' groups described themselves as 'very well' or 'blooming' compared with 57% of 'post' and 69% of 'neither'. The 'ante' and 'both' groups were also much more likely than the other two groups to describe themselves as very tired or exhausted (75% and 70% compared with 40%), and were more likely to have been admitted to hospital during pregnancy: 21% and 22% versus 9% of 'neither' and 15% of 'post'. The same two groups were also significantly more likely to report problems with weight gain and blood pressure.

During the course of pregnancy some women were told of possible foetal abnormalities picked up on scans or alpha fetoprotein screening tests. Others were told of problems that did not have direct implications for the baby's health but which might affect delivery, such as a low lying placenta. Unfortunately, our data from these women are often incomplete because a disproportionate number of them delivered before 35 weeks.

We do, however, have complete data from 49 women who were told of possible foetal abnormalities and 108 who were warned of delivery complications. Women with suspected 'baby' problems were significantly more likely to score above cut-off on at least one occasion, but no such relationship was observed for women warned of delivery problems. 'Ante' women were the least confident about their baby's health and the 'neither' group most confident.

TABLE 12.6
Mean scores on feelings about pregnancy and motherhood at 35 weeks for groups scoring above EPDS cut-off at different points

	Neither (*n* = 1016)	Ante (*n* = 81)	Post (*n* = 109)	Both (*n* = 66)	Significance
Pregnancy (max. 20)	14.6	10.6	13.4	10.1	0.0001
Motherhood (max. 30)	21.9	19.6	19.6	18.4	0.001

The 35-week questionnaire also included questions modified from the Maternal Adjustment and Attitudes (MAMA) questionnaire (Kumar *et al*, 1984) scale. There were two groups of questions. One assessed feelings about pregnancy (4 items) and the other feelings about motherhood (6 items). Each item could score from 0 (most negative) to 5 (most positive). Thus the maximum score on the pregnancy scale was 20 and on the motherhood scale, 30. Scores for the four groups are shown in Table 12.6. It will be seen that the 'neither' group scored highest on both scales, and 'both' scored lowest. The scores of the 'ante' group were not significantly different from those of the 'both' group on either scale. However, the 'post' group are of interest because, while their attitude to pregnancy is significantly higher than that of the 'ante' and 'both' groups, it is still significantly lower than the 'neither' group. Furthermore their 'attitude to motherhood' score is not only significantly lower than the 'neither' group, it is just as low as the 'ante' and 'both' groups. It would therefore appear that these questions may have a predictive value.

The 35-week questionnaire concluded with a section on attitudes to antenatal care. The 'ante' and 'both' groups were more likely to be critical of their care, for example, feeling that they had not been given enough information and rating it as less useful than the other two groups. There were no differences between the groups in the number of women who said that they had never attended antenatal classes (6%). However, women in the 'both' group were, rather surprisingly, most likely to say that they had attended classes in both the current and previous pregnancies (40% compared with 17% of the other groups).

Differences at around the time of birth

As Table 12.7 shows, there were a number of differences between the groups in what happened at around the time of birth. Many of these have to do with women's feelings, particularly their feelings of control. This confirms the findings of Green *et al* (1988, 1990). For example, feeling in control of one's behaviour, in control during contractions, and in control of what staff were doing were all highly significant with the 'neither' group always reporting most control, and the 'both' group least (Table 12.7). The same pattern is seen for various adjectives that women chose to describe themselves

TABLE 12.7
Differences at around the time of birth (reported 6 weeks postnatally) between groups scoring above EPDS cut-off at different points

	Neither (n = 1016)	Ante (n = 81)	Post (n = 109)	Both (n = 66)	Significance
Admitted to hospital (other than to give birth)	13%	24%	22%	17%	0.01
Suggestion of foetal distress	26%	29%	36%	31%	0.05
Baby problems at birth	18%	30%	31%	23%	0.01
Admitted to SCBU	7%	11%	14%	9%	NS
Caesarean	13%	12%	17%	11%	NS
Not able to get comfortable in labour	16%	28%	26%	34%	0.001
Felt in control of behaviour during labour	52%	37%	48%	36%	0.05
Felt in control during contractions	56%	42%	42%	31%	0.0001
Felt in control of what staff doing	64%	58%	48%	46%	0.0001
Satisfaction with birth (marks out of 10)	7.30	6.78	6.70	6.64	0.01*
Mean birth weight (grammes)	3446	3434	3292	3349	0.01**

*'Neither' significantly different from other three groups.
**Only 'neither' and 'post' significantly different from each other.
SCBU, special-care baby unit.

during labour and overall satisfaction with the birth (Table 12.7). 'Neither' and 'ante' women had significantly longer gestations: less than half of them delivered before their EDD, compared with two-thirds of the other two groups. (This analysis necessarily excludes women who delivered before 35 weeks since we have no antenatal EPDS scores for them.) This is reflected in the weight of their babies (Table 12.7). Multivariate analysis suggests that birth weight rather than gestation is the important factor.

Perceptions of the baby and motherhood

As in an earlier study (Green *et al*, 1991*b*), we found that high scoring women were much more likely to use negative words to describe their babies. The groups who were above cut-off antenatally were less likely to attempt breast-feeding and both the 'post' and 'ante' groups were less likely to persist. The result was that only in the 'neither' group were as many as half the women still breast feeding at six weeks. There had been no differences between the groups antenatally in their inclination to breast feed. The 'both' and 'post' groups were more likely to perceive their babies as more difficult than other babies, and also perceived life as more difficult since the birth. A postnatal 'experience of motherhood' scale was devised which matched that used antenatally. 'Both' and 'post' women had significantly lower scores than the other two groups (Table 12.8). Scores of the 'ante' group were not significantly lower than those of the 'neither' group.

TABLE 12.8
Differences at 6 weeks after delivery between groups scoring above EPDS cut-off at different points

	Neither (n = 1016)	Ante (n = 81)	Post (n = (109)	Both (n = 66)	Significance
Breast-fed:					
not at all	25%	32%	24%	36%	
gave up	24%	35%	39%	27%	0.001
still	50%	33%	38%	36%	
Mother's health:					
no problems	56%	54%	36%	30%	
minor problems	43%	43%	54%	61%	0.0001
major problems	1%	3%	10%	9%	
Feel very tired/exhausted	33%	48%	63%	68%	0.0001
5-day blues	51%	46%	80%	76%	0.0001
Feel life much more difficult	15%	18%	44%	49%	0.0001
Husband understands feelings	58%	50%	32%	22%	0.0001
No one can talk to	4%	15%	16%	29%	0.0001
Practical help	77%	71%	69%	71%	NS
Like more help	23%	34%	43%	42%	0.0001
Experience of motherhood score (max. = 30)	23.3	22.8	18.6	19.3	0.0001

Maternal health

As antenatally, there was a strong relationship between scoring above the
EPDS cut-off and reporting physical problems (Table 12.8). The 'ante' group
were no more likely than the 'neither' group to report physical problems,
although they did rate themselves as somewhat more tired. The '5 day blues'
were widely experienced by all groups, but the 'ante' group were no more
affected than 'neither'. Women scoring over cut-off were very much more
likely to rate themselves as depressed on a 0 to 5 scale. The adjectives that
women chose to describe themselves again showed a strong relationship with
EPDS categorisation. The total score (Figure 12.3) showed no significant
difference between 'neither' and 'ante', nor between 'post' and 'both'.

Social support

Twenty-three women reported having no partner at this stage, but this was
unrelated to their EPDS scores. For those with partners, there was, as
antenatally, a strong relationship between perceived support and EPDS score
(Table 12.8). 'Both' women were the most likely to say that they had no
one with whom they could discuss their problems and 'neither' the least
likely. Three-quarters of the women had received some practical help since

the birth from someone other than their partner, but this did not relate to EPDS score. However, those scoring over cut-off were more likely to want more help.

Discussion

We have shown in this chapter, on the evidence of both published and new data, that antenatal depression ranks with postnatal depression as an important health problem. It would seem to be just as prevalent and in the majority of cases is probably as severe and prolonged. For some, but by no means all women, it may continue into the postnatal period.

The data presented here confirm previously reported associations between depression scores and physical symptoms, tiredness, social support and marital relationship. The patterns were similar before and after delivery. The only specific associations with antenatal dysphoria were negative feelings about being pregnant and anxieties about the health of the foetus. By separating out groups with different trajectories it was hoped that light might be shed on differences between them and, in particular, on why scores change when they do. It was found that the group who were consistent high scorers do seem to have more social disadvantages and generally scored at the extreme on all identified correlates. Nearly half had not been pleased to find themselves pregnant. It is particular cause for concern that 29% said that they had no one they could talk to postnatally and only 25% of this group were getting the support that they wanted from their partners at the end of pregnancy. Clearly then, these women form a more vulnerable group.

The two groups who were high EPDS scorers on only one occasion appear very similar to each other on many of the variables investigated. They share many of the characteristics of the persistent high scorers, but to a lesser extent; for example, they were less pleased to be pregnant, less supported by their partners and less likely to have a confidante. In early pregnancy they are already showing significantly lower emotional well-being (as measured by the adjective checklist) than women whose EPDS scores were consistently low, and indeed are not significantly different from the persistent high scorers. Women who scored above cut-off only antenatally still had high EPDS scores postnatally (albeit below cut-off), and were scoring lower than women with consistently low scores on a number of other postnatal measures. The same, in reverse, is true for women whose EPDS scores were above cut-off only at the postnatal measurement. Both of these groups had worse birth experiences than women who were never above cut-off and were less successful at establishing breast-feeding. Both of these findings could, of course, be a cause of depression as well as a result. The findings reported here suggest an additive model of multiple factors throughout pregnancy and the puerperium combining to raise EPDS scores. This is consistent with our own earlier findings (Green, 1990). There is thus no single factor which can be identified as a 'cause' of either antenatal or postnatal depression.

Implications for practice

In summary, there is a strong correlation between antenatal and postnatal scores but there is a large group whose postnatal dysphoria is not predictable from antenatal EPDS. Groups who are dysphoric on only one or other occasion have very similar characteristics: what distinguishes them from each other are only events specific to the antenatal/postnatal period. So, what are the implications for practice?

Firstly, we can recognise the reality of antenatal depression and allow women to admit to it. There is a widespread assumption that women should 'bloom' while pregnant, which makes it that much more difficult for women to talk about their feelings. For many of them, particularly those with clear pregnancy-related reasons for low emotional well-being (e.g. nausea, uncertainty about the health of the baby), life *will* improve after delivery. The women who are at highest risk for continuing depression are those with poor marital relationships and no one to talk to. We were greatly encouraged to obseve in our data that women who felt unsupported by their partners received significantly more home visits from midwives during pregnancy. Clearly this is one way in which midwives are already responding to the issue. Such measures seem like common sense, but should we go beyond this to mass screening for antenatal depression?

Before widespread introduction into use, a screening test should be valid, ethical, acceptable, confer cost benefit (in the broadest sense), be well organised and aimed at an important problem the natural history of which is known (Wilson *et al*, 1991).

It might reasonably be argued that the EPDS is valid, ethical and acceptable and aimed at an important problem whose natural history we know at least something about. Further assessment of the cost benefit and organisational issues regarding screening for antenatal depression will, however, be required.

Organisationally the antenatal care setting in the UK provides opportunities for mass screening; most women attend a hospital clinic at least twice, as well as making several visits to their general practitioner. A computerised version of the EPDS is now available (Glaze & Cox, 1991) and repeated administrations on a number of occasions throughout pregnancy would be feasible and has been shown to be acceptable to women attending GP antenatal clinics (Ancill *et al*, 1986). The big organisational issue arises after the screening.

In a district with 6000 deliveries per year, for example, if all women attending the antenatal clinic were screened once, using a cut-off of 14/15, there would be 600 high scorers; 360 would be found to have RDC major depression and 120 would have minor depression and 120 would not be depressed. RDC major depression corresponds for the most part with mild to moderate depression and will require treatment. Intervention strategies appropriate to pregnancy will need to be devised. Increasing the psychological awareness and counselling skills of antenatal care-givers would seem an appropriate aim but would require careful evaluation. What kind and how much counselling will help? Who would do such work? Referral for more specialised psychological treatment may be required and prescription of antidepressants will often be necessary. Social interventions and help with housing and benefits will need to be addressed.

The EPDS is an appropriate tool for use in pregnancy, but the benefits of mass screening need to be established and weighed against the costs, especially the human costs. In particular we should guard against increasing midwives' workloads with yet another routine test until its benefits can be demonstrated.

We have demonstrated in this chapter that antenatal depression is an issue for a substantial number of women. The phenomenon is of interest both as a predictor of postnatal depression and in its own right. We have gone some way towards unravelling its aetiology, but much more needs to be known about interventions in pregnancy that might alter the course of events. The EPDS will undoubtedly be a valuable tool in the process of acquiring that knowledge.

References

ANCILL, R., HILTON, S., CARR, T., *et al* (1986) Screening for antenatal and postnatal depressive symptoms in general practice using a microcomputer-delivered questionnaire. *Journal of the Royal College of General Practitioners*, **36**, 276–279.

ATKINSON, K. A. & RICKEL, A. U. (1984) Postpartum depression in primiparous parents. *Journal of Abnormal Psychology*, **93**, 115–119.

BECK, A. T., WARD, C. H., MENDELSON, M., *et al* (1961) An inventory for measuring depression. *Archives of General Psychiatry*, **4**, 561–567.

BRAGONIER, J. R., CUSHNER, I. M. & HOBEL, C. J. (1984) Social and personal factors in the etiology of preterm birth. In *Preterm Birth: Causes, Prevention and Management* (eds F. Fuchs & P. G. Stubblefield). New York, NY: Macmillan.

COOPER, P. J., CAMPBELL, E. A., DAY, A., *et al* (1988) Non psychotic psychiatric disorder after childbirth. *British Journal of Psychiatry*, **152**, 799–806.

COX, J. L., HOLDEN, J. M. & SAGOVSKY, R. (1987) Detection of postnatal depression: Development of the 10-item Edinburgh Postnatal Depression Scale. *British Journal of Psychiatry*, **150**, 782–786.

——, CONNOR,Y. & KENDELL, R. E. (1982) Prospective study of psychiatric disorders of childbirth. *British Journal of Psychiatry*, **140**, 111–117.

CUTRONA, C. E. (1983) Causal attributions and perinatal depression. *Journal of Abnormal Psychology*, **92**, 161–172.

ESQUIROL, E. (1845) *Mental Maladies: a Treatise on Insanity* (trans. E. K. Hunt). Philadelphia: Lea & Blanchard.

GLAZE, R. & COX, J. L. (1991) Validation of a computerised version of the 10-item (self report) Edinburgh Postnatal Depression Scale. *Journal of Affective Disorders*, **22**, 73–77.

GOLDBERG, D. P. (1972) *Detection of Psychiatric Illness by Questionnaire*, Maudsley Monographs, No. 21. Oxford: Oxford University Press.

——, COOPER, B., EASTWOOD, M. R., *et al* (1970) A standardised psychiatric interview for use in community surveys. *British Journal of Preventive and Social Medicine*, **24**, 18–23.

GOTLIB, I. H., WHIFFEN, V. E., MOUNT, J. H., *et al* (1989) Prevalence rates and demographic characteristics associated with depression in pregnancy and the postpartum. *Journal of Consulting and Clinical Psychology*, **57**, 269–274.

GREEN, J. M. (1990) 'Who is unhappy after childbirth?': Antenatal and intrapartum correlates from a prospective study. *Journal of Reproductive and Infant Psychology*, **8**, 175–183.

——, COUPLAND, V. A. & KITZINGER, J. V. (1988) *Great Expectations: A Prospective Study of Women's Expectations and Experiences of Childbirth.* University of Cambridge Child Care and Development Group.

——, —— & —— (1990) Expectations, experiences and psychological outcomes of childbirth: a prospective study of 825 women. *Birth*, **17**, 15–24.

——, STATHAM, H. E. & SNOWDON, C. (1994) *Pregnancy: A Testing Time.* Report of the Cambridge Prenatal Screening Study. University of Cambridge Centre for Family Research.

——, SNOWDON, C. & STATHAM, H. E. (1991*a*) EPDS by post. *British Journal of Psychiatry*, **158**, 865.

——, RICHARDS, M., KITZINGER, J., *et al* (1991*b*) Mothers' perceptions of their 6-week-old babies: Relationship with intrapartum and postnatal factors. *Irish Journal of Psychology*, **12**, 133–144.

HAMILTON, M. (1960) A rating scale for depression. *Journal of Neurology, Neurosurgery and Psychiatry*, **23**, 56–62.

KENDALL, P. C., HOLLON, S. D., BECK, A. T., *et al* (1987) Issues and recommendations regarding use of the Beck Depression Inventory. *Cognitive Therapy and Research*, **11**, 289–299.

KUMAR, R. (1982) Neurotic disorders in childbearing women. In *Motherhood and Mental Illness* (eds I. F. Brockington & R. Kumar), pp. 71–118. London: Academic Press.

—— & ROBSON, K. (1984) A prospective study of emotional disorders in child-bearing women. *British Journal of Psychiatry*, **144**, 35–47.

——, —— & SMITH, A. M. R. (1984) Development of a self-administered questionnaire to measure maternal adjustment and maternal attitudes during pregnancy and after delivery. *Journal of Psychosomatic Research*, **28**, 43–51.

MONTGOMERY, S. A. & ÅSBERG, M. (1979) A new depression scale designed to be sensitive to change. *British Journal of Psychiatry*, **134**, 382–389.

MURRAY, D. & COX, J. L. (1990) Screening for depression during pregnancy with the Edinburgh Depression Scale (EPDS). *Journal of Reproductive and Infant Psychology*, **8**, 99–107.

MURRAY, L. & STEIN, A. (1991) Postnatal depression and infant development. *British Medical Journal*, **302**, 978–979.

NILSSON, A. & ALMGREN, P. (1970) Paranatal emotional adjustment; a prospective investigation of 165 women. *Acta Psychiatrica Scandinavica* (suppl. 220).

NOTT, P. N. & CUTTS, S. (1982) Validation of the 30-item General Health Questionnaire in postpartum women. *Psychological Medicine*, **12**, 409–413.

O'HARA, M. W. (1986) Social support, life events and depression during pregnancy and the puerperium. *Archives of General Psychiatry*, **43**, 569–573.

——, ZEKOSKI, E. M., PHILLIPS, L. H., *et al* (1990) Controlled prospective study of postpartum mood disorders: comparison of childbearing and nonchildbearing women. *Journal of Abnormal Psychology*, **99**, 3–15.

PITT, B. (1968) 'Atypical' depression following childbirth. *British Journal of Psychiatry*, **114**, 1325–1335.

REES, W. D. & LUTKINS, S. G. (1971) Parental depression before and after childbirth: an assessment with the Beck Depression Inventory. *Journal of the Royal College of General Practitioners*, **21**, 26–31.

SHARP, D. (1988) Validation of the 30-item General Health Questionnaire in early pregnancy. *Psychological Medicine*, **18**, 503–507.

—— (1989) Emotional disorders during pregnancy and the puerperium – a longitudinal prospective study in primary care. *Marcé Society Bulletin*, Spring.

SPITZER, R. L., ENDICOTT, J. & ROBINS, E. (1978) Research Diagnostic Criteria: rationale and reliability. *Archives of General Psychiatry*, **35**, 773–782.

STEIN, A., GATH, D. H., BUCHER, J., *et al* (1991) The relationship between postnatal depression and mother–child interaction. *British Journal of Psychiatry*, **158**, 46–52.

UDDENBERG, N. (1974) Reproductive adaptation in mother and daughter. A study of personality development and adaptation to motherhood. *Acta Psychiatrica Scandinavica* (suppl. 254).

WATSON, J. P., ELLIOTT, S. A., RUGG, A. J., *et al* (1984) Psychiatric disorder in pregnancy and the first postnatal year. *British Journal of Psychiatry*, **144**, 453–462.

WILSON, J. M. G. (1991) The worth of screening. *Proceedings of the Royal College of Physicians of Edinburgh*, **21**, 288–310.

WOLKIND, S. (1981) Prenatal emotional stress – effects on the foetus. In *Pregnancy: a Psychological and Social Study* (eds S. Wolkind & E. Zajicek). London: Academic Press.

——, ZAJICEK, E. & GHODSIAN, M. (1980) Continuities in maternal depression. *International Journal of Family Psychiatry*, **1**, 167–182.

ZIGMOND, A. S. & SNAITH, R. P. (1983) The Hospital Anxiety and Depression Scale. *Acta Psychiatrica Scandinavica*, **67**, 361–370.

ZUCKERMAN, B., AMARO, A., BAUCHNER, H., *et al* (1989) Depressive symptoms during pregnancy: Relationship to poor health behaviours. *American Journal of Obstetrics and Gynecology*, **160**, 1107–1111.

13 Beyond the Edinburgh Postnatal Depression Scale: other rating scales and standardised interviews of use in assessing disturbed parents and their children

DAVID FOREMAN

Postnatal mental illness affects the whole family. Fifty per cent of spouses (Foreman *et al*, 1992; Lovestone & Kumar, 1993) suffer concurrent mental illness, usually depression. The marital relationship may suffer, and children are also adversely affected in many ways (O'Hara & Zekoski, 1988). The range of measures that address these issues is too large to be covered in a single chapter. Therefore, this chapter will concentrate on observer- and self-rated interview scales, as these are most likely to be used concurrently with the Edinburgh Postnatal Depression Scale (EPDS).

Measures suitable for children

There are four factors that make the measurement of children different from the measurement of parents. An individual child is likely to change much more over a given period than a parent will over the same period. A homogeneous group of children of a given age are likely to resemble each other more than a homogeneous group of adults with an equivalent age-range (making differences more difficult to detect). Child psychiatric disorders tend to express themselves as quantitative differences from the norm, rather than qualitative differences. 'Self-rated' measures are in fact frequently parent-rated, as parent ratings are mostly more reliable (Edelbrock *et al*, 1985).

The concept of development underpins all of the available measures for children. Although it is an inescapable part of childhood, there exists no one theory that encompasses it. The key measurement issue resulting from this is that of construct validity. Any theory that organises data is a construct, and so any theory of development (such as temperament or attachment) is a construct. Construct validity assesses the extent to which a measure reflects the construct it supposes. It may be assessed in three main ways: factor analysis, the multimethod–multitrait matrix, and predictive validity.

Factor analysis groups the various items of a scale together. The resulting factors should reflect the constructs underpinning the scale. The 'multimethod–multitrait matrix' of Campbell & Fiske (1959) relies on the assessment of multiple measures. Some of these should correlate positively with the construct (convergent validity), and some negatively with it (divergent validity). This leads to the concept of predictive validity: one *predicts* the behaviour of the measures based on one's views of the construct. It is frequently the case that two measures should associate with each other, but do not share a common construct. This form of mutual validation, called concurrent validity, needs to be distinguished from convergent validity, as it does not validate the construct of any individual measure. However, it does support the general relevance of the measures to the subject under investigation.

While adult measures may cover an age range of 40 years or more, no child measure can be so extensive, given the importance of development. Available measures tend to fall into three broad bands: the first two years of life; the 'pre-school/toddler' period, from the second to the fourth year of life inclusive; and school-age children. Within the school-age group, at least some measures make a further distinction between pre-pubertal and teenage children.

Detecting symptomatology

Unsurprisingly, children exhibit quite different symptoms to adults, and so different measures must be used. In principle, the same phenomenological/ diagnostic approach is used in children as in adults. In practice, the need to take developmental differences into account has resulted in a variety of approaches. There are no structured interviews, and surprisingly few rating scales designed simply to assess the general behaviour of children in the first two years of their life. Most behavioural studies of this group rely on an ethological paradigm, using systematised observations of naturalistic settings. Ainsworth *et al*'s 'Strange Situation' (Ainsworth *et al*, 1978), Trevarthen *et al*'s (Trevarthen *et al*, 1981) and Murray's (Murray, 1988) investigations of infant behaviour all fall into this category. This methodology is beyond the scope of this chapter. However, such methods are even more demanding than structured interviews, and therefore there is considerable need for easier measures that are useful in this group. Murray (1992), Stein *et al* (1991), and Ghodsian *et al* (1984) have all attempted to adapt Richman & Graham's Behavioural Screening Questionnaire (Richman & Graham, 1971) to this age-range, but this adaptation has shown poor predictive validity. None of these authors have been unequivocally successful in demonstrating differences between different groups of infants using this adaptation, even when differences have been shown by ethological techniques.

More measures are available for pre-school children. The Behaviour Screening Questionnaire of Richman & Graham (Richman & Graham, 1971) mentioned above is an observer-rated, semi-structured checklist for behaviour problems that has good validity and reliability and has been widely used. It places less emphasis on emotional difficulties, and also identified difficulties in hearing, speech, locomotion and sphincter (bowel and bladder) control. It has good convergent validity with ethological approaches used in a similar population (Cox *et al*, 1987). It takes, typically, 40 to 60 minutes to complete. It may be used to estimate severity of disturbance, as well as giving a cut-off value. It is particularly effective at estimating the prevalence of child psychiatric disorder in community populations, and can detect differences in the children of disturbed parents (Cox *et al*, 1987; Ghodsian *et al*, 1984; Wrate *et al*, 1985).

Achenbach & Edelbrock's Child Behaviour Checklist (CBCL) (Achenbach & Edelbrock, 1983, 1986, 1987*a,b*) is probably the most widely used measure of child behaviour for pre-school and school-age children. It comprises a whole family of measures, being child-, observer-, parent- or teacher-rated for several different ages of children from the second year of life onwards (Achenbach *et al*, 1987*a*). Its validity, as well as its reliability, has been repeatedly tested, and is good for its estimates of problems, but less good for its estimate of children's competencies (Fombonne, 1991). It not only supplies absolute symptom counts, but also allows the development of a symptom profile. In some observer-rated versions repeated observations may be required, and the number of individual items can be large.

Measuring 'caseness' and associated concepts

The relative paucity of diagnostically or symptomatologically based behavioural measures for very young children and infants reflects the dominance of two developmentally based constructs for behaviour in these age-groups: temperament and attachment.

Temperament: definition and measurement

Personality has never been a useful concept for children. Its classic definition, embodying enduring psychological characteristics of the individual, is simply not applicable to a developing organism. However, even young babies do exhibit systematic differences in how they interact with the world. These differences in behavioural style are better called temperament (Prior, 1992). For largely historical reasons, temperamental measures are parent-rated scales rather than direct observational assessments. The scales consist of descriptions of the child's behaviour that are rated by the parent: these descriptions are analysed to give differing temperamental dimensions, which can then be classified further into temperamental types. The best-known model of temperament is that of Thomas & Chess (1977), which identified nine dimensions: activity; rhythmicity (regularity of eating and sleeping); emotionality (fussiness); distractibility; persistence (the ability to maintain an activity); intensity of expression; threshold (the level of stimulation that elicits a response); and ease of adaptation to novel stimuli or situations. These dimensions may, in their turn, be used to diagnose three different temperamental types: easy; difficult; and slow-to-warm-up.

The questionnaires derived from their work have been the most commonly used measures of temperament. Though primarily contrived for school-age children, the measures have been modified for use with both pre-school children and infants (Carey, 1970; McDevitt & Carey, 1981). Test–retest reliability over short periods is good, suggesting that these measures reliably report child behaviour, but there is doubt over their construct validity. First, the predictive validity of these differences over periods as short as 12 months can be quite low (Rothbart & Derryberry, 1981). Secondly, contextual variables (such as marital satisfaction or maternal psychological status) have a considerable influence on reported temperament in some studies (Lancaster *et al*, 1989), but not others (Wolkind & De Salis, 1982). Furthermore, authors other than Thomas & Chess have identified alternative factor structures for temperament (Buss & Plomin, 1984; Rothbart, 1987, 1989), which further challenges the idea that temperament represents an unequivocal construct. Two main constructs of temperament have evolved. Some authorities regard temperament as reflecting intrinsic biological, and especially genetic, determinants of the child. Others emphasise that temperament reflects continuities of behavioural style within a transaction, and thus environmental influences represent an integral part of the construct.

Evidence exists to support both the first view (Saudino & Eaton, 1991) and the second (Belsky *et al*, 1991). Thus, temperament is a complex construct, which must result in multidimensional measures. This, in turn, makes universal validation difficult, as precise criteria for construct validity remain unclear. For example, it is unclear whether some differences result from measurement error or the nature of temperament itself (Carey & McDevitt, 1989; Gibbs *et al*, 1989). Nonetheless, the temperamental types, and some sets of characteristics identified, have modest predictive validity in identifying subsequent behavioural difficulty in children and even adults (Rutter, 1987). So, they are valuable for identifying behavioural abnormalities in young children that may have long-term significance. There is a relationship between children's temperamental scores and maternal mental state (Cutrona & Troutman, 1985; Wolkind & De Salis, 1982). As the ratings are by parents, mental disturbance in a parent might be expected to generate bias in the resultant score, and is therefore important to the assessment of families with disturbed parents. We have already seen that there is equivocal evidence regarding this (Lancaster *et al*, 1989; Wolkind

& De Salis, 1982), but the problem can be minimised by asking each parent to record temperament independently. Provided the mental state of all the parents (both husbands and wives) is known, any bias from this source can be estimated statistically.

The problems with construct validity discussed above make the use of observer-rated measures equally beset with problems of meaningful reliability and inter-rater agreement (Matheny *et al*, 1987). When working with families with a disturbed parent, it probably makes most sense to use questionnaires, such as those derived from the work of Thomas & Chess, that emphasise the interactional nature of temperament. This should maximise the sensitivity of the measure to the area of interest.

Attachment and its disturbances

Attachment theory has probably been the single most influential theory of child development to emerge since the 1960s. It proposes that children develop and maintain an affectional bond with their mothers (Bowlby, 1978), using many behavioural strategies to do so. Failure to maintain such a bond results both in an increase in the frequency of those behavioural strategies required to maintain it, and subsequent difficulties in emotional and social relationships. As well as an explanatory theory, it has generated a test with intrinsic criterion validity, Ainsworth's 'strange situation' (Ainsworth *et al*, 1978). This is an experimental test, where the infant or young child is confronted by either a novel situation, a stranger, or a combination in the presence or absence of the mother. The child's responses are systematically noted. Ainsworth's original study suggested a tripartite classification. Most children were securely attached to their mothers, in that they showed slight distress on parental departure, but recovered swiftly, and swiftly greeted their parents on reunion. Some children showed 'insecure avoidant attachment', which meant that they showed indifference to their mother on reunion. Other children showed 'insecure resistant attachment', which meant that they both clung to and pushed away their mother on reunion. The mothers of insecurely attached children had to increase their nurturing in response, until the child relented. These two latter categories of insecure attachment have proved to predict subsequent behavioural difficulties (Erickson *et al*, 1985), or parental disturbance (Murray, 1992; Stein *et al*, 1991), further supporting the validity of the test. However, like temperament, the construct validity of the test has been eroded. The tripartite classification has become unstable, with some authorities preferring a fourth category to include cases of insecure attachment that are neither anxious or avoidant (Main & Cassidy, 1988). The boundary between attachment and the very different construct of temperament has become increasingly unclear, in that the concept of security is closely related to both (Belsky & Rovine, 1987; Vaughn & Waters, 1990).

Both these problems, and the test's inconvenience, have highlighted a need for alternative measures of attachment. This led Waters & Deane (1985) to develop a Q-sort alternative to the strange situation. Cards are used which carry descriptions of various behaviours (some with their opposites), and the rater sorts the cards into nine piles, ranging from 'very like' to 'very unlike'. The factor loading for each card on a 'security dimension' has been calculated, and so the level of security typical of the child may be estimated. In their original paper, Waters & Deane reported good inter-rater reliability with pairs of student observers, and developed an extensive argument to support its construct validity. Subsequently, it has been both suggested and used as a parent-rated scale. Vaughn & Waters (1990) found it had good convergent validity with the strange situation when used as an observer-rated measure. However, Van Dam & Von Ijzendoorn (1988) found its convergent validity was rather less when used as a parent-rated measure. It has the advantage of being usable in a naturalistic setting. In this author's experience, it is usable between eight months and five years. Parents seem to find it a very difficult measure to use as the sorting procedure is complex and time-consuming, being about 45 minutes per child. As an observer-rated instrument, the measure seems very acceptable to parents: many will tolerate an observer spending time in their homes to perform a Q-sort but not agree to a 'strange situation' test.

The Separation Anxiety Test (Klagsbrun & Bowlby, 1976) is an alternative measure of security suitable for older children, though its age-range does overlap with that of the strange situation. In it, a child is asked to comment on a series of separation-related pictures in a structured manner, and the child's responses scored from typed verbatim transcripts. In principle, it may be used in either naturalistic or laboratory settings. A recent study (Shouldice & Stevenson-Hinde, 1992) has shown that it has criterion validity when compared with the 'strange situation' in that its various items related predictably to a 'strange situation' classification. However, it is not suitable for children younger than 4.5 years.

The Adult Attachment Interview (George *et al*, 1985), now in its third revision, seeks to classify the attachment status of adults (with respect to their own parents) by making an observer-rated assessment of adults' parenting experiences. It identifies three attachment types: autonomous; dismissing; or preoccupied. These are determined from both the content and the style of the answers given to the interviewer's probes. Training in administration and scoring is required (Main & Goldwyn, 1994). In an unselected community sample, it may take between 30 minutes and 2 hours, but is reliable (Fonagy *et al*, 1991). There may be a relationship between its attachment types and those found in the strange situation (Main *et al*, 1985). So far, predictive validity has been demonstrated for the autonomous and dismissive categories in mothers. These associate, respectively, with the secure and avoidant strange situation categories of their infants (Fonagy *et al*, 1991; Zeanah *et al*, 1993). It may also predict interactional styles in mothers' reactions with their older children (Kobak *et al*, 1993).

The Parental Bonding Instrument (PBI) is a self-report scale that gives both valid and reliable data about the respondent's experience of parenting along two dimensions: degree of care and degree of protection (Parker, 1981; Parker *et al*, 1979, 1982). In adolescents, bonding difficulty measured on this instrument covaries with psychiatric disorder (Burbach *et al*, 1989), and so it makes a simple and acceptable measure for this group, with concurrent validity.

There are thus some measures available for estimating behaviours associated with the child's maintenance of child-caretaker relationships over a wide age-range. These are of clear value in assessing the impact of psychiatrically disturbed caretakers on their children. However, the doubts indicated above over the construct validity of attachment measures suggests that positive findings from these measures should not be taken as necessarily supporting attachment theory.

Psychiatric 'caseness' in children

The attachment and temperament classifications detailed above are not diagnoses of psychiatric 'caseness'. Child psychiatric disorder may be defined as a disturbance of behaviour, thought, emotions or relationships, that is out of keeping with the child's developmental status or sociocultural milieu, and does the child harm (Hersov, 1977). As with adults, there are two ways of deriving caseness: (semi-) structured interviews and rating scales with cut-offs.

The Child Assessment Schedule (CAS; Hodges & Fitch, 1979; Hodges *et al*, 1982*a*,*b*) and the Schedule for Affective Disorders and Schizophrenia for School-Aged Children (K–SADS; Puig-Antich & Chambers, 1978) are probably the best-known interview measures of child psychiatric disorder. The K–SADS is a semi-structured diagnostic interview for school-age children and their parents, and has versions to cover lifetime as well as current diagnoses. Early versions were deficient in reliability in anxiety disorders, and characterised behaviour problems poorly outside common conduct disorder. Recent revisions appear to have resolved these difficulties (Ambrosini *et al*, 1989), and the reliability is now equivalent to the adult SADS. Additionally, there is good convergent validity. With adolescents there is good agreement between ratings obtained from mothers and assessment of the teenagers themselves (Apter *et al*, 1989). In younger children, though there was a marked difference in the rates of symptoms reported between parents and children, this did not markedly affect the clinician's subsequent diagnosis (Ivens & Rehm, 1988).

The latter study also demonstrated that depressed mothers were as accurate as non-depressed mothers in reporting their children's symptoms, suggesting that the K–SADS is especially valuable in this area. It requires clinically trained interviewers, and can take as long as two hours per subject. The CAS has roughly equivalent validity and reliability to the K–SADS (Hodges *et al*, 1982*b*; Hodges, 1993), and indeed shows good concordance with it (Hodges *et al*, 1987). Like the K–SADS, it is long, and training in its use is recommended. It has the advantage over the K–SADS of offering several quantitative estimates of the intensity of its diagnoses. However, unlike the K–SADS it does not have a version that covers past episodes of psychiatric caseness.

Highly structured interview scales for use by raters without clinical training also exist. The best known are the Diagnostic Interview Schedule for Children (DISC; Costello *et al*, 1984), and the Diagnostic Interview for Children and Adolescents (DICA; Herjanic *et al*, 1975).

Further information available for the DISC includes the following. While it can distinguish between psychiatric and non-psychiatric patient groups (Costello *et al*, 1985) it continues to have difficulties in reliability and discriminant validity between specific diagnoses, despite revisions (Costello *et al*, 1984; Shaffer *et al*, 1988). These difficulties are particularly acute with computer-generated diagnoses, such as would be required with untrained interviewers. The DICA appears to give better results (Vitiello *et al*, 1990; Welner *et al*, 1987) but with clinician-generated diagnoses, and so would give only limited resource advantage over a semi-structured interview. Thus, they appear to suffer from equivalent criticisms to the Adult DISC (Edelbrock *et al*, 1986). There may be a specific reason to prefer semi-structured child diagnostic interviews in assessments of children. Semi-structured parental interviews are more sensitive to the child's symptomatology as directly observed or reported than highly structured parental interviews (Verhulst *et al*, 1987). So, the use of a suitable semi-structured interview may reduce the likelihood of disagreement between parent and child about symptomatology. However, the amount of agreement varies with the type of symptomatology reported (Edelbrock *et al*, 1986; Hodges *et al*, 1990). One should therefore interview the child as well as the parents in any interview schedule, whenever possible.

If one does not wish to make use of structured interviews, there are some rating scales that may be used with cut-offs to define caseness. The original standardisation of the Behavioural Screening Questionnaire (Richman & Graham, 1971) included such a cut-off suitable for pre-school children. In Rutter's Isle of Wight study, two questionnaires were used with school-age children in large community populations, one for parents ('Rutter A') (Rutter, 1970) and one for teachers ('Rutter B') (Rutter, 1967). The study gave them impressive reliability and validity, and they are quick (5 minutes), acceptable and easy to use. They allow the identification of children with emotional disorders, behaviour disorders, or mixtures of the two.

The symptom profile generated by the CBCL may be used to supply diagnoses at various levels of refinement. The CBCL gives two major subscores, 'internalising' and 'externalising', corresponding roughly with the Rutter scales' distinction between behavioural and emotional disturbances. In fact, good concurrent validity exists between these two measures (Fombonne, 1989). Additionally, the CBCL subscale scores may be analysed further to give seven specific syndromes: aggressive; delinquent; depressed; hyperactive; social withdrawal; somatic complaints; and non-communication (Achenbach *et al*, 1987*a*,*b*). The names of these syndromes suggest close links with both ICD and DSM criteria. However, despite good construct validity demonstrated by factor analysis, they will only have concurrent validity with respect to the diagnoses of the two main classification systems. This is because the CBCL is dimensionally based, whereas both ICD and DSM are categorical taxonomies.

As with adults, one may also use specific individual measures to detect a specific individual problem in children. Detailed discussion of them is beyond the scope of this chapter. However, it is important to note that self-report scales for children may result in over-reporting of emotional disorders (Asarnow & Carlson, 1985), and under-reporting of behavioural disturbance (Patterson, 1986).

Measuring familial interactions

As disturbed mental states are likely to affect relationships as well as individuals, it is important to have measures that specifically address interactions. These measures can be divided into three groups: those that measure the marital relationship; those that measure the parent–child relationship; and those that consider the family as a whole.

Measures of the marital relationship

The Short Marital Adjustment Test (SMAT; Locke & Wallace, 1959) is a 15-item questionnaire which yields a linear score reflecting the spouse's level of adjustment in the marriage. It covers disagreements, communication, leisure time activities, and regrets about having married one's spouse. Its validity and reliability are good (Gottman *et al*, 1976), and it is sensitive to changes in family functioning that include child disturbance (Howes & Markman, 1989), thus making it especially useful in this area. However, its item weighting may leave it open to bias from families' concerns to give socially desirable answers. Therefore, other ratings may be necessary to exclude this, if it is likely to influence the results (Harrison & Westhuis, 1989). Spanier's Dyadic Adjustment Schedule (Spanier, 1976) is a more comprehensive self-report questionnaire, with norms. It can reliably detect marital dysfunction for families coping with sickness, but its norms for the general population cannot be assumed (Walker *et al*, 1992). Its factor structure seems to vary markedly between studies (Eddy *et al*, 1991; Kazak *et al*, 1988), and so there is some doubt over what it measures. In particular, the scale may confuse the relationship between 'adjustment' and 'satisfaction'. The marital measure with the best psychometric properties is the Marital Satisfaction Inventory. However, its daunting length makes it unsuitable for use as part of the battery of questionnaires which are likely to be used in this field (Burnett, 1987).

An alternative to the above is the Waring Intimacy Questionnaire (Waring & Reddon, 1983). It focuses on an operationalised definition of marital intimacy, which is more restrictive than the broader definition of 'adjustment'. This may have more clinical relevance, especially in the development of psychiatric disorder in women (Brown & Harris, 1978; Costello, 1982). Its construct and concurrent validity and reliability are all acceptable (Waring, 1985).

Measures of parenting

Probably the best single questionnaire for parent–child interaction is the Parenting Stress Index (PSI; Abidin, 1990). This includes scales for attachment, childhood temperament, tolerance of parental role, and parental relations. As such, it comes close to being a summary measure of family functioning, but the focus is on those areas that are likely to impede effective parenting. Though it has 101 items in its full form, it takes no more than 25 minutes to complete. Age-ranges are not specified, but, being parent-reported, it is better with younger children. Its reliability is now well established, and it has both construct and criterion validity (Kline *et al*, 1991; Mash & Johnston, 1983). As it includes a 'social desirability' scale, it works well with the SMAT discussed above, and the two have been used together with success (Cowan & Cowan, 1988). For adolescents, attitude scales towards each parent are reliable estimators of the child's perception of problems in the parental relationship. They have both construct and concurrent validity in relation to psychiatric caseness (Saunders & Schuchts, 1987).

Unlike the PSI, the Maternal Adjustment and Maternal Attitudes (MAMA) questionnaire (Kumar, 1984) was designed specifically for pregnant and postnatal women. It is acceptable, very reliable, and its symptom scores agree with those made concurrently by interviewers. More detailed testing of its validity is currently unavailable. A modification for fathers (PAPA) is also available, but as yet has not been validated independently. However, Lovestone & Kumar (1993) found the latter's marital adjustment subscales unable to distinguish between psychiatrically ill and well spouses, though marital adjustment and spousal psychiatric status may be related (Harvey & McGrath, 1988).

Family measures

When choosing measures of family functioning, it is important to realise that many of the best-known measures have resulted from specific theories about family functioning or therapy. This can therefore have a bearing on the choice of measure in one's own investigation.

Olson's 'Circumplex' model of family functioning (Olson *et al*, 1979) has resulted in the development of a series of questionnaires to measure family functioning in terms of that model. Generically known as FACES (Family Adaptation and Cohesion Evaluation Scales), version IV is now being piloted (Green *et al*, 1991*b*). It already shows high reliability. Olson *et al*'s basic construct assumes that family functioning can be organised along two axes: adaptability and cohesion. The most extensively researched version to date is FACES III, which is a self-report scale of 20 items, making it a very brief and acceptable measure. Unfortunately, although it has good criterion validity, its construct validity is suspect, as empirical findings give only partial support for the circumplex model that underpins it (Green *et al*, 1991*a*).

The Family Assessment Device (FAD; Epstein *et al*, 1983) is based on the McMaster model of family functioning (Epstein & Bishop, 1981). It is a self-rating scale consisting of 60 items covering six dimensions of family functioning: problem solving; communication; affective involvement; affective responsiveness; behaviour control; and family roles. Additionally, a seventh scale gives a global estimate of functioning. It appears to have good concurrent validity in distinguishing between families containing patients versus non-patients (Sawyer *et al*, 1988). However, its convergence with other family measures is limited (Perosa & Perosa, 1990), suggesting impaired construct validity, and it also seems culturally bound (Morris, 1990).

The Family Assessment Measure (FAM; Skinner *et al*, 1983) is both conceptually and structurally very similar to the FAD. It differs from the FAD in that there is an additional dimension of 'values and norms', which is explicitly designed to include cultural issues. It also includes social desirability and denial scales. It investigates three levels of functioning: the individual's perceptions of the family as a whole; family dyads; and the individual's self-perception within the family. It may be given to children as young as 10–12 years. Like the FAD, it has good concurrent validity in distinguishing clinic from non-clinic families. It also produces results (comparing husbands and wives) that parallel those of the FACES system, suggesting more convergence (Skinner, 1987). However, it is less widely tested than the FAD, and the multiplicity of possible questionnaires (it also rates the family's constituent dyads) may make the full form unsuitable. Nonetheless, the cultural elements and the dyadic element make a useful addition in certain circumstances, and its reliability and concurrent validity are as good as the FAD.

The Family Environment Scale (Moos & Moos, 1986) is a 100-item self-report scale that assesses family relationships, personal growth, and system maintenance across 10 categories. These are: cohesion; expressiveness; conflict; independence; achievement orientation; intellectual/cultural orientation; active/relational orientation; moral/religious emphasis; organisation; and control. Many of its dimensions are therefore conceptually similar to those of the FAM and FAD. It has been used with success in the assessment of families of depressed patients (Billings *et al*, 1985; Billings & Moos, 1985), and so has good criterion validity for this group. This may be sufficient for many studies (Moos, 1990). However, both its reliability and construct validity are more suspect. There are conflicting reports regarding agreement of the scale with observer-rated measures (Glass, 1993; Nelson *et al*, 1992; Roosa & Beals, 1990), and its conceptual structure is suspect (Loveland-Cherry *et al*, 1989; Roosa & Beals, 1990) in at least some populations.

Conclusions

The impact of mental illness on families requires multiple measures to explore it thoroughly. Many interviews and rating scales are available to investigate problems at the individual, dyadic and family level, and their validity and reliability make them useful tools. However, no measure is perfect, and one's final choice of measure should be based on the question one wishes to ask. It is important to realise that there are many questions that cannot be answered by either standardised interviews or rating scales. Important investigations I have *not* been able to cover in this chapter include genetic assessment, assessments of biological functioning, quality-of-life estimation, and cognitive assessments of both adults and children as well as the ethological investigations that have only been alluded to. Finally, no measure can be valid if it does not answer the right question, whatever its psychometric properties or practical convenience.

References

ABIDIN, R. (1990) *Parenting Stress Index*. Charlottesville, VA: Pediatric Psychology Press.
ACHENBACH, T. & EDELBROCK, C. (1983) *Manual for the Child Behavior Checklist and Revised Child Behavior Profile*. Burlington, VT: University of Vermont Department of Psychiatry.
—— & —— (1986) *Manual for the Teacher's Report Forma and Teacher Version of the Child Behavior Profile*. Burlington, VT: University of Vermont Department of Psychiatry
—— & —— (1987) *Manual for the Youth Self-report and Profile*. Burlington, VT: University of Vermont Department of Psychiatry.
——, —— & HOWELL, C. (1987*a*) Empirically-based assessment of the behavioral/emotional problems of 2–3-year-old children. *Journal of Abnormal Child Psychology*, **15**, 629–650.

———, VERHULST, F., BARON, G., *et al* (1987*b*) A comparison of syndromes derived from the Child Behavior Checklist for American and Dutch boys aged 6–11 and 12–16. *Journal of Child Psychology and Psychiatry*, **28**, 437–454.

AINSWORTH, M., BLEHAR, M., WATERS, E., *et al* (1978) *Patterns of Attachment: a Psychological Study of the Strange Situation*. Hillsdale, NJ: Lawrence Erlbaum.

AMBROSINI, P., METZ, C., PRABUCKI, K., *et al* (1989) Videotape reliability of the Third Revised Edition of the K–SADS. *Journal of the American Academy of Child Psychiatry*, **28**, 723–728.

APTER, A., ORVASCHEL, H., LASEG, M., *et al* (1989) Psychometric properties of the K–SADS-P in an Israeli adolescent inpatient population. *Journal of the American Academy of Child Psychiatry*, **46**, 61–65.

ASARNOW, R. & CARLSON, G. (1985) Depression self-rating scale: utility with child psychiatric inpatients. *Journal of Consulting and Clinical Psychology*, **53**, 491–499.

BELSKY, J. & ROVINE, M. (1987) Temperament and attachment security in the strange situation: An empirical rapprochement. *Child Development*, **58**, 787–795.

———, FISH, M. & ISABELLA, R. (1991) Continuity and discontinuity in infant negative and positive emotionality: family antecedents and attachment consequences. *Developmental Psychology*, **27**, 421–431.

BILLINGS, A., CRONKITE, R. & MOOS, R. (1985) Social environmental factors in unipolar depression: Comparison of depressed patients and nondepressed controls. *Journal of Abnormal Psychology*, **92**, 119–133.

——— & MOOS, R. (1985) Psychosocial processes of remission in unipolar depression: Comparing depressed patients with matched community controls. *Journal of Consulting and Clinical Psychology*, **53**, 314–425.

BOWLBY, J. (1978) *The Making and Breaking of Affectional Bonds*. London: Tavistock.

BROWN, G. & HARRIS, T. (1978) *Social Origins of Depression: A Study of Psychiatric Disorder in Women*. London: Tavistock.

BURBACH, D., KASHANI, J. & ROSENBERG, K. (1989) Parental bonding and depressive disorders in adolescents. *Journal of Child Psychology and Psychiatry*, **30**, 417–430.

BURNETT, P. (1987) Assessing marital adjustment and satisfaction: a review. *Measurement and Evaluation in Counseling and Development*, **20**, 113–121.

BUSS, A. & PLOMIN, R. (1984) *Temperament: Early Developing Personality Traits*. Hillsdale, NJ: Erlbaum.

CAMPBELL, D. & FISKE, D. (1959) Convergent and discriminant validation by the multimethod–multitrait matrix. *Psychological Bulletin*, **54**, 81–105.

CAREY, W. (1970) A simplified method for measuring infant temperament. *Journal of Pediatrics*, **77**, 188–193.

——— & MCDEVITT, S. (1989) Technical note: comment on Paper by Gibbs *et al*. *Journal of Child Psychology and Psychiatry*, **30**, 639–642.

COSTELLO, A., EDELBROCK, L., DULCAN, M., *et al* (1984) *Report on the NIMH Diagnostic Interview Schedule for Children (DISC)*. Washington, DC: National Institute of Mental Health.

COSTELLO, C. (1982) Social factors associated with depression: a retrospective community study. *Psychological Medicine*, **12**, 329–340.

COSTELLO, E., EDELBROCK, C. & COSTELLO, A. (1985) Validity of the NIMH diagnostic interview schedule for children: a comparison between psychiatric and pediatric referrals. *Journal of Abnormal Child Psychology*, **27**, 579–595.

COWAN, C. & COWAN, P. (1988) Who does what when partners become parents: Implications for men, women and marriage. *Marriage and Family Review*, **12**, 105–132.

COX, A., PUCKERING, C., POUND, A., *et al* (1987) The impact of maternal depression in young children. *Journal of Child Psychology and Psychiatry*, **28**, 917–928.

CUTRONA, C. & TROUTMAN, B. (1985) Social support, infant temperament and parenting self-efficacy: a mediational model of postpartum depression. *Child Development*, **57**, 1507–1519.

EDDY, J., HEYMAN, R. & WEISS, R. (1991) An empirical evaluation of the Dyadic Adjustment Scale: exploring the differences between marital "satisfaction" and "adjustment". *Behavioral Assessment*, **13**, 199–220.

EDELBROCK, C., COSTELLO, A., DULCAN, M., *et al* (1985) Age-differences in the reliability of the psychiatric interview of the child. *Child Development*, **56**, 265–275.

———, ———, ———, *et al* (1986) Parent–child agreement on child psychiatric symptoms assessed by structured interview. *Journal of Child Psychology and Psychiatry*, **27**, 181–190.

EPSTEIN, N. & BISHOP, D. (1981) Problem-centred systems therapy of the family. In *Handbook of Family Therapy* (eds A. Gurman & D. Kniskern). New York: Brunner/Mazel.

———, BALDWIN, L. & BISHOP, D. (1983) The McMaster Family Assessment Device. *Journal of Marital and Family Therapy*, **9**, 171–180.

ERICKSON, M., SROUFE, L. & EGELAND, B. (1985) The relationship between causality of attachment and behaviour problems in preschool in a high risk sample. In *Growing Points in Attachment Theory and Research* (eds I. Bretherton & E. Waters). Chicago: University of Chicago Press.

FOMBONNE, E. (1989) The Child Behaviour Checklist and the Rutter Parental Questionnaire: a comparison between two screening instruments. *Psychological Medicine*, **19**, 777–785.

——— (1991) The use of questionnaires in child psychiatry research: measuring their performance and choosing an optimal cut-off. *Journal of Child Psychology and Psychiatry*, **32**, 677–694.

FONAGY, P., STEELE, H. & STEELE, N. (1991) Maternal representations of attachment during pregnancy predict the organization of infant–mother attachment at one year of age. *Child Development*, **62**, 891–905.

FOREMAN, D., HACKNEY, M. & COX, J. (1992) The impact of postnatal depression on new infants and their older siblings – preliminary results from a controlled study. (Conference paper.) Edinburgh: Marcé Society.

GEORGE, C., KAPLAN, N. & MAIN, M. (1985) *The Adult Attachment Interview*. University of California at Berkeley, Department of Psychology.

GHODSIAN, M., ZAJICEK, E. & WOLKIND, S. (1984) A longitudinal study of maternal depression and child behaviour problems. *Journal of Child Psychology and Psychiatry*, **25**, 91–109.

GIBBS, M., CUNNINGHAM, C. & REEVES, D. (1989) Technical note: reply to Carey and McDevitt. *Journal of Child Psychology and Psychiatry*, **30**, 643–648.

GLASS, C. (1993) The impact of home-based ventilator dependence on family life. *Paraplegia*, **31**, 93–101.

GOTTMAN, J., NOTARIUS, C., MARKMAN, H., *et al* (1976) Behavior exchange theory and marital decision taking. *Journal of Personality and Social Psychology*, **34**, 14–23.

GREEN, R., HARRIS, R., FORTE, J., *et al* (1991*a*) Evaluating FACES III and the circumplex model: 2,440 families. *Family Process*, **30**, 55–73.

———, ———, ———, *et al* (1991*b*) The wives' data and FACES IV: making things appear simple. *Family Process*, **30**, 79–83.

HARRISON, D. & WESTHUIS, D. (1989) Rating scales for marital adjustment. *Journal of Social Services Research*, **13**, 87–105.

HARVEY, I. & MCGRATH, G. (1988) Psychiatric morbidity in spouses of women admitted to a mother and baby unit. *British Journal of Psychiatry*, **152**, 506–510.

HERJANIC B., HERJANIC, M., BROWN, F., *et al* (1975) Are children reliable reporters? *Journal of Abnormal Child Psychology*, **3**, 41–48.

HERSOV, L. (1977) Emotional disorders. In *Child Psychiatry: Modern Approaches* (eds M. Rutter & L. Hersov). Oxford: Blackwell.

HODGES, K. (1993) Structured interviews for assessing children. *Journal of Child Psychology and Psychiatry*, **34**, 49–68.

——— & FITCH, P. (1979) Development of a mental status examination interview for children. (Conference paper.) Kansas City: Missouri Psychological Association.

———, KLINE, J., FITCH, P., *et al* (1982*a*) The development of a child assessment interview for research and clinical use. *Journal of Abnormal Child Psychology*, **10**, 173–189.

———, ———, CYTRYN, L., *et al* (1982*b*) The Child Assessment Schedule (CAS) diagnostic interview: a report on reliability and validity. *Journal of the American Academy of Child and Adolescent Psychiatry*, **21**, 468–473.

———, MCKNEW, D., BURBACH, D., *et al* (1987) Diagnostic concordance between the Child Assessment Schedule (CAS) and the Schedule for Affective Disorders and Schizophrenia for School-age Children (K–SADS) in an outpatient sample using lay interviewers. *Journal of the American Academy of Child and Adolescent Psychiatry*, **26**, 654–661.

——, GORDON, Y. & LENNON, M. (1990) Parent–child agreement on symptoms assessed via a clinical research interview for children: the Child Assessment Schedule (CAS). *Journal of Child Psychology and Psychiatry*, **31**, 427–436.

HOWES, P. & MARKMAN, H. (1989) Marital quality and child functioning: a longitudinal investigation. *Child Development*, **60**, 1044–1051.

IVENS, C. & REHM, L. (1988) Assessment of childhood depression: correspondence between reports by child, mother, and father. *Journal of the American Academy of Child and Adolescent Psychiatry*, **27**, 738–741.

KAZAK, A., JARMAS, A. & SNITZER, L. (1988) The assessment of marital satisfaction: an evaluation of the Dyadic Adjustment Scale. *Journal of Family Psychology*, **2**, 82–91.

KLAGSBRUN, M. & BOWLBY, J. (1976) Responses to separation from parents: a clinical test for young children. *Projective Psychology*, **21**, 7–26.

KLINE, M., COWAN, P. & COWAN, P. (1991) The origins of parenting stress during the transition to parenthood: a new family model. *Early Education and Development*, **2**, 287–305.

KOBAK, R., COLE, H., FERENZ-GILLIES, R., *et al* (1993) Attachment and emotion regulation during mother-teen problem solving: a control theory analysis. *Child Development*, **64**, 231–245.

KUMAR, R., ROBSON, K. & SMITH, A. (1984) Development of a self-administered questionnaire to measure maternal adjustment and maternal attitudes during pregnancy and after delivery. *Journal of Psychosomatic Research*, **28**, 43–51.

LANCASTER, S., PRIOR, M. & ADLER, R. (1989) Child behaviour ratings: the influence of maternal characteristics and child temperament. *Journal of Child Psychology and Psychiatry*, **30**, 137–149.

LOCKE, H. & WALLACE, K. (1959) Short marital adjustment and prediction tests: their reliability and validity. *Marriage and Family Living*, **21**, 251–255.

LOVELAND-CHERRY, C., YOUNGBLUT, J. & LEIDY, N. (1989) A psychometric analysis of the Family Environment Scale. *Nursing Research*, **38**, 262–266.

LOVESTONE, S. & KUMAR, R. (1993) Postnatal psychiatric illness: the impact on partners. *British Journal of Psychiatry*, **163**, 210–216.

MAIN, M. & CASSIDY, J. (1988) Categories of response to reunion with the parent at age six: predicted from infant attachment classifications and stable over a one-month period. *Developmental Psychology*, **24**, 415–426.

——, KAPLAN, N. & CASSIDY, J. (1985) Security in infancy, childhood and adulthood: A move to the level of representation. In *Growing Points of Attachment Theory and Research* (eds I. Bretherton & E. Waters). Chicago: University of Chicago Press.

—— & GOLDWYN, R. (1994) Adult attachment rating and classification systems. In *Behavioural Development – A Representational Model* (ed. M. Main). New York: Cambridge University Press (in press).

MASH, E. & JOHNSTON, C. (1983) Sibling interactions of hyperactive and normal children and their relationship to reports of maternal stress and self esteem. *Journal of Clinical Child Psychology*, **12**, 91–99.

MATHENY, A., WILSON, R. & THOBEN, A. (1987) Home and mother: relations with infant temperament. *Developmental Psychology*, **23**, 323–331.

MCDEVITT, S. & CAREY, W. (1981) Stability of ratings vs perception of temperament from early infancy to 1–3 years. *American Journal of Orthopsychiatry*, **51**, 342–345.

MOOS, R. (1990) Conceptual and empirical approaches to developing family-based assessment procedures: Resolving the case of the Family Environment Scale. *Family Process*, **29**, 199–208.

—— & MOOS, B. (1986) *Family Environment Scale*. Palo Alto: Consulting Psychologists Press.

MORRIS, T. (1990) Culturally sensitive family assessment: an evaluation of the Family Assessment Device used with Hawaiian–American and Japanese–American families. *Family Process*, **29**, 105–116.

MURRAY, L. (1988) Effects of postnatal depression on infant development: direct studies of early mother–infant interactions. In *Motherhood and Mental Illness* (eds R. Kumar & I. Brockington). London: Wright.

—— (1992) The impact of postnatal depression on infant development. *Journal of Child Psychology and Psychiatry*, **33**, 543–562.

NELSON, M., RUCH, S., JACKSON, Z., *et al* (1992) Towards an understanding of families with physically disabled adolescents. *Social Work in Health Care*, **17**, 1–25.

O'HARA, M. & ZEKOSKI, E. (1988) Postpartum depression: a comprehensive review. In *Motherhood and Mental Illness 2: Causes and Consequences* (eds R. Kumar & I. Brockington). London: Wright.

OLSON, D., SPRENKLE, D. & RUSSELL, C. (1979) Circumplex model of marital and family systems. 1. Cohesion and adaptability dimensions, family types, and clinical applications. *Family Process*, **18**, 3–28.

PARKER, G. (1981) Parental reports of depressives: an investigation of several explanations. *Journal of Affective Disorders*, **3**, 131–140.

——, FAIRLEY, M., GREENWOOD, J., *et al* (1982) Parental representations of schizophrenics. *British Journal of Psychiatry*, **141**, 573–581.

——, TUPLING, H. & BROWN, L. (1979) A parental bonding instrument. *British Journal of Medical Psychology*, **52**, 1–10.

PATTERSON, G. (1986) Performance models for antisocial boys. *American Psychologist*, **41**, 432–444.

PEROSA, L. & PEROSA, S. (1990) Convergent and discriminant validity for family self-report measures. *Educational and Psychological Measurement*, **50**, 855–868.

PRIOR, M. (1992) Childhood temperament. *Journal of Child Psychology and Psychiatry*, **33**, 249–280.

PUIG-ANTICH, J. & CHAMBERS, W. (1978) *The Schedule for Affective Disorders and Schizophrenia for School-Aged Children*. New York, NY: New York State Psychiatric Institute.

RICHMAN, N. & GRAHAM, P. (1971) A behavioural screening questionnaire for use with three-year old children: preliminary findings. *Journal of Child Psychology and Psychiatry*, **12**, 5–33.

ROOSA, M. & BEALS, J. (1990) Measurement issues in family assessment: The case of the Family Environment Scale. *Family Process*, **29**, 191–198.

ROTHBART, M. (1987) A psychobiological approach to the study of temperament. In *Temperament Discussed* (eds G. Kohnstamm & J. Bates). Lisse: Swets and Zeitlinger.

—— (1989) Temperament and development. In *Temperament in Childhood* (eds G. Kohnstamm, J. Bates & M. Rothbart). Chichester: John Wiley.

—— & DERRYBERRY, D. (1981) Development of individual differences in temperament. In *Advances in Developmental Psychology* (eds M. Lamb & A. Brown). Hillsdale, NJ: Lawrence Erlbaum.

RUTTER, M. (1967) A children's behaviour questionnaire for completion by teachers: preliminary findings. *Journal of Child Psychology and Psychiatry*, **8**, 1–11.

—— (1970) Appendix 6. A children's behaviour questionnaire for completion by parents. In *Education, Health and Behaviour* (eds M. Rutter, J. Tizard & K. Whitmore). London: Longman.

—— (1987) Temperament, personality, and personality disorders. *British Journal of Psychiatry*, **150**, 443–458.

SAUDINO, K. & EATON, W. (1991) Infant temperament and genetics: an objective twin study of motor activity level. *Child Development*, **62**, 1167–1174.

SAUNDERS, B. & SCHUCHTS, R. (1987) Assessing parent–child relationships: a report of normative scores and revalidation of two clinical scales. *Family Process*, **26**, 373–381.

SAWYER, M., SARRIS, A., BAGHURST, P., *et al* (1988) Family assessment device: reports from mothers, fathers and adolescents in community and clinic families. *Journal of Marital and Family Therapy*, **14**, 287–296.

SHAFFER, D., SCHWAB-STONE, M., FISHER, P., *et al* (1988) *Results of a Field Trial and Proposals for a New Instrument (DISC–R)*. Washington, DC: National Institute of Mental Health.

SHOULDICE, A. & STEVENSON-HINDE, J. (1992) Coping with security distress: the Separation Anxiety Test and Attachment Classification at 4.5 years. *Journal of Child Psychology and Psychiatry*, **33**, 331–348.

SKINNER, H. (1987) Self-report instruments for family assessment. In *Family Interaction and Psychopathology* (ed. T. Jacob). New York: Plenum.

——, STEINHAUER, P. & SANTA-BARBARA, J. (1983) The Family Assessment Measure. *Canadian Journal of Community Mental Health*, **2**, 91–105.

SPANIER, G. (1976) Measuring dyadic adjustment: new scales for assessing the quality of marriage and similar dyads. *Journal of Marriage and the Family*, **38**, 15–28.

STEIN, A., GATH, D., BUCHER, J., *et al* (1991) The relationship between postnatal depression and mother–child interaction. *British Journal of Psychiatry*, **158**, 46–52.

THOMAS, A. & CHESS, S. (1977) *Temperament and Development*. New York: Brunner/Mazel.

TREVARTHEN, C., MURRAY, L. & HUBLEY, P. (1981) Psychology of infants. In *Scientific Foundations of Paediatrics* (eds J. Davis & J. Dobbing). London: Heinemann.

VAN DAM, M. & VAN IJZENDOORN, M. (1988) Measuring attachment security. *Journal of Genetic Psychology*, **149**, 447–457.

VAUGHN, B. & WATERS E. (1990) Attachment behavior at home and in the laboratory: Q-sort observations and Strange Situation classifications of one-year-olds. *Child Development*, **61**, 1965–1973.

VERHULST, F., ALTHAUS, M. & BERDEN, G. (1987) The Child Assessment Schedule: parent–child agreement and validity measures. *Journal of Child Psychology and Psychiatry*, **28**, 455–466.

VITIELLO, B., MALONE, R., BUSCHLE, P., *et al* (1990) Reliability of DSM–III diagnoses of hospitalized children. *Hospital and Community Psychiatry*, **41**, 63–67.

WALKER, J., MANION, I., CLOUTIER, P., *et al* (1992) Measuring marital distress in couples with chronically ill children: the Dyadic Adjustment Scale. *Journal of Pediatric Psychology*, **17**, 345–357.

WARING, E. (1985) Editorial: Measurement of intimacy. *Psychological Medicine*, **15**, 9–13.

—— & REDDON, J. (1983) The measurement of intimacy in marriage: the Waring Intimacy Questionnaire. *Journal of Clinical Psychology*, **39**, 53–57.

WATERS, E. & DEANE, K. (1985) Defining and assessing individual differences in attachment relationships: Q-methodology and the organization of behavior in infancy and early childhood. In *Growing Points in Attachment Theory and Research* (eds I. Bretherton & E. Waters). Chicago: University of Chicago Press.

WELNER, Z., REICH, W., HERJANIC, B., *et al* (1987) Reliability, validity and parent–child agreement studies of the Diagnostic Interview for Children and Adolescents (DICA). *Journal of the American Academy of Child and Adolescent Psychiatry*, **29**, 627–634.

WOLKIND, S. & DE SALIS, W. (1982) Infant temperament, maternal mental state and child behavioral problems. In *Temperamental Differences in Infants and Young Children* (eds R. Porter & G. Collins). London: Pitman/Ciba Foundation.

WRATE, R., ROONEY, A., THOMAS, P., *et al* (1985) Postnatal depression and child development: a 3-year follow-up study. *British Journal of Psychiatry*, **146**, 622–627.

ZEANAH, C., BENOIT, D., BARTON, M., *et al* (1993) Representations of attachment in mothers and their one-year-old infants. *Journal of the American Academy of Child and Adolescent Psychiatry*, **32**, 278–286.

Part III. Workshop reports

Introduction

The conference at Keele which provided much of the stimulus for this book was called "Prevention of depression after childbirth: use and misuse of the Edinburgh Postnatal Depression Scale". The chief characteristics of the conference were informality and innovation. This was particularly apparent in the ten workshops, which ranged from teaching counselling skills to the use of antidepressants and progesterone in prophylaxis. Two of the workshops are described in this section by their conveners.

The chapter by Mike Watson and David Foreman sadly has another dimension. Mike Watson, Chairman of the National Psychodrama Association, and who contributed substantially to mental health services in North Staffordshire, suddenly died in January. His collaboration with David Foreman, a child and adolescent psychiatrist, and their joint exploration of new boundaries between psychodrama and Rogerian counselling are symbolic of the workshop which Mike Watson directed. Participants were encouraged to explore the role of the postnatal mother and its derivations. In his introduction to the workshop, Mike wrote: "very often there are generational factors that have helped to create this postnatally depressed mother; behind her there is probably at least one more mother who was also unfulfilled". The workshop was planned to develop these ideas further and to demonstrate psychodramatic ways of working.

Chapter 14, by Sandra Elliott, was also based on a workshop, and demonstrates the need for caution before the EPDS is used routinely in clinical and research practice – especially by inexperienced health professionals. Sandra Elliott correctly points out that the EPDS is not a magic wand.

The Editors

14 Uses and misuses of the Edinburgh Postnatal Depression Scale in primary care: a comparison of models developed in health visiting

SANDRA A. ELLIOTT

Any problems with use of the Edinburgh Postnatal Depression Scale (EPDS) in routine practice derive primarily from the myth that introducing the EPDS will solve all a health authority's problems *vis-à-vis* postnatal disorders rather than from the EPDS itself. Perhaps the fact that the EPDS outstrips other questionnaires for face validity and acceptability has allowed it to run too far ahead of its knowledge base.

This chapter outlines some concerns regarding the way the EPDS is sometimes adopted, then evaluates a variety of EPDS-based systems which could be adopted in primary care. It concludes with a section on my own philosophy and practice arising out of a multicentre research project on training health visitors in the management of postnatal depression (Elliott, 1989; Gerrard *et al*, 1993). The issues raised apply to any primary care health professionals wishing to adopt the system, although it was developed and piloted with health visitors since the philosophy and practice fit most closely with this group.

Problems of the EPDS in routine practice

The first and most salient point is that the EPDS is often used without any clear idea as to what it is being used for, so inappropriate decisions are made on administration and scoring. It is necessary to be clear about differences between the general population and the population being tested and between those who should be referred on and those who should not. Decisions of time, place and frequency of administration as well as cut-off points are dependent on these facts.

The system for referring on is often not in place. In such circumstances considerable stress is generated for those doing the scoring as the detection rate increases through its use. The EPDS does not make a differential diagnosis, so it trawls in all sorts of problems health visitors or other

221

screening professionals might prefer not to be aware of. The boundaries for responsibility for such professionals tend not to be clear and the problem is exacerbated if the secondary services beyond the boundaries (in this case, mental health services) are poor, scarce or inaccessible to the screening professional. Health promotion professionals such as health visitors have responsibility for the total population and are, appropriately, spread thinly. They cannot afford to find themselves following up too many serious problems for which the responsibility remains with them. Furthermore, health professionals' anxiety is raised by the self-harm question. Once again, their ability to tolerate this anxiety is dependent on their access to secondary care for the client as well as supervision for themselves.

If the EPDS is administered once only it pulls in transient problems, especially if administered early on in the puerperium. On the other hand, there is a lack of clarity on the moral, ethical and legal position of not acting on one high score and waiting four weeks for a second one before taking action. Implementing research findings was further complicated by the fact that the routine practice, which the original EPDS system (Holden *et al*, 1989) was designed to fit into, was not nearly as routine as descriptions of the health visitor service at the time implied. In practice sick leave, unfilled posts, pressures to provide a crisis intervention service, etc., push the routine contacts system of health promotion to the bottom of priorities.

Individuals should always have the right to protect their privacy by declining to complete the forms or to 'falsify' the responses. It is important to realise, though, that the person administering the forms can influence the extent to which this happens by the manner in which they present the questionnaire and its purpose. For example, in a deprived area of Stoke, word got around that you shouldn't score high on that questionnaire or you'll get the health visitor turning up every week! A hospital midwife in Edinburgh exerted considerable pressure on a woman to fill in the EPDS at her six-week postnatal check-up despite her reluctance, partly related to her having filled one in the week before for the health visitor. This changes the message from one of real concern about her as a woman to one of invasive 'big brother' service systems. This rather negates the anxiety-reducing intentions of an EPDS-based system.

Many health professionals remain unclear as to the difference between feeling depressed (as indicated by self-report, health professionals' observation and/or high EPDS score) and 'having depression' (i.e. would be classified as clinically depressed by a psychiatrist using a standardised interview technique). This is hardly surprising since the distinction, although now more reliably made, was derived fairly arbitrarily (with the cut-off defined by that which a psychiatrist would not be surprised to see in out-patients). While the grey area may be wider and murkier than in physical medicine, there is a clinically meaningful distinction to be made between feeling depressed and suffering from depression, i.e. where the negative affect itself generates somatic, intrapsychic and/or interpersonal problems. In any event, many treat the EPDS as if it were a diagnostic instrument. They use it only where they feel a client may be depressed in order to confirm that they 'have postnatal depression'. Clearly, this is technically incorrect, and pre-empting the diagnosis could alienate the medical staff. It is understandable that pressure of work may restrict the numbers given the EPDS, but care should be taken to use the EPDS score only as an additional piece of information on how the client feels, not as a diagnostic tool. For example, if the EPDS is used only when a health visitor already suspects depression, a high score can add to confidence in reporting depressive symptomatology to the GP (or, preferably, persuading the woman herself to report it to the GP).

Technical accuracy is not the only issue in the labelling dilemma. Women who are irritable, not coping with children, having relationship problems and so on are often relieved to be given a label 'postnatal depression' since it provides an explanation for their experience. This explanation is usually preferable to those that the woman or her partner may have already entertained. These typically entail a fear that they are going mad or the conviction that her lack of feelings confirm that she is a bad mother or a sign that she no longer loves her husband. Yet, despite the fact that Esther Rantzen and others have worked hard to get postnatal depression recognised as an acceptable label, so that it is now preferred to psychiatric labels given less media attention, it is still 'a label' and therefore carries stigma. Labelling may also in itself stultify the process of change that the depressed mood should be heralding (Alibhai, 1989; Bennett, 1981; Elliott, 1984; Elliott *et al*, 1983; Oakley, 1980; Nicolson, 1990; Welburn, 1980) since the label is widely misunderstood. That is, the fact that the term is often taken to imply a physical illness, aetiologically rooted in the birth process manifesting as a mood disorder, may block what should have been a prompt to looking at what is troublesome in a woman's life. It does this by shifting the focus to hormones or other bodily functions over which she has no direct control.

To put it another way, for those who have reached the bottom of the spiral in clinical depression, the label may point the way out and bring in some badly needed care and attention as well as the medication which may be necessary since at this level physical processes are affected (e.g. appetite and sleep disturbance). However, for the majority of those scoring say ten or above at the six-week health visitor-administered EPDS, what is required to halt the down-spiralling is validation of their emotions, some normalisation of their experience of parenting and not a pathologising of them via labelling. Properly explained 'postnatal depression' labelling, when at the bottom of the spiral, may remove 'depression about depression', the maintaining factor referred to by cognitive therapists such as Teasdale (1985). Labelling when at the early depressed mood or subclinical depression level of the spiral may actually create 'depression about depression' if the label is perceived as representing failure. It may simultaneously medicalise emotions which warrant freer expression and further analysis followed by a problem-solving approach applied to the sources of discontent.

Options for the use of the EPDS in routine practice

It should be clear by now that, far from being a magic wand, the EPDS by itself is just a piece of paper. The power of the EPDS in clinical practice is invested in the system within which it functions. The EPDS is at its best when adopted for its face validity and acceptability by those wishing to introduce a 'good practice initiative' to their health district. A variety of such systems are possible. The workshop on 'Uses and Abuses of the EPDS in Primary Care' took six such systems (A–F, below) for small group discussions. The group leaders were required to report back from a brainstorming on the advantages and disadvantages of their allocated system which participants had to imagine was to be introduced to their district 'tomorrow'.

(a) Using the EPDS only to confirm the suspicion that a woman is depressed

Advantages

It dramatically cuts the number of EPDS administrations required so permits introduction even where resources are severely limited. 'Confirmation makes you feel safe.'

Disadvantages

The system will miss women who are depressed. The EPDS would be less acceptable than if done routinely and clients may feel stigmatised simply by being asked to complete it. Other clients may feel left out. It is a non-preventative procedure which could allow the undetected development of severe depression. Intervention may be delayed, thus reducing the opportunity for secondary prevention of breakdown of the family unit and/or delayed development and emotional deprivation of the child and therefore greater time and cost to management in the long term. The system gives no indication of the action to be taken or the criteria for intervention.

Comment

This group was not impressed by their remit, discussed the proposal fairly rapidly, and moved on to discussing other things.

(b) Computerised EPDS routinely at six weeks postnatal only – score 12 + offered four half-hourly listening visits

Advantages

Single, computerised administration reduces demand on staff time, permitting introduction even where staffing levels are low. Data collection would be convenient since the score results would automatically be recorded onto floppy disk for easy transportation and storage. Data can be easily viewed and examined statistically without fear that the necessary details had been incorrectly copied from paper to computer and without data loss (since a computer is harder to lose than numerous pieces of paper). Data collected can easily be transformed into an audit report to support requests for resources from managers. Hardware purchased for EPDS purposes could be made available for other important uses by the primary care team.

Disadvantages

Computer anxiety by some postnatal women and staff was anticipated. Staff would require training in the use of the computer. There may be additional concerns about the security of data and about the Data Protection Act if computers are used. Computers would need to be purchased and, for use in the field, this would mean expensive laptops. The absence of laptops could lead to the restriction of EPDS testing to a specific venue conducting routine postnatal examinations, thus increasing the chances of missing high risk women. Single administration could lead to too many interventions and was not considered viable. Repeat administration after two weeks and prior to action was advocated. The system was judged to be dependent on support from a psychiatrist and close liaison with the GP. These were considered crucial but previous experience of participants raised anxieties about the practicality of setting this up.

Comment

The group leader was surprised by the enthusiasm of his randomly allocated group for the use of computerised systems and by their detailed technical knowledge. In contrast he was disheartened to learn of their anxieties about the liaison with psychiatric services and primary health care workers.

(c) Using EPDS routinely at six months postnatal only – score 12 + and discuss possibility of referral to mental health services with GP

Advantages

Single administration requires fewer resources, making implementation less costly and more practical. Six-month postnatal screening will pick up on the later-onset postnatal depression missed by a system using single administration at six weeks. It will detect and focus on more serious, longer lasting depression. It will not be confounded by the more short-lived depressions/new baby anxieties as in the early postnatal weeks. It will restrict referrals to the mental health services to a level with which it should be able to cope. A system of liaison with the GP (and hopefully with mental health services) would be negotiated as a prerequisite to implementation.

Disadvantages

Administration at six months misses the opportunity for primary or secondary prevention. Single administration, even at six months, could allow transient depressed mood to lead to a case conference with the GP. Referral as the only intervention option denies the potential of a short series of 'listening visits' from the screening health professional with an existing relationship with the woman. The message that the health visitor is interested in the mother's emotional well-being as well as the child's physical health comes too late.

Comment

This group's main preoccupation was one which was echoed in various comments made by the other groups. Several criticisms were made of the notion that management could introduce a new system overnight without consultation. They were particularly concerned that there had been no apparent thought given to training, support, and supervision for the primary care workers or about the availability and accessibility of secondary care.

(d) Using EPDS routinely at six weeks, three and six months (score 12 + requires another EPDS after 7–14 days, if still 12 + offer four half-hour weekly listening visits)

Advantages

Three administrations reduces the number of missed episodes of depression. Repeat administration allows exclusion of transient depressions from the costly intervention phase. Intervention is specified. The need for training on postnatal depression, non-directive counselling principles of listening visits and EPDS administration is explicit. Setting up the system could lead to future preventive work via antenatal explanations of the process.

Disadvantages

Three routine administrations is labour intensive and demands a fully resourced service. Management may not support the introduction of this system. Management may support but not understand the system. The system is dependent on cooperation from GPs.

Comment

This group wanted to compare how they fared with this option to the deliberations of the other groups. They proposed a vote on the options at the end of the feedback session.

(e) Using EPDS routinely in late pregnancy and six weeks postnatal

Advantages

Antenatal administration provides opportunities for prophylactic action in relation to postnatal problems. Antenatal administration permits detection of antenatal depression. Choice of six weeks as the time of the single postnatal administration was judged sufficiently early for an early detection and intervention programme. Antenatal administration contributes to familiarity and acceptability as a routine procedure rather than as stigmatising.

Disadvantages

The directive was given in a vacuum and there was a danger it would be administered in a similar vacuum without explanation or follow-up reassurance for low scorers. No criteria for action were specified. No intervention was recommended antenatally or indeed postnatally. No referral mechanism was in place. GPs had not been informed. No instructions on the avoidance of stigmatising were provided. There was a suspicion that very low scorers may be false negatives. The absence of policy for this group was seen as a potential problem. Information was lacking as to which score range antenatally predicted scores above 12 postnatally or on how well it did so.

Comment

This group felt constrained by their remit and wanted to construct an ideal option by combining with others.

(f) Using EPDS routinely at six weeks and ten weeks postnatal – score 12 + leads to eight-week counselling and informing GP

Advantages

This system is the same as that researched and reported in the original Edinburgh study (Holden *et al*, 1989). Timing of administration fits in with the routine contacts of many health visitors. It makes a specific point of informing the GP (i.e. after two high scores). A rigid system focuses you on what should be done and things are less likely to slip through. This system may provide the opportunity to pick up on other things. The process says to women that there is time purely for them. Routine administration would not raise women's anxiety about why they were asked to fill it in. Adoption of this system may force health professionals to raise the subject early on and explain the system. This makes it easier for health visitors who are uncomfortable with the topic. Requirement for high score to be present on two occasions four weeks apart before intervention is offered reduces the counselling workload. More episodes of depression go undetected if the system is not in use. A set number of listening visits makes it easier to negotiate time for the system from a manager. The pre-fixed number of visits allows the health visitor to end 'counselling' and return to health visiting.

Disadvantages

The timing of administration does not fit in with the routine contacts of some health visitors. Allocation of eight visits per depressed client takes too much health visitor time. The health visitor's appearance for a repeat administration at ten weeks might raise anxiety if it was unanticipated. The system uses only the EPDS as the prompt to treat. It was considered preferable to also have a discussion with the GP or catchment CPN/ psychologist. Health professionals could experience discomfort at leaving high scorers for four weeks before assessment to treat. If the six-week high score was not just the result of a 'bad' day, a high scoring client may feel 'let down' if nothing happens and may not even respond again at ten weeks. Some clients improve after only a few weekly visits so eight seems too long. It may be preferable to transfer the time to more desperate cases. Pre-fixed number of sessions overrides the notion of the client setting the agenda which is part of the non-directive approach.

Comment

This group pointed out that several pros and cons raised for this system could equally apply to other options but could not constrain their comments to specific points since they were not informed of the alternative options.

The trainers in the multicentre trial (Jeni Holden, Janice Gerrard and Sandra Elliott) were denied a vote on the options. Votes were split between option E (8 votes) and D (11 votes) while the other four options did not get any votes at all. In the closing minutes of the debate better options were sought and group E offered the solution they had prepared earlier – a combination of D and E. When added as a seventh choice all 19 chose it as the most preferred option. A comment was made, however, that those present were all practitioners and that the result may not be replicated among a sample of managers responsible for budgetary control.

Translating research into practice: a philosophical shift

The feedback from these small group discussions of just 20 minutes' deliberation illustrates just how complex is the decision process required. The EPDS is a short and simple tool. Its introduction into primary care is anything but simple. In its wake it carries widespread system change as well as a new philosophy. When the multicentre trial of training health visitors began in Lewisham, I envisaged adopting the philosophy of the Edinburgh project (Holden *et al*, 1989) alongside that of the Lewisham primary prevention programme (Elliott *et al*, 1988). The Edinburgh project seemed to be demonstrating that health visitors could take on detection and treatment in mental health. Indeed, the Lewisham project had been deliberately designed to complement the Edinburgh study by covering instead the fields of prediction and prevention. However, when I began to teach health visitors, I felt compelled to make a shift away from selection for 'treatment'. In the original Edinburgh study the research psychiatrist, Ruth Sagovsky, made the 'decision to treat' and the discharge from treatment process or referral. For a variety of reasons, including those given earlier in the chapter, the knowledge that a second high EPDS score is a good predictor of psychiatric diagnosis of depression, treatable by counselling, was not sufficient to make health visitors confident about their role in 'decision to treat' in individual cases. The shift was also prompted by an increasing understanding of health visiting philosophy and practice. Health visitors in Britain provide a universal service to families with under 5s with the emphasis being on health promotion and on screening. They are not a treatment agency although pressure of work, combined with the unavailability of social workers or secondary care health professionals, often finds them operating a crisis intervention or treatment service.

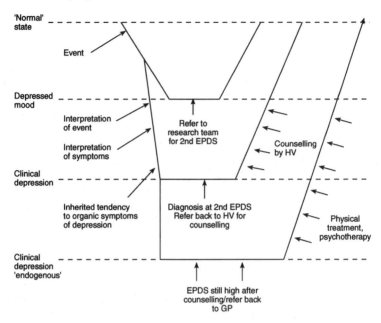

Fig. 14.1. Interventions in response to high EPDS in Edinburgh study (Holden et al, *1989)*

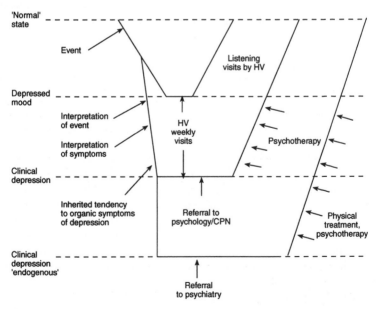

Fig. 14.2. Interventions dependent on stage in depression at which first high EPDS score obtained by health visitors

For health visitors it may be better to shift from the notion of selection for 'treatment' to what is almost prevention. That is, the original use of the EPDS at six and ten weeks, has high scores at both functioning as the prompt for offering non-directive counselling. This represents giving formal treatment to women who almost certainly meet Research Diagnostic Criteria for depression. Is this what health visitors should be doing? On the other hand, taking a high score at six weeks by itself is probably picking up women who are experiencing depressed mood and for whom what we call 'listening visits' can prevent the spiral into diagnosable depression. Also, a report at the six-week administration that depression had been long lasting and/or severe would be taken to indicate that immediate referral was required. The figures illustrate the various levels of depression, the routes down and the possible points of intervention to bring a person back up again. Figure 14.1 shows the point of intervention used by health visitors in the original Edinburgh study. The one that I would recommend on the basis of our experience in trying to utilise this method in practice is shown in Figure 14.2. This shows mental health professionals taking on the type of clients that were treated by the health visitors in the Edinburgh study while the health visitors concentrate on preventing episodes of depression becoming this severe via earlier but briefer interventions in addition to antenatal preventive interventions. GPs, however, may opt to function at either or both of these levels according to the gaps in the other services as well as in response to their own personal skills and interests, not to mention the availability of a waiting-room computer in EPDS mode.

Acknowledgements

I would like to thank the other group leaders in the workshops – Anna Robinson, Robin Glaze, Janice Gerrard, Jeni Holden and Jo Green – for supplying me with the notes from their discussions, and Janice Gerrard and Tessa Leverton for comments on an earlier draft. The multicentre research project on which my ideas were tested was funded by the Gatsby Charitable Foundation. The combined text was typed by Yvonne Hedderman.

Thanks are also due to Marjorie Jackson, Marion Sanjack and health visitors in the Jenner and Jews Walk Health Centres who were in the first group trained in Lewisham who suffered from our naivety but were very generous in their evaluations of the programme.

References

ALIBHAI, Y. (1989) Burning in the cold. In *Balancing Acts: On Being a Mother* (ed. K. Gieve), pp. 24–40. London: Virago.

BENNETT, E. A. (1981) Coping in the puerperium: The reported experience of new mothers. *Journal of Psychosomatic Research*, **25**, 13–21.

ELLIOTT, S. A. (1984) Pregnancy and after. In *Contributions to Medical Psychology* (ed. S. Rachman) Vol. 3, pp. 93–116. Oxford: Pergamon.

—— (1989) Psychological strategies in the prevention and treatment of postnatal depression. *Baillière's Clinical Obstetrics and Gynaecology*, **3**, 879–903.

——, RUGG, A. J., WATSON, J. P., *et al* (1983) Mood changes during pregnancy and after the birth of a child. *British Journal of Clinical Psychology*, **22**, 295–308.

——, SANJACK, M.. & LEVERTON, T. J. (1988) Parents' groups in pregnancy: A preventive intervention for prenatal depression? In *Marshalling Social Support: Format, Processes and Effects* (ed. B. J. Gottlieb), pp. 87–110. California: Sage.

GERRARD, J., HOLDEN, J. M., ELLIOTT, S. A., *et al* (1993) A trainer's perspective of an innovative training programme to teach health visitors about the detection, treatment and prevention of postnatal depression. *Journal of Advanced Nursing*, **18**, 1825–1832.

HOLDEN, J. M., SAGOVSKY, R. & COX, J. L. (1989) Counselling in a general practice setting: Controlled study of health visitors intervention in treatment of postnatal depression. *British Medical Journal*, **298**, 223–226.

NICOLSON, P. (1989) Postnatal depression: Implications for clinical research and practice. *Clinical Psychology Forum*, **22**, 15–18.

—— (1990) The meaning of postnatal depression a further comment. *Clinical Psychology Forum*, **25**, 48–49.

OAKLEY, A. (1980) *Women Confined – Towards a Sociology of Childbirth*. Oxford: Martin Robertson.

TEASDALE, J. D. (1985) Psychological treatments for depression – how do they work? *Behavioural Research and Therapy*, **23**, 157–165.

WELBURN, V. (1980) *Postnatal Depression*. London: Fontana.

15 Diminishing the impact of puerperal neuroses: towards an expressive psychotherapy useful in a community setting

MIKE WATSON and DAVID FOREMAN

"The real issue is not exhausted by stating it as an aim, but by carrying it out, nor is the result the actual whole, but rather the result together with the process through which it came about."

(Hegel, 1807)

Postnatal depression: a family matter

Ten per cent or more of all mothers will experience postnatal depression after the birth of their child (Kumar & Robson, 1984). The distress to the mothers is obvious. Additionally, the fathers and the children of affected families (for this is a family problem) will suffer. The children may show a variety of problems in their development or adjustment (Murray, 1992; Stein *et al*, 1991). Strain will be put on the marriage (Foreman *et al*, 1992; Nettlebladt *et al*, 1985), while the fathers themselves may suffer 'postnatal' mental illness, most typically depression or anxiety (Foreman *et al*, 1992; Harvey & McGrath, 1988; Lovestone & Kumar, 1993). Thus, postnatal depression leads to an additional experiential change for the sufferer as these various problems reveal themselves. Coming to terms with experiences such as these are very much a matter for psychotherapy. Such therapy should therefore be seen as an integral part in the treatment of postnatal depression, even if one is using pharmacotherapy to achieve symptomatic change. However logical it may seem, a 'family therapy' approach may not be the most suitable psychotherapeutic intervention. Some reports (Beer, 1992; Nicol, 1989) suggest that patterns of service delivery associated with family therapy may result in reduced satisfaction with therapy and non-attendance in mothers with pre-school children. A major concern of many postnatally depressed women is guilt at the burden their illness places on their spouses, even as they feel cut off from them and their family. Several mothers have told us that they found relief and comfort in knowing that, for once, therapy was directed to themselves as people, rather than them as mothers or

233

members of a family. They expressed relief that their partners or children were not specifically involved. The husbands (or partners) of postnatally depressed mothers frequently have the double burden of caring for both their children and their companions (Cox, 1988), while maintaining their employment to cope with the additional economic burdens a new child brings. For them, finding the time for such therapy would be difficult, even if they found the will.

In these circumstances, group therapy holds several advantages. First, it uses therapists' time economically. Secondly, in bringing together women with a similar experience, it can reintroduce a sense of 'belonging' without imposing the demands of duty that follow from being a mother in a family. Psychodramatic group therapy (see below), which is mainly used with adjustment or behavioural disorders (Kellerman, 1987), seems especially suited to treat postnatally depressed women. It focuses on social roles, and concern over the maternal role is an essential element in the fears and anxieties expressed by postnatally depressed women. It places primacy on individual validation, and so overlaps the person-centred counselling that has been shown by Holden *et al* (1987) to improve up to two-thirds of postnatally depressed women. It has recently been shown to have long-lasting beneficial effects on other emotional disorders in a community setting (Arn *et al*, 1989).

Despite such potential, the application of psychodrama to postnatally depressed women seems new. A survey of some recent applications of psychodrama with a variety of client groups did not include postnatally depressed women (Holmes & Karp, 1991). We believe this chapter to be the first account of the use of psychodrama in this patient group.

Psychodrama is a powerful method of psychotherapy, so we stress the importance of therapists taking care when they use its techniques, and paying especial attention to the context in which they are employed. However, we do endorse its efficacy and usefulness in a community-based setting. We hope readers will be encouraged to obtain training in these skills and begin to apply them in similar settings.

The theory of psychodrama

For many readers, the word 'psychodrama' will be associated with all that was worst about the 'alternative' therapy movement of the 1960s and 1970s. To others, the word may be almost completely unfamiliar. In fact it is neither new, disorganised nor esoteric. Psychodrama was developed in Vienna and America between 1921 and 1950, making it possibly the first application of group psychotherapy (Moreno, 1934). Furthermore, ideas first proposed in the theory of psychodrama have since found expression in systems theory, family therapy and community therapy (Blatner & Blatner, 1988;

Marineau, 1989). Psychodrama has been well known in the United States for many years. In the United Kingdom, only isolated pioneers worked with it in the 1960s and 1970s. However, a professional organisation for psychodramatists, the British Psychodrama Association, was founded in 1984. It created well defined codes of training and practice, and became a full member of the United Kingdom Standing Conference for Psychotherapy in 1991.

Psychodrama was 'invented' and developed by Jacob Levy Moreno (Moreno, 1934, 1946, 1969; Moreno & Moreno, 1956), a Romanian physician and psychiatrist. He trained and first practised in Vienna. His varied client group included children, actors and prostitutes, and he rapidly saw that many of their complaints and problems were related to their psychosocial circumstances. This led to his evolving a variety of novel procedures to deal with these issues. In 1919 he moved to a small town, Bad Vöslau, outside Vienna to take up a practice as a family doctor. During those early years in Bad Vöslau he built up a reputation as a doctor who both cared about his patients and used an original approach to treating them. He went into people's homes, which was not common then. There he explored new ways of helping people emerge from difficult psychological situations. He would call upon members of the immediate family and the larger community to re-enact situations that had initially brought pain. He found that such re-enactment could lead to de-dramatisation, that the psychological effects could be reduced, and that liberation often occurred through laughter (Marineau, 1989). He was exploring this field with no preconceived model: as a man of action and intuition, he produced results that won him a following in the community without yet being able to systematise his work (Marineau, 1989). It is not inconceivable that he encountered mothers with psychological difficulties following parturition. However, his work as a small-town family doctor was short-lived. He became absorbed in other projects and emigrated to the United States in 1925, where he devoted the rest of his life to developing his method. He died in 1974, having seen psychodrama accepted and his reputation as a pioneer in the field of group psychotherapy established for all time.

Unlike Freud, Moreno had considerable difficulty in systematising his discoveries into a coherent metapsychology (Marineau, 1989). However, a central organising idea in his work is that of the 'spontaneous/creative matrix', which defines people's ability to develop new roles to cope with their circumstances. Moreno started with the idea that this could be made the central focus of people's worlds, not only as an underlying foundation to life, but on the very surface of daily existence.

Psychodrama has as its goal the enhancement of the client's 'spontaneity'. Moreno considered spontaneity to be the capacity to take up adequate new roles within the network of social interaction between the client and those closest to him or her – the 'social atom' of the client (Williams, 1989).

First the client must be alerted to the possibility of making such a change: Williams (1989) calls this giving the client 'news of difference'. Secondly, to achieve such a change, the client must undergo a process of catharsis – a term that is frequently misunderstood. Catharsis is *not* a dramatic display of emotion, although intense emotions may be associated with it. It *is* the accurate expression of an emotional awareness of one's situation. Frequently, such expression may be associated with a sense of liberation or relief since new role possibilities are revealed by such a carefully constructed representation of one's emotional world. This is why Moreno was able to observe that laughter was a useful marker for the success of this process (Marineau, 1989). In fact, Moreno was able to distinguish between two types of catharsis; 'action' catharsis and 'integrative' catharsis. While 'action' catharsis may provide some relief through the honest expression of feelings associated with a client's stituation, it is 'integrative' catharsis, where new possibilities are realised, that is most likely to generate long-term change (Kipper, 1986).

The rather non-intuitive definition of spontaneity used in psychodrama (see above) comes from Moreno's conception of role. Most of us think of a role as a part played by someone. Moreno extended this idea to suggest that we symbolise the multifarious actions of everyday life as 'parts', to give us a language of social intercourse between people. In his definition, a role is the symbolisation of the functioning form that the individual assumes in the specific moment he reacts to a specific situation in which other persons or objects are involved. This 'functioning form' is created by past experiences and the cultural patterns of the society in which the individual lives, as a fusion of both private and collective elements (Fox, 1987).

Though each individual is composed of many such roles, they form three great classes (Blatner & Blatner, 1988). Psychosomatic roles are those concerned with biological self-maintenance, for example, eating and sleeping. Social roles are, unsurprisingly, one's public roles of occupation, social class, racial or family role. Psychodramatic roles are those that people one's inner life, perhaps one's idea of oneself as 'the successful mother' or another as 'the cherished daughter'. Moreno proposed that these various roles could compete, both with reality and with each other, leading to both distress and disorientation. This idea has much in common with, and can draw experimental support from, Festinger's theory of cognitive dissonance (Festinger, 1957; Wickland & Brehm, 1976).

The 'integrative' element to catharsis described above refers to the elimination of contradictions between competing roles. As well as spontaneity, two key processes are essential in this programme, respectively called creativity, and warming up. Creativity refers to the clients' ability to create and transform roles. Warming up involves bringing the clients' emotional resources to bear on their roles, which otherwise remain perceived as abstract ideas, rather than lived realities. Of course, roles have a context, and therefore Moreno identified an additional factor the therapist must consider – 'cultural conserves'. These are those aspects of a society that are invariable elements of that society. It is important to ensure that any new or changed roles mesh with the conserves of the society in which the client must survive.

A psychodrama group resembles a play, in that there will be protagonists playing roles significant to themselves or other group members (when they are called 'auxiliaries'), and an audience of observing group members. All group members (excluding the leaders) can be either protagonist or audience. Kipper (1986) has classified the major techniques into two levels, which he called 'basic' and 'general'. The former refers to ways in which the protagonists are encouraged to interact, while the latter refers to the focus given to such interactions. Table 15.1, below, illustrates this.

TABLE 15.1
Basic (above) and general (below) psychodrama techniques

Basic techniques	
Self-presentation	Person describes in the first person the essential qualities of self or of another
Role-playing	Interaction between two or more roles using self or auxiliaries
Dialogue	Vocal interaction between two or more roles *in situ*
Soliloquy	Person talks aloud his thoughts, feelings or reactions *in situ*
Double (may be multiple)	Person's unexpressed thoughts or feelings expressed by other(s) in role of the person
Aside	Person expressed to group, but not to other roles present, his thoughts and feelings
Role-reversal	Person changes roles with significant others
Empty chair	Use of an unoccupied chair to represent significant other or role
Mirror	Use of auxiliary to portray protagonist in manner, feeling, tone, etc.
General techniques	
Future projection	Portrayal of anticipated events, enacting what has not yet happened
Time regression	Enactment of significant events from the past as if they occur in the present
Spontaneity test	Protagonist confronted unexpectedly with new situation. Role playing structured by therapist using auxiliaries without the knowledge of the protagonist
Dream technique*	Enactment of a dream through role-playing, making sense of it and training the dreamer to dream better
Psychodramatic shock technique*	Treatment of psychotic attacks through role-playing the hallucinatory experience afterwards
Role playing under hypnosis*	Role playing while person is under hypnosis for diagnostic or therapeutic purposes

*Not used in postnatal depression.

The safe application of these various techniques within the theoretical frame already outlined makes up the art of psychodrama. We now describe such an application for postnatal depression.

Psychodrama with postnatally depressed women

This work derives from an ongoing relationship between a general psychiatrist with an interest in postnatal depression (Professor J. L. Cox) and the first author, a practising psychodramatist. It entailed several referrals of postnatally depressed women to an open, mixed, out-patient psychodrama group over some time, the number increasing as it became apparent that the women benefited from this approach. The postnatally depressed women thus formed a variable proportion of the psychodrama group. Though not purely for postnatal depression, such a group is the easiest to set up in a NHS setting, and thus represents a 'real', if not 'ideal', community psychotherapy setting for postnatal depression. As we shall see, it is entirely possible to conduct therapy for postnatally depressed women in such a group, provided the *therapists* are aware of the special needs of these women. When we looked at the experiences of these postnatally depressed women, we could identify four general areas that might be helped by psychodrama.

First, their social roles seemed to exert an intensely constricting effect on them.

> "I had totally unrealistic expectations." "I could never work out why I felt so awful struggling to cope with being a Mum, with what I thought a Mum should be like."

Secondly, the role played by the depressed woman's own mother was experienced by these women as an unavoidable cause of their difficulties.

> "I never had a good enough example of a Mum – I was probably raised by a depressed mother."

The third difficulty was closely related to the second, but associated with the depressed woman's own feelings of being 'fatally flawed'. As one woman commented:

> "If I was a better child, my mother would treat me better."

The above idea was usually expressed more subtly, as an idea that there was something 'genetic' about the depression, with the woman being 'different' from other people. This led to much anxiety over whether it was 'right' for them to have children.

The fourth difficulty concerned the role played by the women's spouses. They were perceived by the women as attempting to stifle their expressions of emotion, becoming emotionally unavailable to the women, or treating the women's emotions as signifying only psychopathology. There may have been some justification in this view, as one husband commented:

"It was quite good to be able to get out of it all and go to work"

though other husbands reported how their spouses seemed impervious to their concern, or how stressful they found their own lives during the period of their wives' depression.

From this analysis of their experiences, it might be thought that being unable to supply a monotypical group for postnatal depression would be detrimental to these women. The women's sense of unique aloneness, combined with the priority they gave to matters of motherhood, might cause them to be cut off from a mixed group, leaving them unable to benefit from the group experience. However, this was not so. In practice, other women in the group were able to identify with the postnatally depressed women's experiences of personal inadequacy, fear of motherhood and poor parental relationships. This had the beneficial effect of reducing the feeling of flawed uniqueness that burdened our postnatally depressed women. Yalom (1975) has identified some factors relating to effective group therapy. Many of these, including catharsis, imitative behaviour, corrective emotional experiences, and group cohesion, are subject to direct manipulation in psychodrama groups. Such manipulation may have allowed us to integrate these women successfully into a mixed group; however, a further implication is that our positive results may not generalise to mixed groups that are less prescriptive in these areas.

Although they blended well into a mixed group, their special needs required some techniques specific to their own difficulties. Two techniques proved to be especially useful: the 'expert witness' and the 'good enough mother'. Both these techniques are a kind of role reversal, where the protagonist, here the postnatally depressed mother, takes on another role within the psychodrama.

In the 'expert witness' (based on the ideas of Alice Miller, the Swiss psychoanalyst) the protagonist takes on the role of a child care expert. The role might be that of a senior social worker or child psychologist or psychiatrist, or even a named expert (Anna Freud has proved effective on occasion!). In that expert role, she then makes a measured judgement about the situation being enacted. For example, if the enaction concerns the protagonist as a child, she tells her 'child self' (played by an auxiliary) that she has tried really hard, but she is bound to fail, that the difficulty is not her fault, that she can be angry with the parent who has hurt her, and she has a right to move on and seek more rewarding relationships for herself, not taking responsibility for her parents' inadequacies. The protagonist will usually make these sorts of comments with very little prompting from the therapist. When these words are repeated back to the protagonist when they have returned to their own role, it has additional subjective impact.

In the role-reversal of 'good enough mother' the protagonist plays a mother figure, while an auxiliary plays the protagonist's child self, in a particular situation. The protagonist then acts as she believes her own mother should have done, rather than as her mother actually did. The mother and auxiliary then reverse roles, so that the protagonist can then directly experience her own idea of positive mothering from the auxiliary.

Both of these techniques directly address the matter of having been ruined for life by one's own mother. In 'expert witness' the protagonist is brought straight to the contradiction between the standards she judges she should have and the standards she feels she must accept. One must be wrong, and by definition, it cannot be her own 'expert judgement'. When this technique is used in its proper context, with an adequately warmed-up group, the sense of liberation it may produce is profound. The depressed mother discovers she has judged herself and found herself innocent of blame in her relationship with her own mother. In 'good enough mother' the depressed mother comes to realise that any damage inflicted by her own past may undergo restitution. Within a group setting, this idea is further sustained by the succour given to the protagonist by the group, which is usually extremely intense.

The 'good mother' technique has an additional value. It challenges the postnatally depressed mother's belief that she is inadequate as a mother in the most direct way possible – she experiences the adequacy of her mothering on herself.

The expressed memories of the depressed women's interactions with their own mothers have connotations of unmet need being transferred through successive generations. Direct experiential confirmation of this came in one psychodrama. A scene was enacted that needed to include the postnatally depressed mother herself, her own mother, and her grandmother, before the protagonist (the postnatally depressed mother) could move on and meet her own needs alone. This proved therapeutically as well as theoretically interesting, as the postnatally depressed mother was only able to feel anger at her own mother, after she had felt angry on behalf of her mother at her grandmother.

Postnatally depressed mothers are also depressed women. Therefore, many psychodrama techniques of general use in depression are also useful in this group. Such techniques include 'concretising'; mirroring; doubling; and choosing one's action in the 'core scene'.

'Concretising' is a method of making an emotion (especially guilt) tangible. In many psychodramas (a relevant example might be the 'expert witness' described above) guilt is discovered to be an unjust acceptance of blame from another person, typically the protagonist's mother. By symbolising it as an object (perhaps a cushion), the protagonist may enact returning it to an auxiliary playing the mother, experiencing appropriate relief in consequence.

Helping a client to forgive themselves may be especially important in postnatal depression, where one's inner sense of failure from the depression is magnified by a manifest failure in achieving the prototypical role of vibrant motherhood. The technique of 'mirroring' is a useful way of achieving this. An auxiliary enacts the role of the protagonist, usually with despondency and lack of spontaneity. The protagonist is then encouraged to see that anyone in their position would have trouble coping with the situation being enacted. In particular, factors are brought to the protagonist's attention that she might have overlooked when she began blaming herself. Thus, in postnatal depression, it becomes apparent that no one could adequately cope with any baby when the circumstances are fully considered, opening the way for the women to stop compounding their unhappiness with blame.

'Doubling' may be an effective way of both overcoming the depressed woman's sense of isolation, and giving permission for the depressed woman to hold socially unacceptable thoughts as a prerequisite to raising self-esteem. It can be performed either by the therapist or a group member, though to be successful a high level of intimacy must already have been reached. The person doubling for the protagonist stands alongside but slightly behind her, and expresses some unspoken thought or feeling that the protagonist might have inside. The very fact that another group member has the same feeling and can express it so supportively and directly is one of the great benefits of psychodramatic group therapy.

Psychodramatists frequently find that all the difficulties that beset a person may be symbolised in a single enactment – the 'core scene' – usually relating to childhood. The restrictive boundaries to a postnatally depressed woman's perception of her role have already been identified, together with the lack of choice and powerlessness that follow in their train. An essential element of the psychodramatic enactment of the 'core scene' is that, at the climax of the scene, the protagonist has the right to choose their response. In particular, if the 'core scene' relates to childhood, the protagonist both perceives the lack of choices available to the child and recognises, as an adult, that new choices are now possible. The protagonist discovers the ability to choose at the heart of her being, and is thus empowered.

These techniques have been described as isolated, encapsulated interventions. While it is possible to use them in other therapeutic settings, or even within other therapies, it is important to understand that their success depends to a large extent on the context given to them by the therapist. One essential element is that the techniques are carried out in an atmosphere where clients' personal expression may be honest, full and therefore possibly passionate. This is a more demanding criterion than the conventional 'confiding relationship', which aims for accuracy of substance, but not necessarily accuracy of intensity. Achieving a therapeutic milieu that allows accuracy of intensity involves the process Moreno called 'warming up'. Psychodramatists are taught warming-up exercises as part of their training, and these are beyond the scope of this chapter. However, training in other therapies have their own equivalents to warming up, and even careful, non-judgemental and accepting listening may serve as an adequate warming up technique. It is important to recognise that the process of warming up takes time, even when correctly done. Therefore, it is important to review the progress made in therapy before carrying out these techniques, and only implement them if it can be said that the group, family or individual has been adequately prepared.

It is important that a realistic and supportive milieu is used to keep a relevant frame of reference for the protagonist. Within psychodrama groups, this is frequently done by a period of discussion after the psychodrama itself. Group members share their reactions, and talk about what the psychodrama has meant for them. Besides the value this has for the group process, it also serves to maintain appropriate connections between the psychodrama and the real world. New roles developed in psychodramas are used in the everyday life of the protagonist, and the effects of these reported to the group, who give further comment or advice as necessary. This retains the group in an auxiliary position to everyday life. Failure to maintain cultural conserves can either result in the client coming to live for the group, with consequential excess dependency, or even using catharsis inappropriately in the real world to achieve personal relief.

Ensuring that intense emotional expression results in true catharsis may require the skilled help of the therapist. This is because intensity and the ability to reflect both need to be retained for catharsis to occur. Several methods may be used to achieve this dual goal. Props may be used to make the feelings more concrete and easily acted upon, as described above. The protagonist may be asked to repeat an action, putting more emotion into it each time. However, and simultaneously with this, self-monitoring by the protagonists will be emphasised, with the therapist requiring them to take note of their feelings, together with the thoughts and incidents connected with them.

One psychodramatic technique used to ensure integrative catharsis (see above) is that of 'surplus reality'. This is an encounter or scene that has not yet happened or could not happen in reality (for instance, if the other person is dead or absent). Perhaps they might move to a scene of what it might be like the next time their mother tries to direct their life for them. One such psychodrama ended with a scene at an airport, where the protagonist's mother, on returning from her holiday that is the usual 'disappointment' for her, is met by quite a different daughter. It is not the overburdened child-daughter, feeling responsible for mother's unhappiness. Instead, a more assertive adult-daugher is quite unmoved by the mother's critical ruminations and recounting of the many ailments that had flared up because the hotel had not been right.

Women's experience of therapy

With its emphasis on action techniques and intense emotional displays, one might have expected that psychodrama would not be acceptable to a group of working class women from a city in the north of England, where the tradition is for sobriety, reticence, and acceptance of one's lot in life. However, postnatally depressed women both attended and kept attending. Moreover, the vast bulk of their comments were extremely positive. Thus, when used in a slow, open group, psychodrama appears acceptable to people who might not be expected to tolerate its intensity.

Psychodrama's emphasis is on encouraging people to find new ways of interpreting and living their lives. It does not focus simply on symptom reduction; its philosophy implies rather that symptomatology results from its client's unhelpful roles. We do not therefore believe that psychodrama or its techniques offer a complete treatment for postnatal depression. However, there is more to the experience of depression than specific symptoms, and psychodrama seeks to encourage women to renegotiate that experience. Our preliminary impressions are both that psychodrama helps postnatally depressed women to do this, and that they find such a renegotiation valuable. This renegotiation represents the successful application of the principles of spontaneity and creativity discussed above.

First, their attitude to their symptoms appeared to change. They found their discoveries in our group had enabled them to assign their experience to a manageable place in their lives and so cope with and grow from it. As one mother succinctly put it:

"It gave me a kick start."

Secondly, women seemed to benefit from the groups, whether they were active or passive within them. A typical comment was:

"Listening to and seeing others makes you think about yourself – you find out why."

It certainly could surprise the women with the novel insights it brought.

"You can say the most amazing things and bring out all your inner feelings."

The therapy was not seen as entirely pleasant. In particular, there was a sense of psychological purging that, while bringing great relief in retrospect, was frightening at the time. As one said, using the analogy of herself as a dustbin filled with rubbish:

"It felt like being tipped upside down and shaken out."

However, the women found it valuable in helping them face the painful issues in their lives, and resolve them.

> "It makes you stick with it", said one woman, who had to come to terms with an ambivalent relationship with her mother, "You can't wriggle out."

It seemed that postnatally depressed women used their experience in psychodrama for two purposes. First, they were able to link their current depression to previous life experiences in a way that made sense of both. Williams & Wood (1986) have pointed out that this is an important component of coming to terms with even physical illness. Secondly, they were able to use this understanding (or insight) to mobilise their determination to overcome their depression. In short, the psychodrama group seemed to improve the women's belief in their ability to recover, with consequentially improved motivation. This is consistent with Carlson-Sabelli's (1989) finding that psychodramatic techniques produce changes in both opinions, which are people's expressed beliefs, and attitudes, which are those beliefs that predispose actions.

Psychodramatic techniques in other psychotherapies

Only a small minority of therapists have undergone the long and intense training necessary to become fully qualified psychodramatists. However, many of the techniques are adaptable for use in other therapeutic methods and settings.

Both Williams (1989) and Guldner (1982) describe how psychodrama may be used successfully with whole families. Holmes (1992) formulates a theoretical synthesis between psychodrama and object relations theory, allowing freer communication between these two disciplines. In its emphasis on action-orientated techniques, rehearsal and feedback, it also relates to the behaviour therapies, which recommend very similar techniques, especially in relation to problems involving self-concept behaviours such as assertiveness (Wolpe, 1990). Wolpe has in fact referred to these techniques as 'behavioural psychodrama'. The relationship between psychodrama and person-centred counselling will be treated in more detail, as this method has been used successfully with postnatally depressed women already (Holden *et al*, 1987).

In Rogers' (1961) description of person-centred counselling, he identified six elements to the client's experience of the method. These were: (1) the experiencing of responsibility; (2) experiencing of exploration; (3) the discovery of denied attitudes; (4) the reorganisation of the self; (5) a sense of progress; and (6) ending. It can be seen above that the second, third, fourth and fifth of these elements have been expressed by the postnatally depressed women experiencing psychodrama. The matter of 'ending' in psychodrama has not been previously discussed in this chapter but, as with person-centred counselling, it involves encouraging the client to overcome his or her fears of managing alone.

Furthermore, Rogers' (1961) account of the therapeutic process in his method suggests that its stages are closely mirrored by the key elements of psychodrama, illustrated in Table 15.2 below.

TABLE 15.2
Psychodrama according to Rogerian principles

Rogerian stage	*Psychodramatic equivalent*
Loosening of feeling	Warming up
Change in the manner of experiencing	Effected by many techniques, especially role reversal
A shift from incongruence (difference between real and ideal self-perceptions) to congruence	Integrative catharsis
Changing the manner and extent to which the individual is willing to communicate himself in a receptive climate	Role play, spontaneity training, surplus reality, doubling
A loosening of the cognitive maps of experience	Role-reversal, future projection
Changing the individual's relationship to his problem	Experimentation with new roles, concretisation, doubling
Changing the individual's manner of relating	Transactions in the psychodrama group between group members, being generalised into new roles or patterns of behaviour in the outside world

Thus, there are close similarities between psychodrama and person-centred counselling in both the client's experience of therapy, and in the intended goals of therapy. It is therefore not surprising that psychodrama was found to be of benefit in postnatal depression.

The differences between the two seem to lie in two areas. First, psychodrama seems to be experienced as a directive process. Secondly, it employs a wider range of specific techniques to promote personal change. These differences, as well as the similarities, may have been of benefit.

The postnatally depressed women attending the group, though treated in a community setting, were different to those examined by Holden and her colleagues (Holden *et al*, 1987). They were all deemed sufficiently ill by their general practitioners to require psychiatric assessment. They seemed to find the therapy's directive quality a valuable, if uncomfortable, aspect of their therapy, as might be expected if they experienced disability through depressive anergy. Furthermore, we have already seen that these postnatally depressed women had an intense experience of personal responsibility for their duties and difficulties, that they found overwhelming. The introduction of specific techniques by the therapist allows the therapist to share responsibility for the women's experiences in therapy, a position difficult to achieve using the Rogerian method of simply accepting the women's experiences for what they are. It is tempting to speculate that psychodramatic techniques may be able to act as a complement to more conventional person-centred approaches in postnatally depressed women, possibly on that third that Holden found did not respond to her approach.

In any event, the very considerable overlap between the two approaches suggests that an eclectic approach to therapy, combining elements of both, will not produce an incoherent experience for the client, despite the enormous contrast in methods between them.

Psychodrama is a therapy that moves people, in the fullest sense of that word. It is also a practical and acceptable therapy, that easily fits within conventional treatment programmes for depression. Perhaps most importantly, it seems to address aspects of postnatally depressed women's experience that may not otherwise be confronted. We have not sought to present a systematic outcome study of group psychodrama in postnatal depression, although we believe that many seriously depressed women so treated have improved as a result. Instead, our intention was to convey the theory, techniques and atmosphere of such groups conducted with postnatally depressed women in a community setting. As our initial quote from Hegel implies, this is as necessary as quantitative outcome research in assessing the use of psychodrama in this patient group. If, at the end of the chapter, the reader believes that group psychodrama is a sensible, realisable form of therapy that may be conducted usefully with psychiatrically ill women in their everyday lives, then we will have succeeded in our intention. Any further enthusiasm is up to the reader.

References

ARN, I., THEORELL, T., UVNAS-MOBERG, K., *et al* (1989) Psychodrama group therapy for patients with functional gastrointestinal disorders – a controlled long-term follow-up study. *Psychotherapy and Psychosomatics*, **51**, 113–119.

BEER, R. (1992) A preschool child psychiatric service: predictors of post-assessment default. *Child Care, Health and Development*, **18**, 1–13.

BLATNER, A. & BLATNER, A. (1988) *Foundations of Psychodrama. History, Theory and Practice*. New York: Springer.

CARLSON-SABELLI, L (1989) Role reversal: a concept analysis and reinterpretation of the research literature. *Journal of Group Psychotherapy, Psychodrama and Sociometry*, **41**, 139–152.

COX, J. (1988) The life event of childbirth: sociocultural aspects of postnatal depression. In *Motherhood and Mental Illness: Causes and Consequences* (eds R. Kumar & I.Brockington). London: Wright Scientific.

FESTINGER, L. (1957) *A Theory of Cognitive Dissonance*. Stanford, CA: Stanford University Press.

FOREMAN, D., HACKNEY, M. & COX, J. (1992) The impact of postnatal depression on infants and their older siblings – preliminary results from a controlled study (Conference paper). Edinburgh: Marcé Society.

FOX, J. (1987) *The Essential Moreno. Writings on Psychodrama, Group Method and Spontaneity by J. L. Moreno.* New York: Springer.

GULDNER, C. (1982) Multiple family psychodramatic therapy. *Journal of Group Psychotherapy, Psychodrama and Sociometry*, **35**, 47–56.

HARVEY, I. & McGRATH, G. (1988) Psychiatric morbidity in spouses of women admitted to a mother and baby unit. *British Journal of Psychiatry*, **152**, 506–510.

HEGEL, G. W. F. (1807 (1977)) *Phenomenology of Spirit.* Oxford: Clarendon Press.

HOLDEN, J., SAGOVSKY, R. & COX, J. (1987) Counselling in a general practice setting: a controlled study of health visitor intervention in the treatment of postnatal depression. *British Medical Journal*, **298**, 223–226.

HOLMES, P. (1992) *The Inner World Outside. Object Relations Theory and Psychodrama.* London: Routledge & Kegan Paul.

—— & KARP, M. (1991) *Psychodrama; Inspiration and Technique.* London: Routledge & Kegan Paul.

KELLERMAN, P. (1987) Outcome research in classical psychodrama. *Small Group Behavior*, **18**, 459–469.

KIPPER, D. (1986) *Psychotherapy Through Clinical Role Playing.* New York: Brunner/Mazel.

KUMAR, R. & ROBSON, K. (1984) A prospective study of emotional disorders in childbearing women. *British Journal of Psychiatry*, **144**, 35–47.

LOVESTONE, S. & KUMAR, C. (1993) Postnatal psychiatric illness: the impact on partners. *British Journal of Psychiatry*, **163**, 210–216.

MARINEAU, R. (1989) *Jacob Levy Moreno 1889–1974. Father of Psychodrama, Sociometry and Group Psychotherapy.* International Library of Group Psychotherapy and Group Process. London: Tavistock/Routledge.

MORENO, J. (1934) *Who Shall Survive? A New Approach to the Problem of Human Relations.* Washington, DC: Nervous and Mental Disease Publishing.

—— (1946) *Psychodrama* Vol. I. 1. New York: Beacon House.

—— (1969) *Psychodrama* Vol. III. 3. New York: Beacon House.

—— & MORENO, Z. (1956) *Psychodrama* Vol. II. 2. New York: Beacon House.

MURRAY, L. (1992) The impact of postnatal depression on infant development. *Journal of Child Psychology and Psychiatry*, **33**, 543–562.

NETTLEBLADT, P., UDDENBERG, M. & ENGLESSON, I. (1985) Marital disharmony four and a half years post partum. *Acta Psychiatrica Scandinavica*, **71**, 392–401.

NICOL, A. (1989) Implications for practice of the mother and toddler project. (Conference paper.) London: Royal Society of Medicine.

ROGERS, C. (1961) *On Becoming a Person.* Boston: Houghton Mifflin.

STEIN, A., GATH, D., BUCHER, J., *et al* (1991) The relationship between postnatal depression and mother–child interaction. *British Journal of Psychiatry*, **158**, 46–52.

WICKLAND, J. & BREHM, J. (1976) *Perspectives in Cognitive Dissonance.* New York: John Wiley.

WILLIAMS, A. (1989) *The Passionate Technique. Strategic Psychodrama with Individuals, Families and Groups.* London: Tavistock/Routledge.

WILLIAMS, G. & WOOD, P. (1986) Common-sense beliefs about illness: a mediating role for the doctor. *Lancet*, **ii**, 1435–1437.

WOLPE, J. (1990) *The Practice of Behavior Therapy.* New York: Pergamon.

YALOM, I. (1975) *The Theory and Practice of Group Psychotherapy.* New York: Basic Books.

Appendix. Translations of the Edinburgh Postnatal Depression scale

This appendix gives presently available translations of the Edinburgh Postnatal Depression Scale. Readers are referred to Chapter 9 for notes on the use of the scale, and in particular pages 139–143 for details of its scoring.

All the translations have been back-translated, but to our knowledge only the Swedish and Dutch translations have been specifically validated. When using a translation of the Edinburgh Postnatal Depression Scale it is fundamentally important to consider the precise idiomatic equivalents as far as possible. It may be appropriate, for example, to modify the scale by omitting items or adding others for the scale to be useful in a different culture—especially if this is a non-Western society. For the scale to be recommended for use in research or clinical settings outside the UK, where it was developed, there should be a carefully conducted validation study on a representative sample of postpartum women. The reader is referred to Chapter 10 for a full discussion of the cultural context of the EPDS.

Czech Republic

Vaše pocity v minulém týdnu:

1. Byla jste schopna se smát a vidět věci i z veselé stránky:
   stejně jako dříve
   ne tak často jako dříve
   rozhodně ne tak často jako dříve
   vůbec ne

2. S radostí jsem se těšila na příští věci:
   stejně jako dříve
   poněkud méně mež dříve
   rozhodně méně než dřív
   skoro vůbec ne

3. Zbybečně jsem si vyčítala, když se něco nedařilo:
   ano, většinou
   ano, někdy
   ne moc často
   ne, nikdy

4. Cítila jsem úzkost nebo měla starosti bez přiměřeného důvodu:
   ne, vůbec ne
   skoro vůbec ne
   ano, někdy
   ano, často

5. Měla jsem strach nebo pocit paniky bez podstatného důvodu:
   ano, hodně
   ano, někdy
   ne, moc ne
   ne, vůbec ne

6. Věci mi přerůstaly přes hlavu, nestačila jsem:
   ano, většinou
   ano, někdy
   zcela výjimečně
   ne, vůbec ne

7. Byla jsem tak nešťastná, že jsem měla potíže se spánkem:
   ano, většinou
   někdy
   ne moc často
   ne, vůbec ne

8. Bylo mi smutno nebo mizerně:
   ano, většinou
   ano, dost často
   ne moc často
   ne, vůbec ne

9. Byla jsem tak nešťastná, že jsem plakala:
   ano, většinou
   ano, dost často
   jen sřídka
   ne, nikdy

10. Naspadaly mne myělvenky, že si něco udělám:
    ano, dost často
    někdy
    sotvakdy
    nikdy

Dutch

De volgende vragen hebben betrekking up hoe u zich de afgelopen 7 dagen heeft gevoeld. Kruis dat antwoord aan dat het beste aangeeft hoe u zich voelde.

1. Ik heb kunnen lachen en de zonnige kant van de dingen kunnen inzien:
   Zoveel als ik altijd kon
   Niet zo veel nu als anders
   Zeker niet zo veel nu als anders
   Helemaal niet

2. Ik heb met plezier naar dingen uitgekeken:
   Zoals altijd of meer
   Wat minder dan ik gewend was
   Absoluut minder dan ik gewend was
   Nauwelijks

3. Ik heb mij zelf onnodig verwijten gemaakt als er iets fout ging:
   Ja, heel vaak
   Ja, soms
   Niet erg vaak
   Nee, nooit

4. Ik ben bang of bezorgd geweest zonder dat er een aanleiding was:
   Nee, helemaal niet
   Nauwelijks
   Ja, soms
   Ja, zeer vaak

5. Ik reageerde schrikachtig of paniekerig zonder echte goede reden:
   Ja, tamelijk vaak
   Ja, soms
   Nee, niet vaak
   Nooit

6. De dingen groeiden me boven het hoofd:
   Ja, meestal was ik er niet tegen opgewassen
   Ja, soms was ik minder goed tegen dingen opgewassen dan anders
   Nee, meestal kon ik de dingen erg goed aan
   Nee, ik kon alles even goed aan als anders

7. Ik voelde me zo ongelukkig dat ik er bijna niet van kon slapen:
   Ja, meestal
   Ja, soms
   Niet vaak
   Helemaal niet

8. Ik voelde me somber en beroerd:
   Ja, bijna steeds
   Ja, tamelijk vaak
   Niet erg vaak
   Nee, helemaal niet

9. Ik was zo ongelukkig dat ik heb zitten huilen:
   Ja, heel vaak
   Ja, tamelijk vaak
   Alleen af en toe
   Nee, nooit

10. Ik heb er aan gedacht om mezelf iets aan te doen:
    Ja, tamelijk vaak
    Soms
    Nauwelijks
    Nooit

French

Vous venez d'avoir un bébé. Nous aimerions savoir comment vous vous sentez. Nous vous demandons de bien vouloir remplir ce questionnaire en soulignant la réponse qui vous semble le mieux décrire comment vous vous êtes sentie durant la semaine (c'est-à-dire sur les 7 jours qui viennent de s'écouler) et pas seulement au jour d'aujourd'hui.

Voici un exemple

Je me suis sentie heureuse:
 Oui, tout le temps
 Oui, la plupart du temps
 Non, pas très souvent
 Non, pas du tout.

Ceci signifiera "je me suis sentie heureuse la plupart du temps durant la semaine qui vient de s'écouler". Merci de bien vouloir répondre aux autres questions.

PENDANT LA SEMAINE QUI VIENT DE S'ECOULER

1. J'ai pu rire et prendre les choses du bon côté:
 Aussi souvent que d'habitude
 Pas tout-à-fait autant
 Vraiment beaucoup moins souvent ces jours-ci
 Absolument pas

2. Je me suis sentie confiante et joyeuse, en pensant à l'avenir:
 Autant que d'habitude
 Plutôt moins que d'habitude
 Vraiment moins que d'habitude
 Pratiquement pas

3. Je me suis reprochée, sans raisons, d'être responsable quand les choses allaient mal:
 Oui, la plupart du temps
 Oui, parfois
 Pas très souvent
 Non, jamais

4. Je me suis sentie inquiète ou soucieuse sans motifs:
 Non, pas du tout
 Presque jamais
 Oui, parfois
 Oui, très souvent

5. Je me suis sentie effrayée ou paniquée sans vraiment de raisons:
   Oui, vraiment souvent
   Oui, parfois
   Non, pas très souvent
   Non, pas du tout

6. J'ai eu tendance à me sentir dépassée par les évènements:
   Oui, la plupart du temps, je me suis sentie incapable de faire face aux situations
   Oui, parfois, je ne me suis pas sentie aussi capable de faire face que d'habitude
   Non, j'ai pu faire face à la plupart des situations
   Non, je me suis sentie aussi efficace que d'habitude

7. Je me suis sentie si malheureuse que j'ai eu des problèmes de sommeil:
   Oui, la plupart du temps
   Oui, parfois
   Pas très souvent
   Non, pas du tout

8. Je me suis sentie triste ou peu heureuse:
   Oui, la plupart du temps
   Oui, très souvent
   Pas très souvent
   Non, pas du tout

9. Je me suis sentie si malheureuse que j'en ai pleuré:
   Oui, la plupart du temps
   Oui, très souvent
   Seulement de temps en temps
   Non, jamais

10. Il m'est arrivé de penser à me faire du mal:
    Oui, très souvent
    Parfois
    Presque jamais
    Jamais

German

Nachdem Sie kürzlich ein Baby hatten, würden wir gerne wissen, wie Sie sich fühlen. Bitte, unterstreichen Sie die Antwort, die am ähnlichsten beschreibt, wie Sie sich in den letzten sieben Tagen gefühlt haben, nicht nur wie Sie sich heute fühlen:

Hier ist ein bereits ausgefülltes Beispiel:

Ich war glücklich:
   Ja, die ganze Zeit
   <u>Ja, meistens</u>
   Nein, nicht sehr oft
   Nein, gar nicht

Das würde bedeuten: "Ich habe mich den größten Teil der Zeit glücklich gefühlt, während dieser Woche." Bitte unterstreichen Sie die für Sie zutreffenden Antworten in derselben Weise.

IN DEN LETZTEN SIEBEN TAGEN

1. Ich konnte lachen und die komische Seite von Dingen sehen:
   So viel wie bisher
   Nicht ganz wie früher
   Entschieden nicht so sehr wie bisher
   Überhaupt nicht

2. Ich habe mich auf Dinge im Voraus gefreut:
   So viel wie bisher
   Wohl weniger als gewöhnlich
   Entschieden weniger wie bisher
   Kaum mehr

3. Ich habe mich unnötiger Weise schuldig gefühlt, wenn Dinge schief gingen:
   Ja, meistens
   Ja, gelegentlich
   Nicht sehr oft
   Nein, niemals

4. Ich war ängstlich oder besorgt ohne guten Grund:
   Nein, gar nicht
   Kaum
   Ja, gelegentlich
   Ja, sehr oft

5. Ich habe mich gefürchtet oder war in Panik ohne guten Grund:
   Ja, sehr häufig
   Ja, gelegentlich
   Nein, nicht viel
   Nein, überhaupt nicht

6. Dinge wurden mir zuviel:
   Ja, meistens konnte ich die Situation nicht meistern
   Ja, gelegentlich konnte ich die Dinge nicht so gut meistern wie sonst
   Nein, meistens konnte ich die Situation meistern
   Nein, ich bewältige Dinge so gut wie immer

7. Ich war so unglücklich, daß ich nur schlecht schlafen konnte:
   Ja, meistens
   Ja, gelegentlich
   Nein, nicht sehr häufig
   Nein, gar nicht

8. Ich habe mich traurig oder elend gefühlt:
   Ja, meistens
   Ja, gelegentlich
   Nein, nicht sehr häufig
   Nein, gar nicht

9. Ich war so unglücklich, daß ich weinte:
   Ja, den größten Teil der Zeit
   Ja, sehr häufig
   Nur gelegentlich
   Nein, nie

10. Der Gedanke, mir etwas anzutun, ist mir gekommen:
    Ja, recht häufig
    Gelegentlich
    Kaum jemals
    Niemals

Greek

1. Μπορούσα να γελώ και να βλέπω την αστεια πλευρά της ζωής:
   όπως πριν
   λιγότερο από πριν
   πολύ λιγότερο από πριν
   καθόλου

2. Εβλεπα το αύριο με ενθοθσιασμο:
   όπως και πριν
   μάλλον λιγότερο από πριν
   πολύ λιγότερο από πριν
   καθόλου

3. Κατηγορούσα άδικα τον εαυτό μου, χωρις να χρειάςεται, λια πράγματα που πηγαυ στραβά:
   ναι, όλη την ώρα
   ναι, αρκετά συχνά
   όχι πολύ συχνά
   ποτέ

4. Ενιωθα άγχος ή οτευοχώρια χωρις σοβαρό λόγο:
   όχι, καθόλου
   σχεδόν ποτέ
   ναι, καμιά φορά
   ναι, συχνά

5. Ενιωθα φόβο ή πανικο χωρις, σοβαρό λόγο:
   ναι, πολύ συχνα
   ναι, καμιά φορά
   όχι, όχι συχνά
   όχι, καθόλου

Την περασμένη εβδομάδα

6. Με πήρε η κάτω βόλτα (ένιωθα πολύ πεσμέυη):
   ναι, σχεδόν συνέχεια
   ναι, καμιά φορά
   όχι, σχεδόν ποτέ
   όχι, καθόλου

7. Ημουν τόσο στενοχωρημένη που δεν μπορούσα να κοιμηθώ:
   ναι, σχεδόν συνέχεια
   ναι, καμιά φορά
   πολύ σπάνια
   όχι, καθόλου

8. Ενιωθα θλιμένη ή πως ήμουν για λύπηση:
   ναι, σχεδόν συνέχεια
   ναι, αρκετά συχνά
   όχι, πολύ συχνά
   όχι, καθόλου

9. Ενιωθα τόσο δυστυχισμένη που έκλαιγα:
   ναι, όλη την ώρα
   ναι, αρκετά συχνά
   κάπου-κάπου
   όχι, ποτέ

10. Μου ήρθε να βλάψω τον εαυτό μού:
    ναι, αρκετά συχνά
    καμιά φορά
    σχεδόν ποτέ
    ποτέ

Hindi

'आप कैसा महसूस कर रहीं हैं'

आपके यहां कुछ दिनों पहले बच्चे का जन्म हुआ है, हम यह जानना चाहते हैं कि अब आप कैसा महसूस कर रही हैं। पिछले एक हफ़्ते के दौरान में आपनें जैसा महसूस किया है, उसके सामने निशान [✓] लगा दें, न कि जैसा आप आज महसूस कर रही हैं।

यहाँ हल किया हुआ एक उदाहरण दे रहे हैं
भैने खुश महसूस किया है
हाँ, अधिकांश समय,
हाँ, कुछ समय   ✓
नहीं, अकसर नहीं
नहीं, कभी नहीं

इसका मतलब है कि मैंने कुछ समय खुश महसूस किया है, पिछले एक हफ़्ते के दौरान । कृपया बाकि प्रश्नों का जबाब इसी तरह दें।

पिछले सात दिनों के दौरान'

1. मैं हंस पायी हूँ और बातों का अच्छा पहलू देख पायी हूँ:
जितना मैं सदैव करती पायी हूँ
अब उतना नहीं
निश्चित ही अब कम
बिल्कुल नहीं

2. मैं आने वाली बातों के प्रति खुशी महसूस करती हूँ
जितना मैं पहले कर पायी
जितना पहले कर पाती थी उससे कम
निश्चित रुप से पहले से कम
बिलकुल नहीं के बराबर

3. कुछ भी बिगड़ जाने पर मैं अनावश्यक रुप से अपने को दोषी मानती हूँ।
हाँ, अधिकांश समय
हाँ, कुछ समय
अकसर नहीं
नहीं बिलकुल नहीं

4. पर्यान्त कारण न होने पर भी मैं घबराई या चिंतित महसूस करती रही हूँ:

नहीं बिलकुल नहीं
शायद ही कभी
हाँ, कभी कभी
हाँ, अकसर ही

5. पर्यान्त कारण न होने पर भी मैं भयभीत या अत्याधिक घबराहट महसूस करती रही हूँ:

हाँ, काफी ज्यादा
हाँ, कभी कभी
नहीं, अधिक नहीं
नहीं, कभी नहीं

6. काम मुझे अपने ऊपर बोझ मालूम पड़ता रहा है:

हाँ, अधिकांश समय मैं झेल नहीं पायी हूँ
हाँ, कभी कभी मैं पहले की तरह झेल नहीं पायी हूँ
नहीं अधिकांश समय मैं अच्छे से झेल पायी हूँ
नहीं, मैं हमेशा की तरह ही झेल पायी हूँ

7. मैं इतना उदास महसूस करती रही हूँ कि मुझे नींद आने में परेशानी हुई :

हाँ, अधिकांश समय
हाँ, कभी कभी
अकसर नहीं
नहीं, बिलकुल नहीं

8. मैं उदास या दुखी महसूस करती हूँ:

हाँ, अधिकांश समय
हाँ, अकसर ही
अकसर नहीं
नहीं, कभी नहीं

9. मैं इतना दुखी रही हूँ कि रोती रही हूँ:

हाँ, अधिकांश समय
हाँ, अकसर ही
केवल, कभी कभी
नहीं, कभी नहीं

10. अपने आप को नुकसान/आत्म हत्या/ पहुंचाने का ख्याल मुझे आया है:

हाँ, अकसर ही
कभी, कभी
शायद ही कभी,
कभी नहीं

Japanese

エ ジ ン バ ラ 産 後 う つ 病 調 査 票

ご出産おめでとうございます。ご出産から今までの間にどのようにお感じになったかを
お知らせください。今日だけでなく、過去7日間にあなたが感じられたことに最も近い
答えにアンダーラインを引いてください。必ず10項目に答えてください。

例）　幸せだと感じた。　　　　はい、常にそうだった
　　　　　　　　　　　　　　　<u>はい、たいていそうだった</u>
　　　　　　　　　　　　　　　いいえ、あまり度々ではなかった
　　　　　　　　　　　　　　　いいえ、全くそうではなかった

"はい、たいていそうだった"と答えた場合は過去7日間のことをいいます。この様な
方法で質問にお答えください。

【質問】

1.　笑うことができたし、物事のおかしい面もわかった。

　　　　　　　　　　　　　　　いつもと同様にできた
　　　　　　　　　　　　　　　あまりできなかった
　　　　　　　　　　　　　　　明らかにできなかった
　　　　　　　　　　　　　　　全くできなかった

2.　物事を楽しみにして待った。

　　　　　　　　　　　　　　　いつもと同様にできた
　　　　　　　　　　　　　　　あまりできなかった
　　　　　　　　　　　　　　　明らかにできなかった
　　　　　　　　　　　　　　　ほとんどできなかった

3.　物事が悪くいった時、自分を不必要に責めた。

　　　　　　　　　　　　　　　はい、たいていそうだった
　　　　　　　　　　　　　　　はい、時々そうだった
　　　　　　　　　　　　　　　いいえ、あまり度々ではない
　　　　　　　　　　　　　　　いいえ、そうではなかった

4.　はっきりした理由もないのに不安になったり、心配した。

　　　　　　　　　　　　　　　いいえ、そうではなかった
　　　　　　　　　　　　　　　ほとんどそうではなかった
　　　　　　　　　　　　　　　はい、時々あった
　　　　　　　　　　　　　　　はい、しょちゅうあった

5. はっきりした理由もないのに恐怖に襲われた。

> はい、しょちゅうあった
> はい、時々あった
> いいえ、めったになかった
> いいえ全くなかった

6. することがたくさんあって大変だった。

> はい、たいてい対処できなかった
> はい、いつものようにはうまく対処しなかった
> いいえ、たいていうまく対処した
> いいえ、普段通りに対処した

7. 不幸せなので、眠りにくかった。

> はい、ほとんどいつもそうだった
> はい、ときどきそうだった
> いいえ、あまり度々ではなかった
> いいえ、全くなかった

8. 悲しくなったり、惨めになった。

> はい、たいていそうだった
> はい、かなりしばしばそうだった
> いいえ、あまり度々ではなかった
> いいえ、全くそうではなかった

9. 不幸せなので、泣けてきた

> はい、たいていそうだった
> はい、かなりしばしばそうだった
> ほんの時々あった
> いいえ、全くそうではなかった

10. 自分自身を傷つけるという考えが浮かんできた。

> はい、かなりしばしばそうだった
> 時々そうだった
> めったになかった
> 全くなかった

Portuguese

Como teve recentemente um bebé, gostariamos de saber como se sente. Por favor, sublinhe a resposta que melhor indique o modo como se sente *desde há 7 dias* e näo apenas hoje.

Aqui está um exemplo:

> Senti-me feliz:
> Sim, sempre
> <u>Sim, quase sempre</u>
> Näo, poucas vezes
> Näo, nunca

Isto quereria dizer: "Senti-me feliz quase sempre durante os últimos sete dias". Por favor, complete as outras questöes do mesmo modo.

DESDE HÁ 7 DIAS

1. Tenho sido capaz de me rir e ver o lado-divertido das coisas
   Tanto como dantes
   Menos do que antes
   Muito menos do que antes
   Nunca

2. Tenho tido esperança no futuro
   Tanta como sempre tive
   Bastante menos do que costumava ter
   Muito menos do que costumava ter
   Quase nenhuma

3. Tenho-me culpado sem necessidade quando as coisas correm mal
   Sim, a maioria das vezes
   Sim, algumas vezes
   Raramente
   Näo, nunca

4. Tenho estado ansiosa ou preocupada sem motivo
   Näo, Nunca
   Quase nunca
   Sim, por vezes
   Sim, muitas vezes

5. Tenho-me sentido com medo, ou muito assustada, sem grande motivo
   Sim, muitas vezes
   Sim, por vezes
   Näo, raramente
   Näo, nunca

6. Tenho sentido que säo coisas demais para mim
   Sim, a maioria das vezes näo tenho conseguido resolvê-las
   Sim, por vezes näo tenho conseguido resolvê-las como dantes
   Näo, a maioria das vezes resolvo-as fácilmente
   Näo, resolvo-as täo bem como dantes

7. Tenho-me sentido täo infeliz que durmo mal
   Sim, quase sempre
   Sim, por vezes
   Raramente
   Näo, nunca

8. Tenho-me sentido triste ou muito infeliz
   Sim, quase sempre
   Sim, muitas vezes
   Raramente
   Näo, nunca

9. Tenho-me sentido täo infeliz que choro
   Sim, quase sempre
   Sim, muitas vezes
   Só, às vezes
   Näo, nunca

10. Tive ideias de fazer mal a mim mesma
    Sim, muitas vezes
    Por vezes
    Muito raramente
    Nunca

Spanish

SUS SENTIMIENTOS DURANTE LA SEMANA PASADA

1. He podido reír y ver el lado bueno de las cosas:
   Tanto como siempre
   No tanto ahora
   Mucho menos
   No, no he podido

2. He mirado al futuro con placer:
   Tanto como siempre
   Algo menos de lo que solía hacer
   Definitivamente menos
   No, nada

3. Me he culpado innecesariamente cuando las cosas marchaban mal:
   Sí, la mayor parte de las veces
   Sí, algunas veces
   No muy a menudo
   No, nunca

4. He estado ansiosa y preocupada sin motivo:
   No, nada
   Casi nada
   Sí, a veces
   Sí, a menudo

5. He sentido miedo y pánico sin motivo alguno:
   Sí, bastante
   Sí, a veces
   No, no mucho
   No, nada

6. Las cosas me superaban, me sobrepasaban:
   Sí, la mayor parte de las veces
   Sí, a veces
   No, casi nunca
   No, nada

7. Me ha sentido tan infeliz, que he tenido dificultad para dormir:
   Sí, casi siempre
   Sí, a veces
   No muy a menudo
   No, nada

8. Me he sentido triste y desgraciada:
   Sí, casi siempre
   Sí, bastante a menudo
   No muy a menudo
   No, nada

9. He sido tan infeliz que he estado llorando:
   Sí, casi siempre
   Sí, bastante a menudo
   Sólo ocasionalmente
   No, nunca

10. He pensado en hacerme daño a mí misma:
   Sí, bastante a menudo
   A veces
   Casi nunca
   No, nunca

Swedish

Eftersom Du nyligen fått barn, skulle vi vilja veta hur Du mår. Var snäll och stryk under det svar, som bäst stämmer överens med hur Du känt Dig under de sista 7 dagarna, inte bara hur Du mår idag.

Här är ett exempel, som redan är ifyllt:

> Jag har känt mig lycklig:
> Ja, hela tiden
> <u>Ja, för det mesta</u>
> Nej, inte särskilt ofta
> Nej, inte alls

Detta betyder: Jag har känt mig lycklig mest hela tiden under veckan som har gått. Var snäll och fyll i de andra frågorna på samma sätt:

UNDER DE SENASTE 7 DAGARNA

1. Jag har kunnat se tillvaron från den ljusa sidan:
   Lika bra som vanligt
   Nästan lika bra som vanligt
   Mycket mindre än vanligt
   Inte alls

2. Jag har glatt mig åt saker som skall hända:
   Lika mycket som vanligt
   Något mindre än vanligt
   Mycket mindre än vanligt
   Inte alls

3. Jag har lagt skulden på mig själv onödigt mycket när något har gått snett:
   Ja, för det mesta
   Ja, ibland
   Nej, inte så ofta
   Nej, aldrig

4. Jag har känt mig rädd och orolig utan egentlig anledning:
   Nej, inte alls
   Nej, knappast alls
   Ja, ibland
   Ja, mycket ofta

5. Jag har känt mig strämd eller panikslagen utan speciell anledning:
   Ja, mycket ofta
   Ja, ibland
   Nej, ganska sällan
   Nej, inte alls

6. Det har kört ihop sig för mig och blivit för mycket:
   Ja, mesta tiden har jag inte kunnat ta itu med något alls
   Ja, ibland har jag inte kunnat ta itu med saker lika bra som vanligt
   Nej, för det mesta har jag kunnat ta itu med saker ganska bra
   Nej, jag har kunnat ta itu med saker precis som vanligt

7. Jag har känt mig så ledsen och olycklig att jar har haft svårt att sova:
   Ja, mesta tiden
   Ja, ibland
   Nej, sällan
   Nej, aldrig

8. Jag har känt mig ledsen och nere:
   Ja, för det mesta
   Ja, rätt ofta
   Nej, sällan
   Nej, aldrig

9. Jag har känt mig så olycklig att jag har gråtit:
   Ja, nästan jämt
   Ja, ganska ofta
   Bara någon gång
   Aldrig

10. Tankar på att göra mig själv illa har förekommit:
    Ja, rätt så ofta
    Ja, ganska ofta
    Ja, då och då
    Aldrig

Urdu

آپ کیسی ہیں !

جیسا کہ آپ کا محفوظ آگرم پہلے پڑھائے ۔ اب آپ کیسا محسوس کر رہی ہیں ؟
مہربانی سے اپنے جواب (جو تقریباً آپ کی عادت کے حوالات نمبر میں) کے نیچے لائن
لگائیں کہ مطیعے سات دن سے آپ کی طبیعت کیسی ہے ؟ ۔ ابھی کہ آج کے کیسا محسوس کرتی ہیں ۔

یہ مثال کے طور پر چند سوال ہیں ۔ جو آپ کے تکمیل کیلئے ائیے گئے ہیں ۔ آپ ایسی دیکھ کر اسی طرح
اپنے جواب لکھیں ۔ یعنی اس جواب کے نیچے لائن لگائیں جو آپ کی عادت کے زیادہ قریب ہے ۔
تھکڑ   میں نے اپنے آپ کو خوش محسوس کیا ہے ۔
               اکثر اوقات ۔
               کبھی کبھی دقت ۔
               نہیں اکثر نہیں ۔
               نہیں   بالکل نہیں ۔
اس کا مطلب ہوا کہ مطیعے سننے کے دوران اپنے آپ کو " کبھی کبھی کسی دقت خوشی محسوس کیا ہے "
مہربانی سے دوسرے سوالات کے جواب بھی اسی طرح دیں ۔

پچھلے سات دنوں سے :

1.   چیزوں کے مزامین رُخ کی طرف دیکھ کر میں ہنسی ۔
               جیسا میں پہلے کرتی تھی ۔
               اب سے اتنا میں ہنسی ۔
               یقیناً اب کے اتنا میں ہنسی جتنا پہلے ہنستی تھی ۔
               بالکل نہیں ۔

2.   میں چیزوں کے واقع ہونے کا خوشی سے انتظار کرتی ہوں۔ میں چیزوں کی پرواہ کرتی ہوں ۔
               اتنا ہی جتنا پہلے کرتی تھی ۔
               پہلے سے ذرا کم ۔
               یقیناً اس کے ذرا کم جتنا پہلے کرتی تھی ۔
               بالکل نہیں ذرا بھی پرواہ نہیں کرتی ۔

3.   جب کوئی چیز غلط ہو گئی ۔ تو میں نے اپنے آپ کو قصور دار مانا ئے ۔ بغیر وجہ کے اپنے آپ کو
        کوسائے ؟
        اچھے صفحہ پر دیکھیں ۔

پچھلے سات دنوں سے   (جاری ہے)

               اگر ایسا کرتی ہوں ۔
               تھم گھسار ایسا کرتی ہوں ۔
               میں اکثر اپنے آپ کو برا نہیں کہتی
               بالکل نہیں اپنے کو الزام نہیں دیتی ۔

4. میں نے اپنے آپ کو پریشان اور بغیر خاص وجہ کے مگر منہ محسوس کیا ہے ۔!
- بالکل ہیں
- شاید کبھی
- ہاں کبھی کبھار
- اکثر اوقات

5. میں نے آپ کو خوفزدہ اور گھبرایا ہوا محسوس کیا ہے !
- ہاں بہت زیادہ ۔
- کبھی کبھار ۔
- زیادہ ہیں ۔
- بالکل ہیں

6. چیزیں میرے سر پر سوار رہی ہیں ؟
- ہاں اکثر اوقات میں کئی چیزوں کو بالکل ہیں نمٹ سکی ۔
- ہاں میں کبھی کبھی چیزوں کو اس طرح ہیں نمٹ سکی جیسے پہلے ۔
- بہت اکثر میں چیزوں کو اچھی طرح ہیں کر سکی ۔
- ہیں میں بالکل ٹھیک سے کوئی کام پورا نہ کر سکی ۔

7. میں اتنی ناخوشی ہوئی کہ مجھے اچھی طرح سونے میں مشکل پیش آئی ۔
- بہت دفعہ ایسا ہوا ۔
- کبھی کبھار ایسا ہوا ۔
- کبھی ایسا اکثر ہیں ہوتا ۔
- ایسا بالکل ہیں ہوتا کہ میں سو نہ سکوں ۔

8. میں نے اپنے آپ کو بہت غمگین اور بڑا بڑا محسوس کیا ۔
- اکثر اوقات ؟
- ہاں اکثر ایسا ہوا ۔
- ہیں اکثر میں کبھی کبھار ۔
- ہیں بالکل ہیں ۔

9. میں اتنی ناخوشی ہوئی کہ میں روتی رہی ۔
- ہاں اکثر ایسا ہوا ۔
- ہاں اکثر اوقات ایسا ہوا ۔
- صرف کبھی کبھار ایسا ہوا ۔
- بالکل ہیں ۔ ناخوشی بھی مگر رونے ہیں ۔

10. اپنے آپ پر بہت کفتہ آیا اور اپنے آپ کو نقصان کو جی چاہا ۔
- اکثر ایسا ہوا ۔ اتنا کبھی کبھار ہوا ۔
- شاید ہی کبھی ایسا خیال آیا ہے ۔
- ہیں ایسا بالکل ہیں محسوس کیا ۔

Index

Compiled by JOHN GIBSON